Introduction to Regression and Modeling with R

FIRST EDITION

By Dr. Adam G. Petrie
University of Tennessee – Knoxville

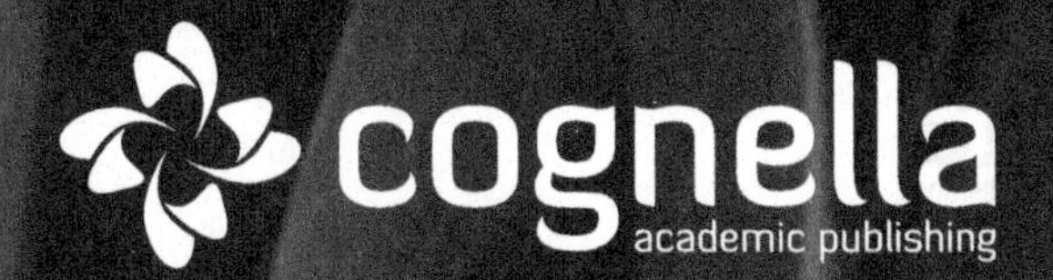

Bassim Hamadeh, CEO and Publisher
Michael Simpson, Vice President of Acquisitions
Jamie Giganti, Senior Managing Editor
Miguel Macias, Graphic Designer
Gem Rabanera, Project Editor
Elizabeth Rowe, Licensing Coordinator

First published in the United States of America in 2016 by Cognella, Inc.

Printed in the United States of America

ISBN: 978-1-63189-250-9 (pbk) / 978-1-63189-251-6 (br)

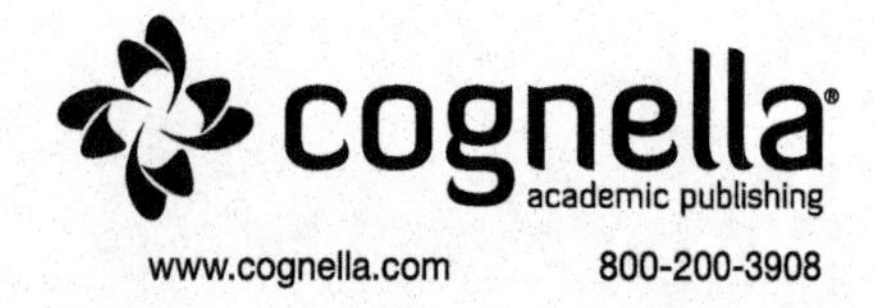

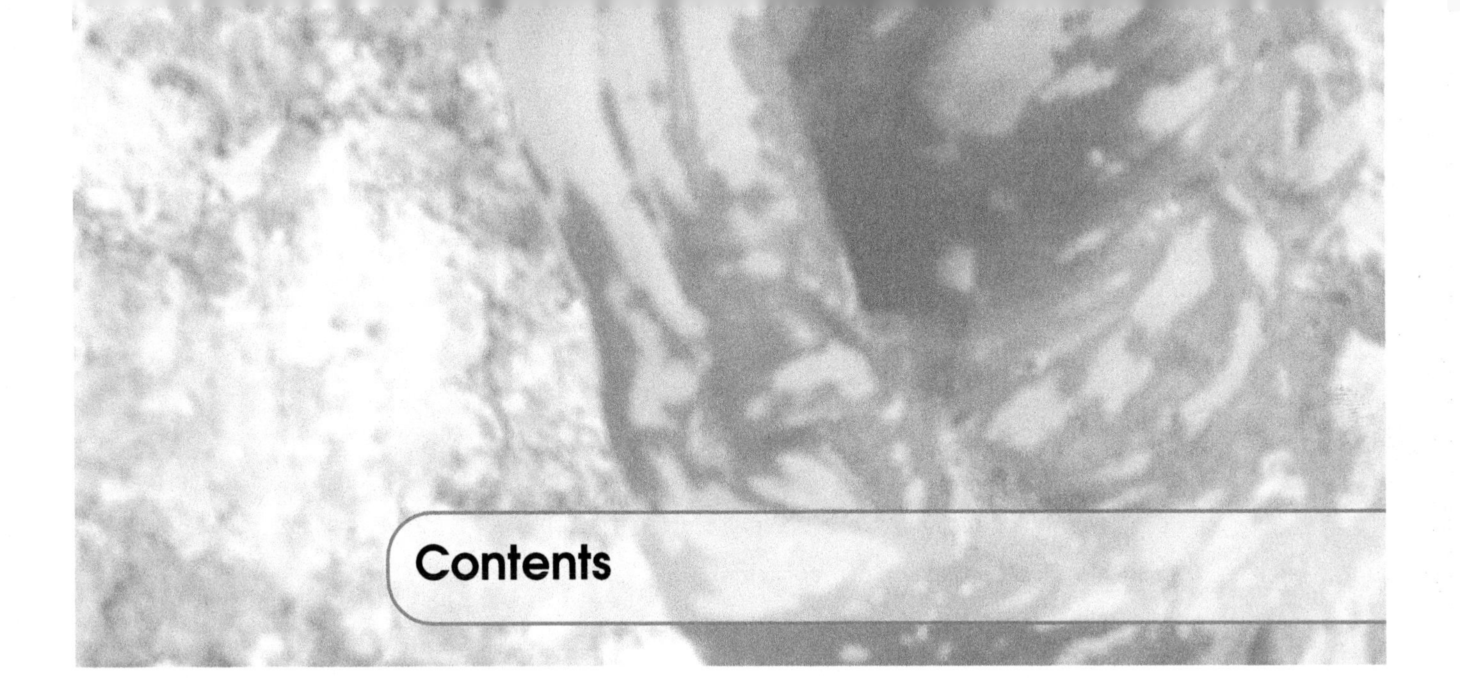

Contents

1 A Brief Introduction 11

1.1 Philosophy of this book **12**

1.2 Target audience **13**

1.3 Outline of topics **13**

1.4 Using R for modeling **14**

1.5 Changes from the preliminary version **14**

2 Associations 15

2.1 Variable types **17**

2.1.1 Categorical variables 17

2.1.2 Quantitative variables 19

2.1.3 Identifier variables 25

2.2 Assigning variables the roles of y and x **25**

2.3 y and x are categorical variables **26**

2.3.1 Visualizing the association with mosaic plots 28

2.3.2 Contingency table 33

2.3.3 Statistical test for association (χ^2 test) 35

2.4 *y* is quantitative and *x* is categorical 39

2.4.1 Visualizations with side-by-side box plots 42

2.4.2 Tests for association 44

2.5 *y* is categorical and *x* is quantitative 49

2.6 *y* and *x* are quantitative variables 52

2.6.1 Visualizing the association with scatterplots 53

2.6.2 Pearson's correlation *r* for linear relationships 57

2.6.3 Statistical significance of linear associations 59

2.6.4 Effect of outliers on correlation 60

2.6.5 Spearman's rank correlation 62

2.7 Causality and lurking variables 63

2.8 Practical significance versus statistical significance 67

2.9 Summary 69

2.10 Exercises 70

3 Simple Linear Regression 75

3.1 Philosophy of Modeling 76

3.2 Regression model and interpretation 78

3.2.1 Interpretation of coefficients 78

3.2.2 Least squares criterion 83

3.2.3 Effect of outliers 84

3.2.4 Assessing the fit: R^2 and RMSE 85

3.3 Inference regarding β_1 87

3.3.1 Standard error of the slope 89

3.3.2 Confidence interval for the slope 91

3.4 Statistical significance of a regression 92

3.4.1 *p*-value approach 93

3.4.2 Confidence interval approach 95

3.4.3 Significance, sample size, and $\mathbf{R}^2$ 95

3.5 Checking assumptions **97**

3.6 Transformations **104**

3.7 Predictions **111**

3.7.1 Predicting average values 112

3.7.2 Predicting individual values 115

3.7.3 Confidence vs. prediction intervals 117

3.7.4 Extrapolation 117

3.8 Simple linear regression using R **118**

3.9 Summary **123**

3.10 Exercises **124**

4 Multiple Regression for Descriptive Modeling 129

4.1 Scatterplot and correlation matrices **131**

4.2 The multiple regression model **133**

4.2.1 Checking assumptions 134

4.2.2 Goodness of fit: $\mathbf{R}^2$ and $\mathbf{R}^2_{\mathbf{adj}}$ 137

4.2.3 Interpretation of coefficients 138

4.2.4 Coefficients are model-dependent 142

4.3 Inference **148**

4.3.1 The standard error of a coefficient 148

4.3.2 Confidence interval for β_i 149

4.3.3 Variance inflation factor and collinearity 151

4.3.4 Examples: salary and body fat data 152

4.4 Statistical Significance **154**

4.4.1 of model 154

4.4.2 of subset of predictors 157

4.4.3 of individual predictors 159

4.4.4 Quirks of coefficients and p-values 160

4.5 Increasing the flexibility of a model 163

4.5.1 Polynomial models 164

4.5.2 Variable creation 167

4.5.3 Interaction variables 171

4.6 Influential points and outliers 176

4.7 Predictions with multiple regression 180

4.8 Summary 183

4.9 Multiple Regression in R 185

4.10 Exercises 189

5 Incorporating Categorical Variables into Regressions 193

5.1 Encoding categorical variables 194

5.1.1 Two levels 194

5.1.2 Three or more levels 195

5.2 Coefficients of indicator variables 195

5.2.1 Categorical variables with two levels 196

5.2.2 Categorical variables with three or more levels 201

5.3 Interactions and categorical variables 206

5.3.1 Categorical variables with two levels 207

5.3.2 Categorical variables with three or more levels 211

5.4 Summary 214

5.5 Using R 215

5.6 Exercises 219

6 Predicting Categorical Responses with Logistic Regression 223

6.1 Logistic regression model 224

6.1.1 Simple logistic regression 224

6.1.2 Logistic curve . . . 225
6.1.3 Multiple logistic regression . . . 226
6.2 Maximum likelihood for finding coefficients **227**
6.3 Coefficients of a logistic regression model **229**
6.3.1 Example: poisoning cockroaches . . . 230
6.3.2 Example: shopping at a chain store . . . 231
6.3.3 Example: Pima diabetes dataset . . . 232
6.3.4 Model dependence of coefficients . . . 233
6.4 Statistical significance **234**
6.5 Confusion Matrix **236**
6.6 Checking Fit **238**
6.7 Interactions in logistic regression **240**
6.8 Categorical variables in logistic regression **242**
6.8.1 Interpretation of coefficients and significance . . . 242
6.8.2 Effect on logistic curve . . . 244
6.9 Summary **247**
6.10 Using R **248**
6.11 Exercises **249**
7 Building a Descriptive Model . . . **253**
7.1 Information criterion for model comparison **254**
7.1.1 AIC . . . 255
7.1.2 BIC and other criteria . . . 256
7.2 Model hierarchy **256**
7.3 Model search and selection **257**
7.3.1 "all possible" procedure . . . 257
7.3.2 Search strategy . . . 259
7.4 Categorical variables and search procedures **263**

7.5 **Building a descriptive logistic regression model** 265

7.6 **Statistical significance and AIC** 266

7.7 **Summary** 266

7.8 **Descriptive Modeling in R** 267

7.9 **Exercises** 268

8 Predictive Modeling with Regression 271

8.1 **Overfitting** 272

8.2 **Assessing predictive performance** 273

8.2.1 Role of a holdout sample 274

8.2.2 Model-building procedure 274

8.2.3 Repeated K-fold cross-validation 275

8.2.4 One standard deviation rule 276

8.3 **Futility of seeking lowest validation error** 277

8.3.1 Example - Body Fat 277

8.3.2 Example - Product Launch 279

8.4 **Search procedure for linear regression models** 281

8.5 **Model building for logistic regression** 283

8.6 **Further issues** 287

8.7 **Summary** 287

8.8 **Using R** 288

8.9 **Exercises** 289

9 Partition Models for Predictive Analytics 291

9.1 **Partition model basics** 294

9.1.1 Terminology 297

9.1.2 Making predictions with a partition model 298

9.2 Building a Tree 300

9.2.1 Choosing a split when y is quantitative . . . 300

9.2.2 Choosing a split when y is categorical . . . 301

9.2.3 Tree construction . . . 303

9.2.4 Determining the number of splits . . . 304

9.3 Variable importance 306

9.3.1 Surrogate splits . . . 308

9.3.2 Connection to variable creation . . . 311

9.4 Random forests 311

9.5 Pros and cons of partition models 312

9.6 Examples and using R 313

9.6.1 Census Analytics . . . 314

9.6.2 NFL analytics . . . 314

9.6.3 Predicting Churn . . . 319

9.6.4 Email analytics . . . 321

9.7 Summary 323

9.8 Exercises 324

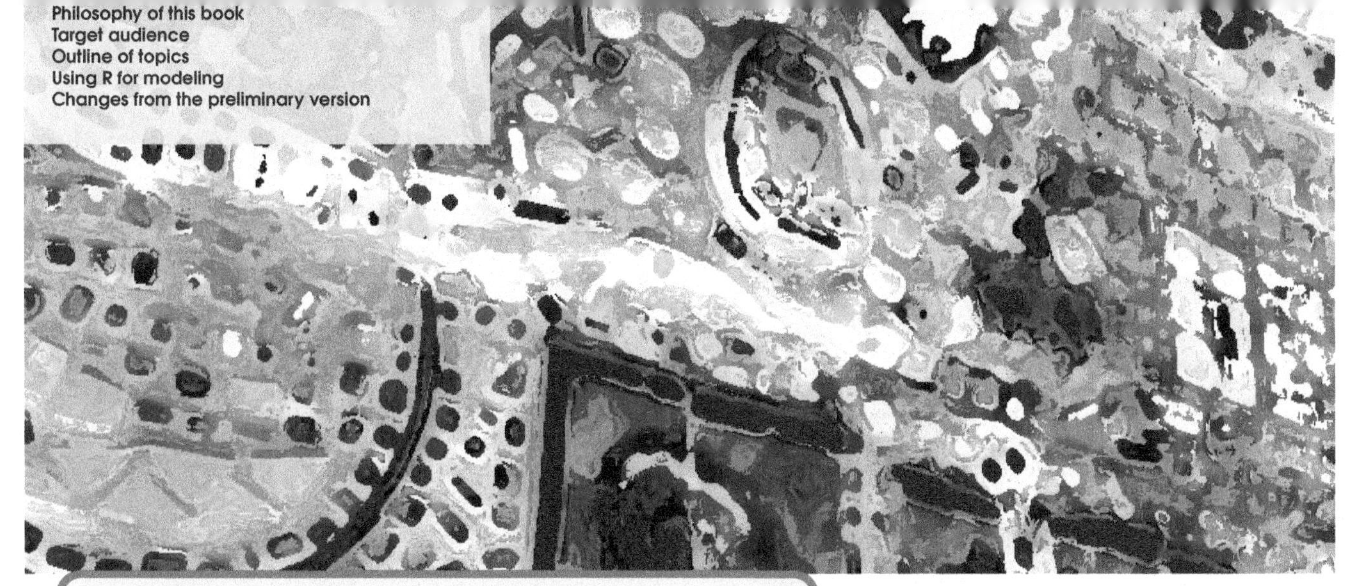

Philosophy of this book
Target audience
Outline of topics
Using R for modeling
Changes from the preliminary version

1. A Brief Introduction

Welcome to the world of statistical modeling, one of the most useful and powerful tools any practitioner can learn, and also one of the most abused as well. A key goal in this work is for you to understand what models *can* and *cannot* do for you. The late George Box said "all models are wrong, but some are useful," and that really is the key mantra in modeling.

The models we will discuss will give you insight into how various quantities are related and will allow you to make predictions about all kinds of things, even the future. Fundamentally, however, these models *never* define physical or natural laws. They are not comments about how quantities are causally linked in the "real world." Now, we may know that a car accelerates faster the further the gas pedal is depressed, and a model may be able to link these two quantities by an equation, but the model can never *establish* a bona fide cause and effect relationship between the two. While a cause and effect relationship will be reflected in the data you collect, your data can never prove a cause and effect relationship exists. For that, you need a theory and scientific analysis.

To become an expert in modeling, you must:

- Understand *when* a particular model can be employed.
- Understand *why* a particular model is used over others (very often the answer is "because it's easier").
- Understand *how* to interpret the findings in your model.
- Understand the *limitations* of your model.

The models you will learn to build throughout this book may lead to great success stories or to dramatic failures; it comes down to how skillfully you can implement a "good" model and how well you know its limitations and assumptions. It is important to be able to explain why the model may have worked and why the model may have failed.

Almost all datasets in this book are taken from or inspired by real-world examples. Many are inspired from websites such as `kaggle.com` (which hosts data competitions), the data repository at the University of California at Irvine (`https://archive.ics.uci.edu/ml/datasets.html`), and the Data and Story Library (`http://lib.stat.cmu.edu/DASL/`). Typically, the original datasets have been reduced in size (both the number of observations and number of variables) to make analysis more tractable, but the fundamental goal of analysis is still the same. These sites also provide a wealth of other data for you to explore and analyze.

1.1 Philosophy of this book

Statistics classes have a bad reputation mainly because people who think they are bad at math think they are going to be bad at statistics. This could not be further from the truth!

While there are academics that are very concerned with the mathematics and theory behind the statistics and models that will be presented in this book, we are not those people. The difference between a mathematics class and a statistics class is that people will (or should) actually be *using* the ideas behind statistics in their everyday lives, i.e., the awareness of randomness and uncertainty has practical implications for how people approach the world.

While there are quite a few equations in this book, they are there to understand the "why" behind modeling. We will study equations and dissect them rather than mindlessly plug in numbers. The reason why mathematics is not emphasized here is that most equations in statistics are extremely tedious to evaluate manually–this is the role of software. Understanding *what* the equations mean is much more important than juggling algebra terms around.

Another reason statistics has a bad reputation is that people think (or have heard) that you can prove anything with statistics, or that "73% of statistics are made up," etc. This is a huge misconception! It's easy to lie and claim to have statistics on your side, but the truth of the matter is that a valid and correct statistical analysis (that is aware of its limitations) really only leads you down one path. The problem is many people use statistics without understanding them, and it's easy to come to the "wrong" conclusion when you use the wrong approach to analyze your data. This is yet another reason why the mathematics behind modeling are less important than motivations and interpretations.

As computers are getting faster and faster, the number of different types of models we can construct has greatly increased. Regression, which is the core topic of this book, is the grandfather of modern techniques. Regression was invented before computers existed and when datasets usually contained only a couple of variables on a few dozen individuals. The assumptions behind the regression model were chosen to make computation easy and simple, and for such datasets (which are still quite common) this type of model can be quite successful.

Modern datasets, on the other hand, are often quite different. Consider any major corporation (Facebook, Walmart, amazon.com, etc.). The data they collect has information on thousands or even millions of individuals or products, and the type of information is extremely diverse and rich. Think about how Facebook might develop a model about what you might like so that it can target ads to you. Not only does it have basic demographic information about you (a few dozen variables itself such as age, gender, school, where you live), but it also knows everything you may have posted (a text analysis could be performed on key words), where you have visited, who your friends are (and what they like and where they have been), etc. Regression provides tools that are somewhat limited in addressing these types of problems, but we will learn techniques that are a bit more flexible and can approach them.

1.2 Target audience

This book is intended for people who, for the most part, plan to deal with observational studies. Nearly all discussion assumes that the analyst has played no part in the collection of the data and is instead in charge of figuring out what story the data has to tell.

When data results from a carefully designed experiment, the types of conclusions that can be reached are more far-reaching than the types we can make from observational studies (i.e., there are no lurking variables and there is a possibility to make statements of causality). Someone working in experimental physics or another science will probably not find this book useful. Those working in social sciences or business should find the discussions most relevant.

Further, much of the statistical theory that justifies the procedure for making inferences and conducting tests is omitted. The goal is to develop an intuitive understanding of how to use a regression model. The interpretation of much of the output of an analysis of associations or of a regression will feel like an oversimplification to pure statisticians. For someone learning the techniques for the first time, this approach is valuable.

1.3 Outline of topics

Modeling is fundamentally about the analysis of relationships and associations (e.g., correlations) between quantities. As such, we will begin with a lengthy discussion about describing and analyzing associations before we even get into modeling them. What does it mean, from a statistical point of view, for two quantities to have an association? How can we measure its strength? What does an association tell us about the fundamental relationship between quantities?

Next, we move into the most basic of models for relationships: linear regression. A regression is nothing more than an equation relating some quantity of interest (the y variable) to other quantities (the x variables). Regression is the cornerstone for the basic analysis of simple relationships. How can I predict my salary based on the amount of work experience and education I have? How should stores be expected to differ in sales if one has two competitors within 10 miles while another has none?

For example, we may want to predict how successful a movie will be based on its opening-weekend gross. However, the success of a movie (as measured by its total domestic gross) is related to more than just its performance opening weekend. It may be necessary to account for the rating of the film (G, PG, R; R movies tend to be less successful since fewer people can see them), the genre of the film, the number of theaters in which the film played opening weekend, the stars of the film, etc., before being able to "isolate" the relationship of interest. Regression models allow us to do this, though the question will always remain: "did I take into account *all* the variables I needed to?" Except under very rare circumstances, you can never quite be sure you've accounted for all other factors that could influence your quantity of interest.

Regression is a phenomenally flexible framework for modeling, and we will explore most of the "neat things" you can do with it, e.g., how to model the case where the strength of the relationship between two quantities depends on a third variable or how to model the probability that something will occur (a customer buys, you are cured by medicine, etc.).

The book concludes by recognizing the limitations of regression and by introducing a different framework for modeling called partition models and random forests. These sort of models are more appropriate for modern datasets where the number of cases and the number of measured quantities is quite large. Statistical modeling is at the stage where the technology and techniques are trying to keep up with the changing nature of the data we are collecting!

1.4 Using R for modeling

Learning how to use R for analysis as opposed to other software such as Excel, SAS, Minitab, etc., has many advantages. First of all, R is free and you will always have it available to you. Second, people *love* R and are constantly submitting new libraries of routines that are specifically focused on tackling a particular problem. The brilliant people behind software development for major vendors simply cannot keep up with the open-source approach for R. If you run into a very specific type of problem, chances are that someone else has already figured out how to solve it and has created a custom set of functions to help you analyze it. Third, companies are beginning to realize how amazing R can be in the hands of a well-trained individual. Becoming familiar with how R works will unlock many opportunities that may not have been otherwise available.

That being said, R is not the easiest piece of software to learn. R is "command-line" based, meaning you have to type in commands to make R do anything (though if you've worked with Excel, you're accustomed to typing in formulas to get the sum, minimum, etc. of groups of cells). Since R is open-source and user-driven, there is no centralized technical support. However, there are many guides and message boards that are freely available to help you out as needed.

One key feature of R is that it lets you write your own code for analysis! In fact, a large chunk of the analysis that you will do in this course uses the `regclass` package (version 1.3)—custom code created by the author. This takes a lot of guesswork out of choosing which procedures are most appropriate, and the code will continue to be useful for many types of problems in the future. However, if something hasn't been done before, you can tell R to do what you want using some basic programming skills. There are online courses (e.g., Coursera) for you to hone your statistical programming skills should you desire.

In this book, snippets of R code are provided that show how to produce the plots and analysis covered in the examples. Using R and the package `regclass` for regression modeling is covered in more detail in the downloadable vignette.

1.5 Changes from the preliminary version

This textbook has greatly expanded upon the material in the preliminary version of the textbook.

- The book has been integrated with the `regclass` package in terms of datasets and code, and code is now visible throughout the book.
- New examples have been added.
- New sections have been added.

Do be aware that the `regclass` package will continue to evolve as new functions are added and existing functions are tweaked. This textbook was printed with `regclass` version 1.3. Future versions of `regclass` will be backwards compatible, and the help files will point out any major changes or additions to functions.

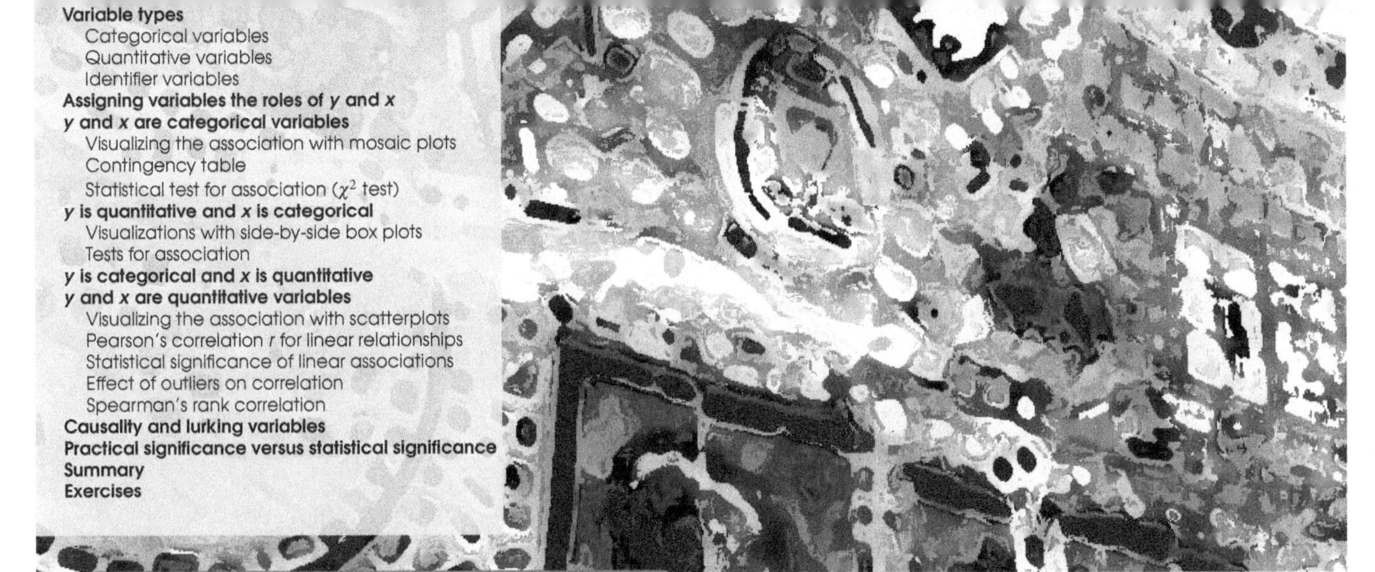

Variable types
Categorical variables
Quantitative variables
Identifier variables
Assigning variables the roles of *y* and *x*
***y* and *x* are categorical variables**
Visualizing the association with mosaic plots
Contingency table
Statistical test for association (χ^2 test)
***y* is quantitative and *x* is categorical**
Visualizations with side-by-side box plots
Tests for association
***y* is categorical and *x* is quantitative**
***y* and *x* are quantitative variables**
Visualizing the association with scatterplots
Pearson's correlation *r* for linear relationships
Statistical significance of linear associations
Effect of outliers on correlation
Spearman's rank correlation
Causality and lurking variables
Practical significance versus statistical significance
Summary
Exercises

2. Associations

"It's all about evaluating skills and putting a price on them. Thirty years ago, stockbrokers used to buy stock strictly by feel. Let's put it this way: Anyone in the game with a 401(k) has a choice. They can choose a fund manager who manages their retirement by gut instinct, or one who chooses by research and analysis. I know which way I'd choose." - Billy Beane

At the turn of the millennium, Billy Beane helped change the way baseball works forever by employing statistical analysis to determine "what matters" when making a winning team. As recounted in the book and film *Moneyball*, the conventional wisdom of picking players based on stolen bases, runs batted in, and batting average turned out not to be the best indicators of a player's success. Rather, to win, players need to get on base, and it turns out on-base and slugging percentages are more strongly associated with a player's scoring. Billy Beane shaped the Oakland Athletics' recruitment strategy based on these (cheaper to find) characteristics, and the approach was likely one of the reasons that brought the Athletics to the playoffs in 2002 and 2003. Now, nearly every baseball team employs these "sabermetrics" to make smart player evaluations.

A similar revolution has taken place in business. The field of business analytics uses statistical modeling, rather than gut instinct, to determine "what matters" when it comes to predicting the sales at a given store or the probability a customer will respond to a promotion. Engineering, science, etc., are also full of investigations regarding known or potentially existing relationships.

- Is there an association between product interest and gender?
- Is there an association between playing video games and showing aggressive behavior?
- Are gender and IQ related?
- Is there a relationship between wine consumption and having a heart attack?

An **association** is a general term used to describe a relationship between two quantities.

> Two quantities are associated when, for whatever reason, knowing the value of one quantity tells you *something* (i.e., provides additional information) about the possible values of the other. In other words, knowing one quantity narrows down the possibilities for the other.

For example, hair and eye color have an association. In one statistics class, the overall distribution of hair color was 18% black, 21% blonde, 48% brown, and 12% red. However, the distribution was different for each eye color.

- Among people with blue eyes, 9% had black hair, 44% had blonde hair, 39% had brown hair, and 8% had red hair.
- Among people with brown eyes, the distribution was 31% black, 3% blonde, 54% brown, and 12% red.

Knowing someone's eye color provides additional information about his or her possible hair color. Overall, 18% of people in the class have black hair. If we know the person has blue eyes, the chance is only 9%. Since the distribution of hair color varies with eye color, these two quantities have an association.

The amount of money consumers spend on DVDs and on Blu-rays also have an association. Typically, people who buy Blu-rays are not in the DVD-buying market, and vice versa. If we know that a person spends more than the average consumer on Blu-rays, we have narrowed down the amount he or she is likely to spend on DVDs: chances are pretty good that this amount is less than the average consumer. In other words, the distribution of the amount a consumer spends on Blu-rays varies based on the amount the consumer spends on DVDs.

Typically, we label the two quantities y and x. To determine if an association exists, we first find the overall distribution of y (e.g., hair color, amount spent on Blu-rays) for all individuals in the data. This is referred to as the marginal distribution of y and is a list of the possible values that y can take along with their relative frequencies. Then, the conditional distribution of y is found for all individuals with some common value of x (e.g., blue eyes, yearly expenditure on DVDs of $50). If any one of the conditional distributions of y differs from the marginal distribution of y, then there is an association—knowing an individual's value of x can provide additional information about his or her value of y.

The **marginal distribution** of y is the overall distribution of y-values of all individuals in the dataset. The **conditional distribution** of y (given x) is the distribution of y-values among individuals who share a common set of characteristics (x). An association exists between y and x if the conditional distribution of y for at least one value of x differs from the others and from the marginal distribution of y.

A formal analysis of an association consists of the following steps:

1. Visualize the relationship with some combination of mosaic plots, box plots, histograms, and/or scatterplots.
2. Numerically measure the strength of the association.
3. Determine whether the association is statistically significant, i.e., unlikely to have arisen by chance. If the association is statistically significant, use the visualization to judge whether the association is strong or of any practical interest to you in the context of the question you wish to answer.

While the three-step procedure will always be the same, both the graphical and numerical analysis depend on what kinds of variables are being studied and how the relationship is approached. Are they categorical variables like gender and opinion or are they quantitative variables like amount spent or weight? Which variable should be assigned the role of y and which should be assigned the role of x? Let us first discuss the different types of variables before moving on to a formal examination and analysis of associations.

2.1 Variable types

Variables come in three major flavors: categorical, quantitative, and identifier. The graphical and numerical analysis of an association proceeds differently depending on the type of variable. Quantitative variables are inherently numerical and typically have units (height, weight, amount, etc.), while categorical variables have possible values that are descriptions (gender, state, color, etc.). An identifier variable is something like a telephone number, order ID, or social security number. These values are used to identify an individual in the data but do not contain any interesting information. A summary can be found in Table 2.1.

Table 2.1 — Variable types. Examples of quantitative, categorical, and identifier variables are as follows. Knowing the type of variable is imperative for doing a correct analysis.

Quantitative	Categorical	Identifier
Amount	Color	Phone Number
Length	Gender	Social Security Number
Mass	Political Party	PIN
Price	Made Purchase	Zip Code
Energy	Emotion	Area Code
Score	Birth State	Purchase Number
GPA	Class Level	Student ID
Percentage	Marital Status	Product ID

2.1.1 Categorical variables

A **categorical** variable has possible values (called **levels**) that are descriptions. For example, gender is a common categorical variable used in marketing and psychology. Typically, it has two levels: male and female. Opinions are also categorical variables. The Likert scale is often used in marketing surveys and typically has five levels: strongly disagree, disagree, neutral, agree, strongly agree. Color is a categorical variable that may be of interest when designing the background or font of a webpage. The number of levels may vary between experiments and could include red, green, blue, etc.

To numerically summarize a categorical variable, we make a **frequency table** of the counts of each level or a **relative frequency table** of the percentages of each level. The table allows us to quickly identify the most and least often occurring levels.

Checking Account

Level	Frequency	Relative Frequency
No	5948	18.4%
Yes	26316	81.6%
Total	32264	100%

Position in Family

Level	Frequency	Relative Frequency
Middle	13	12.5%
Oldest	35	33.7%
Only	24	23.1%
Youngest	32	30.8%
Total	104	100.1% (rounding)

In R

`table()` produces a frequency table. For example, consider the `CALLS` dataset, which contains information on students' cell-phone providers and dropped-call frequency. Dividing the `table()` by the `length()` of the vector containing the values will produce a relative frequency table.

```
data(CALLS)

table(CALLS$DropCallFreq)
Occasionally        Often        Rarely
         105           37           437

table(CALLS$DropCallFreq)/length(CALLS$DropCallFreq)
Occasionally        Often        Rarely
      0.1813       0.0639       0.7647
```

A **segmented bar chart** provides the same information as a frequency table but in graphical form. It is the main tool to visualize the overall distribution of levels of a categorical variable. This plot is essentially the same thing as a pie chart but in the shape of a rectangle. The rectangle is split up into a number of regions equal to the number of levels, and the area devoted to each level is equal to the relative frequency of that level. See Figure 2.1.

Figure 2.1 — Segmented bar chart. A segmented bar chart splits a rectangle into sections whose areas are equal to the fractions of observations with each level. For example, consider the cell-phone providers of students in a statistics class (`CALLS` data). Here, 30% use `ATT`, 7% use `Sprint`, 9.5% use `USCellular`, and 53.5% use `Verizon`. A segmented bar chart of `Provider` would be a rectangle split up into four regions having 30%, 7%, 9.5%, and 53.5% of the total area.

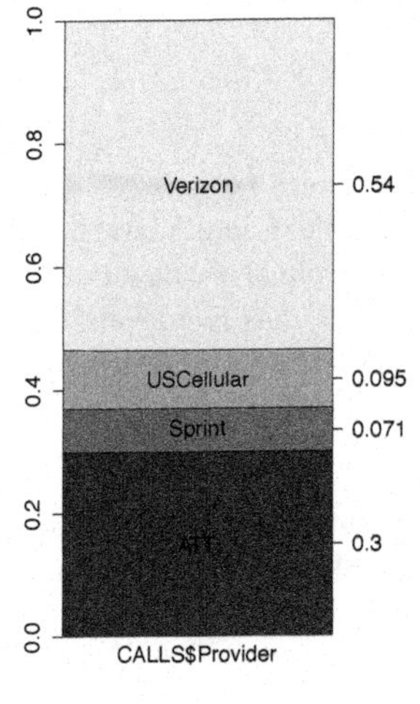

In R

```
data(CALLS)
segmented.barchart(CALLS$Provider)
```

2.1.2 Quantitative variables

A **quantitative** variable has possible values that are inherently numerical. Typically, they have units, e.g., length (inches), weight (kg), amount spent (dollars), etc. Exceptions to this rule are counts (number of purchases at a store) and fractions/percentages (proportion of purchases exceeding $5), which are unitless.

Visualizing the distribution

Histograms and box plots are typically used to graphically summarize the distribution of a quantitative variable. See Figure 2.2.

- **Histogram** - groups values together into categories (e.g., 0-5, 5-10, 10-15, etc.) and plots the number in each category like a bar chart. Use this plot to note where the data is most concentrated (the mode) and to gauge the overall shape of the distribution.
- **Box plot** - the boundaries of the box indicate the range of values of the central 50% of the data values. A horizontal line through the box represents the median value—half the values are smaller and half the values are larger. Whiskers are drawn out to the largest and smallest values that are still "close" to the box (no farther away from the edges than 1.5 times the box's height). Outliers are represented by separate dots and are values that are "unusually" far away from the median.

When describing the distribution, we note the number of peaks/modes, shape, and unusual features. See Figure 2.5 for illustration.

The main features of interest are the number and location of **modes** (peaks). A peak represents a region of relatively high data concentration.

A collection of one or more bars is only considered a peak if it contains a substantial number of cases in them (at least 4 or 5) and contains substantially more cases than surrounding bars (a rough guideline is a factor of two).

Most distributions are unimodal (one peak). Bimodal (two peaks) distributions (or ones with even more peaks) are relatively rare. Small bumps in the histogram rarely indicate a second peak.

The histogram *must* be used to find modes. The box plot cannot reveal the number of peaks in a distribution, but it is very good for summarizing where the values are concentrated (50% of the data is inside the box) for a unimodal distribution.

A secondary feature of interest is the distribution's overall shape. Is the histogram roughly **symmetric** around some value, or is there obvious asymmetry? When there is asymmetry, we say the distribution is **skewed** (toward the "left" when bar heights taper off slowly for smaller values, or toward the "right" when bar heights taper off slowly for larger values). Both the histogram and box plot can be used to assess the overall shape of the distribution.

Evidence for a symmetric distribution when using the box plot consists of the median falling roughly in the center of the box, the whiskers being about the same lengths, and there being about an equal number of **outliers** (points far from the center of the distribution) on both sides of the box.

The box plot for a skewed distribution will have the median much closer to one edge of the box. Further, one whisker will be noticeably longer than the other. The number of outliers beyond each whisker will (likely) be unequal.

Also, take note of any gaps or unusual features. A **gap** separates two peaks and represents a range of values where observations are rare. Unusual features may be a cluster of values far above or below the peak, very sudden high, sharp peaks, etc. Box plots are excellent for finding outliers, while histograms are great for finding gaps.

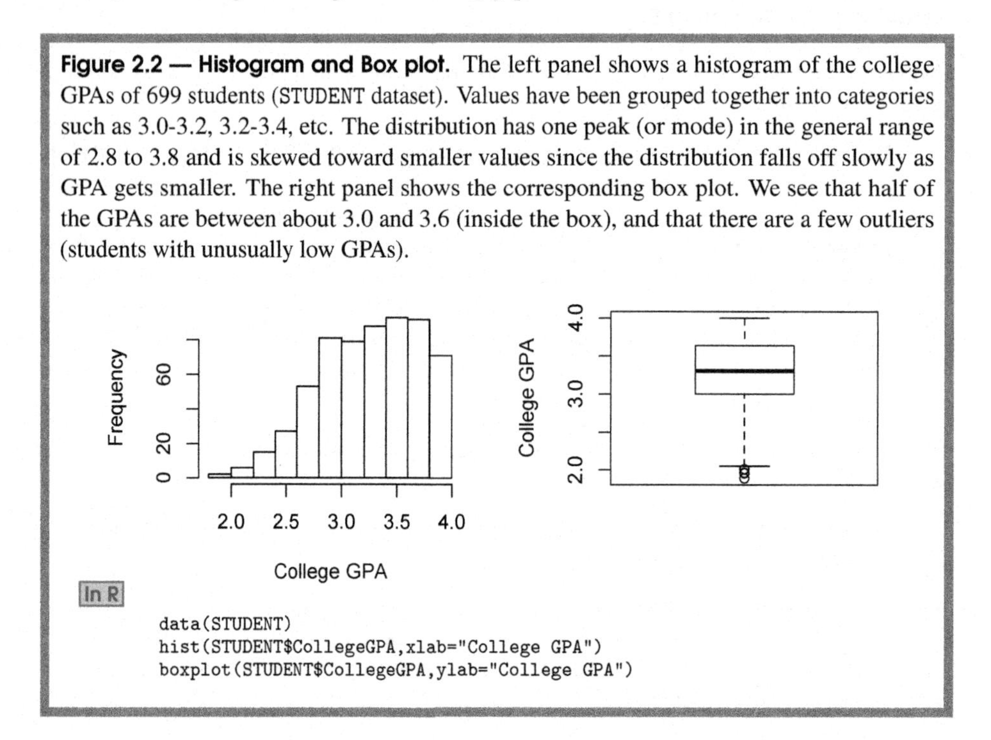

Figure 2.2 — Histogram and Box plot. The left panel shows a histogram of the college GPAs of 699 students (STUDENT dataset). Values have been grouped together into categories such as 3.0-3.2, 3.2-3.4, etc. The distribution has one peak (or mode) in the general range of 2.8 to 3.8 and is skewed toward smaller values since the distribution falls off slowly as GPA gets smaller. The right panel shows the corresponding box plot. We see that half of the GPAs are between about 3.0 and 3.6 (inside the box), and that there are a few outliers (students with unusually low GPAs).

```
data(STUDENT)
hist(STUDENT$CollegeGPA,xlab="College GPA")
boxplot(STUDENT$CollegeGPA,ylab="College GPA")
```

Finally, the distribution is often checked to see how closely its shape resembles a **Normal distribution**, also known as the "bell curve." The Normal distribution is a favorite among statisticians because it is easy to work with mathematically and often describes, at least approximately, the shape of many distributions. Figure 2.3 shows the distribution of students' heights in the STUDENT dataset along with the best-fitting Normal curve.

In R

`qqnorm()` and `qqline()` make a Q-Q plot in R for comparing a distribution to a Normal distribution. `qq()` in package `regclass` will do the same while adding dotted bands to allow for some "wiggle room" in the inevitable departure from the diagonal line. You can manually add a Normal curve to a histogram by adding the argument `freq=FALSE` to `hist()`, then running the command `curve(dnorm(x),desired mean,desired sd),add=TRUE)`, where `desired mean` and `desired sd` are the mean and standard deviation of the Normal curve.

It can be difficult to assess how well a Normal curve describes a distribution from looking at the histogram. The **Q-Q plot** provides another way of looking at the fit. In a Q-Q plot, the observed values of the data are plotted against the expected values had the distribution been exactly Normal.

Figure 2.3 — Checking Normality. The Normal distribution is a bell-shaped curve that roughly describes the shape of many distributions. Shown below is a histogram of students' heights in the STUDENT dataset along with the best-fitting Normal curve. The Normal looks like a good approximation to the distribution.

The Q-Q plot provides a second opinion and shows the observed values of the heights vs. the heights we would have expected students to have if the distribution actually was Normal. Since points fall roughly along the diagonal line and stay, for the most part, within the lower and upper dotted bands, we can say that the distribution of heights is approximately Normal.

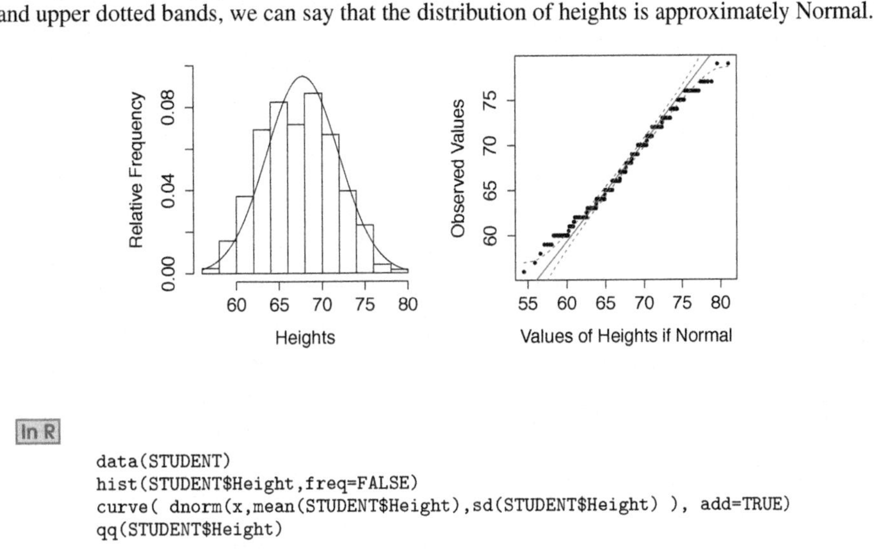

In R

```
data(STUDENT)
hist(STUDENT$Height,freq=FALSE)
curve( dnorm(x,mean(STUDENT$Height),sd(STUDENT$Height) ), add=TRUE)
qq(STUDENT$Height)
```

When the Normal curve is a good description of the shape of the distribution, the observed and expected values should match up and points should fall on a diagonal line. However, since data we collect is a random sample and is never exactly Normally distributed, there is some leeway.

For the Normal curve to be considered a good description of the shape of the distribution, most of the points should fall between the upper and lower dotted bands in the Q-Q plot (it is typically acceptable when a few points near the edges are slightly outside). Further, there should be no global, consistent curvature in the stream of points.

Figure 2.3 shows that the Normal curve provides a good approximation to the distribution of students' heights. Figure 2.4 shows three examples where a Normal curve is not a good approximation for the distribution.

C The Normal distribution *never* exactly describes the distribution of values of any quantity in the real world. It is thus an oversimplification of reality, albeit a useful one. It is tough to specify general conditions when the Normal distribution is "too wrong" to use, so determining whether a distribution is "Normal enough" is a bit of an art.

Figure 2.4 — Non-Normal Distributions. The top plots show the distribution of high school GPAs in the STUDENT dataset. This distribution has longer "tails" (the distribution falls off slowly on either side of the peak) than a Normal distribution. The Q-Q plot has many points outside the upper and lower dotted bands, and there is an obvious, consistent wiggle to the stream of points, showing that the distribution is not well-approximated by a Normal curve.

The middle plots show the distribution of students' weights. There is obvious skewness toward larger values, and this is reflected by a consistent, global curve away from the diagonal line in the Q-Q plot. A Normal curve is not a good approximation for the shape of this distribution.

The bottom plots show the distribution of waiting times between eruptions of Old Faithful (`faithful` dataset). The distribution is clearly bimodal, and the Q-Q plot displays an obvious S shape. While each individual peak may have a shape that is approximately Normal, the distribution of waiting times as a whole is not well-described by a Normal distribution.

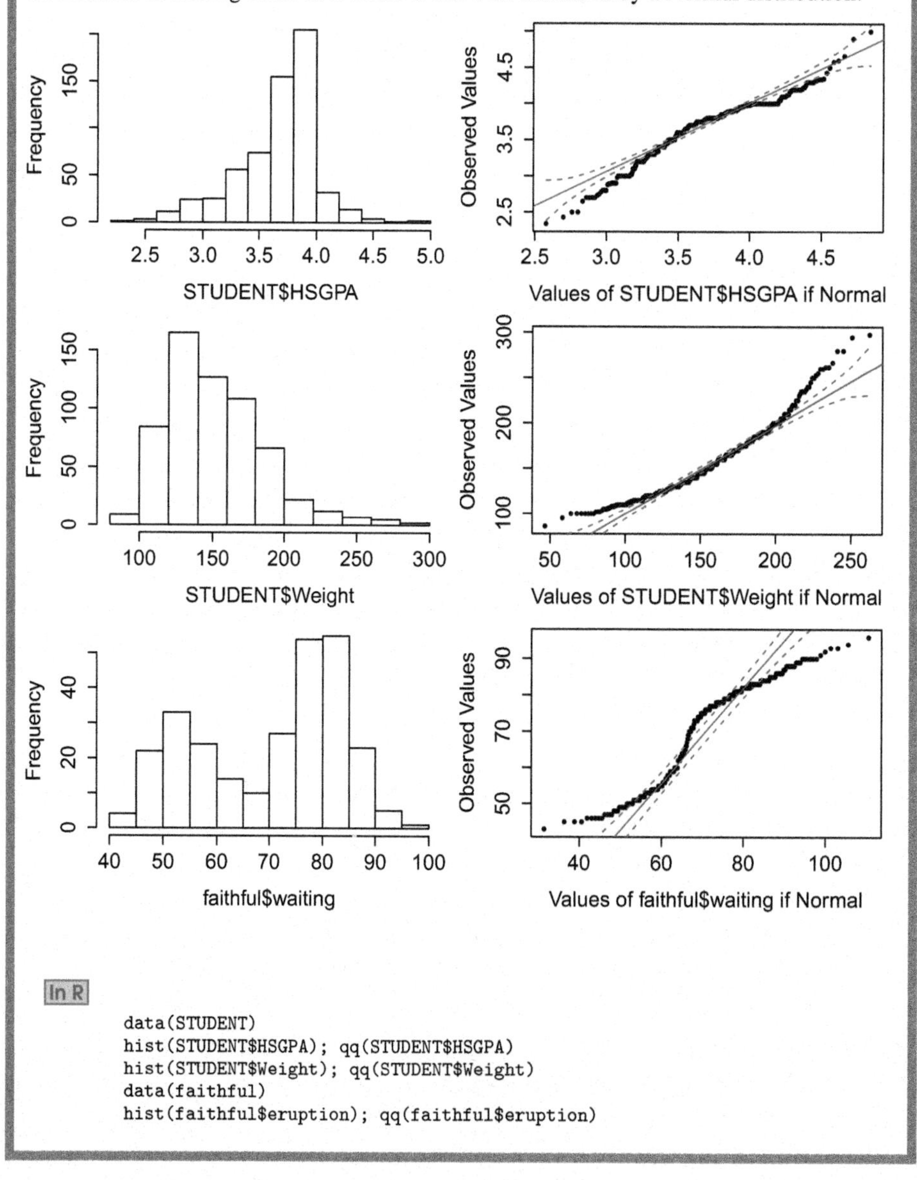

In R

```
data(STUDENT)
hist(STUDENT$HSGPA); qq(STUDENT$HSGPA)
hist(STUDENT$Weight); qq(STUDENT$Weight)
data(faithful)
hist(faithful$eruption); qq(faithful$eruption)
```

Numerically summarizing the distribution

We numerically describe a (unimodal) distribution with two numbers—a "typical" value and the spread around this typical value. Which numbers are used depends on the shape of the distribution.

For roughly symmetric distributions without extreme outliers, the **mean** gives the average (and thus "typical" value) in the dataset. The **standard deviation** tells us the typical difference between the observed values and the average. For example, the distribution of heights of college students is roughly symmetric. The mean is 67.8 inches and the standard deviation is 4.2 inches. This implies that, on average, students are 67.8 inches tall, give or take about 4.2 inches or so.

In R — Numerical summaries are provided by the commands `mean()`, `median()`, `sd()`, `IQR()`, and `summary()`. For example, consider the `AUTO` dataset, which has information on 82 European cars.

```
data(AUTO)
summary(AUTO)
   CabVolume        Horsepower      FuelEfficiency     TopSpeed           Weight
 Min.   : 50.0   Min.   : 49.0   Min.   :13.20   Min.   : 90.0   Min.   :17.50
 1st Qu.: 89.5   1st Qu.: 84.0   1st Qu.:27.77   1st Qu.:105.0   1st Qu.:25.00
 Median :101.0   Median : 99.0   Median :32.45   Median :109.0   Median :30.00
 Mean   : 98.8   Mean   :117.1   Mean   :33.78   Mean   :112.4   Mean   :30.91
 3rd Qu.:113.0   3rd Qu.:140.0   3rd Qu.:39.30   3rd Qu.:114.8   3rd Qu.:35.00
 Max.   :160.0   Max.   :322.0   Max.   :65.40   Max.   :165.0   Max.   :55.00

mean(AUTO$Horsepower)
117.1341

median(AUTO$Horsepower)
99

sd(AUTO$Horsepower)
56.84086

IQR(AUTO$Weight)
10
```

For skewed distributions or ones with extreme outliers, the mean no longer gives a good summary of the "typical" value. Rather, the mean gets "dragged" in the direction of the skewness or location of outliers. Further, the standard deviation no longer gives a good summary of the typical spread in values. Individuals *very* far from the average inflate the value of the standard deviation. Rather, the **median** gives a better idea of the typical value (half the values are smaller and half the values are bigger), and the **interquartile range** gives a better idea of the spread (the interquartile range is the distance between the top and bottom of the box in the box plot).

Consider the numbers 1, 3, 5, 7, and 9. The distribution is symmetric and the mean (which equals 5) provides a summary of the "typical" value. The standard deviation is 3.2, indicating that values are typically 3.2 or so away from the average. Now imagine the 9 is a 90. The average is then 21.2 (not a good summary of a typical value) and the standard deviation is 38.5 (not a good summary of the typical difference between values and the average). The median, however, is 5 and provides a better summary of the typical value. The interquartile range is 4 and gives a good summary of the spread between most values.

Figure 2.5 — More histogram and box plot examples. The left panels show the weights of 699 college students. We would say the distribution is unimodal since there is only one well-defined peak.

While there are a few bars that poke up above their neighbors, these are not separate peaks since they do not contain substantially more cases than the surrounding bars. Likewise, there is a small cluster of bars at around 300 pounds. This does not represent a separate peak since so few cases are contained in these bars. Rather, as the box plot shows, these are outliers.

The box plot also shows the asymmetry in the distribution by having the top whisker be longer than the bottom one and by having all outliers concentrated on one side. The distribution is skewed right (toward larger values).

A truly bimodal distribution can be seen on the right. These are the eruption times of the Old Faithful geyser. Notice how the bars representing the peaks both contain numerous cases and substantially more cases than the bars in the gap between them. This bimodality is hidden in the box plot.

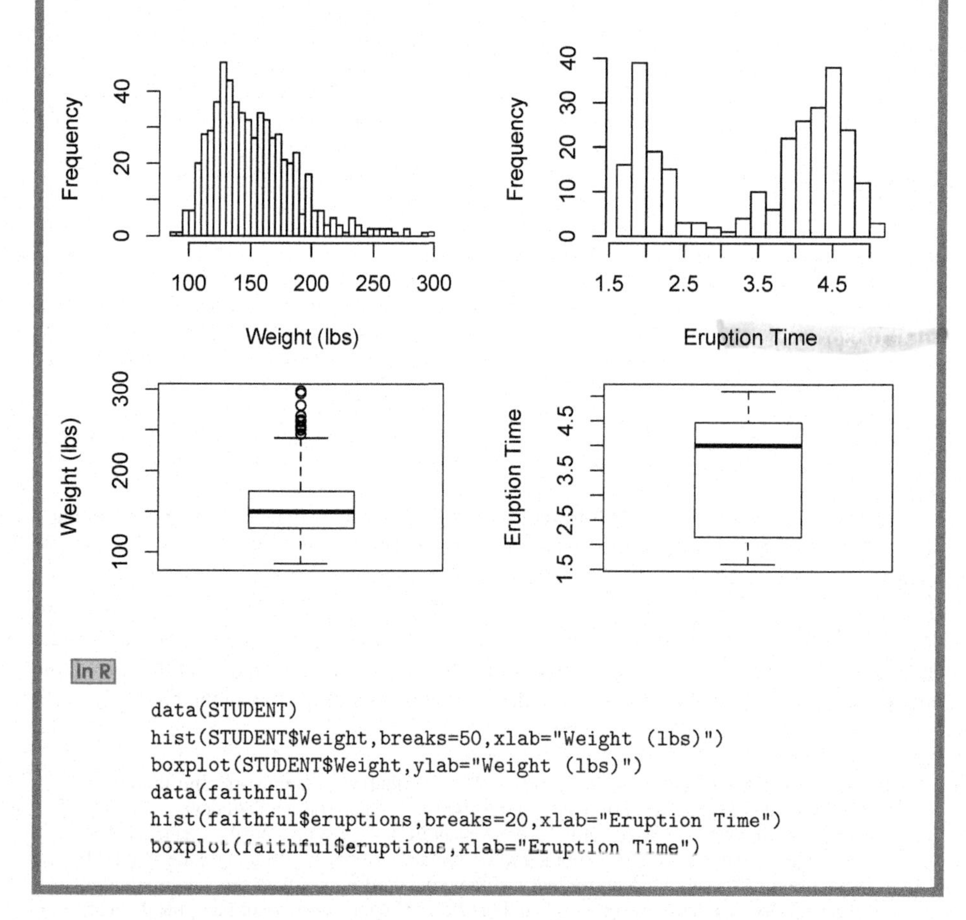

In R

```
data(STUDENT)
hist(STUDENT$Weight,breaks=50,xlab="Weight (lbs)")
boxplot(STUDENT$Weight,ylab="Weight (lbs)")
data(faithful)
hist(faithful$eruptions,breaks=20,xlab="Eruption Time")
boxplot(faithful$eruptions,xlab="Eruption Time")
```

Treating quantitative variables as categorical and vice versa

Any quantitative variable can be treated as a categorical variable if the possible values are grouped together into levels. For example, we could treat the number of weekly purchases of shoppers at a local grocery store as categorical by creating the levels: none (0), a couple (1 or 2), a few (3 to 5), and many (6 or more). We could also treat height as a categorical variable by creating the levels: short (less than 5 feet), average (between 5 and 6 feet), and tall (greater than 6 feet).

It is also sometimes acceptable to treat a categorical variable as a quantitative variable as long as the *ordering* of the levels is meaningful and the *differences* between levels are informative and consistent. For example, if someone's attractiveness is rated on a scale of 1-very unattractive, 2-unattractive, 3-average, 4-attractive, 5-very attractive, then it may be reasonable to treat the ratings as quantitative variables. The ordering is meaningful (lower numbers indicate lower attractiveness). The question is whether the differences between levels is consistent, i.e., is the difference between a 1 and a 2 (very unattractive and unattractive) the same as the difference between a 3 and a 4 (average and attractive), and is the difference between a 1 and a 3 twice as big as the difference between a 1 and a 2, etc. If so, the levels can be treated as actual numbers and as a quantitative variable.

2.1.3 Identifier variables

The last type of variable is an **identifier** variable. These are quantities such as zip codes, social security numbers, PINs, order numbers, etc.

Normally, these quantities are not analyzed because they rarely contain any useful information and exist only for identification or grouping purposes. For instance, it would not make sense to take the average of the last four digits of people's phone numbers because these numbers contain no real information.

That being said, you may be able to determine something useful in rare cases. For example, a zip code is reflective of someone's rough geographic location. A small average zip code implies that the individuals live further east, while a large average zip code implies the individuals live further west.

Since many identifiers are numbers (e.g., zip code), it is easy to mistake them for quantitative variables. However, an analysis of identifier variables is typically meaningless. It is imperative to know what a numerical value represents before conducting any sort of analysis.

2.2 Assigning variables the roles of y and x

To streamline the analysis of an association, the two quantities under study are assigned the generic placeholders y and x. Which variable plays the role of y and which plays the role of x dictates how the graphical and statistical analysis unfolds. By convention:

y is the quantity you wish to predict and x is the quantity used to make predictions.

For example, imagine we are studying a possible association between the selling price of an item on eBay and whether the seller charges for shipping. In this case, selling price would play the role of y while shipping would play the role of x since the question we'd likely want to answer is: "Do auctions with free shipping typically have higher selling prices?" In other words, can we predict the selling price based on whether the auction has free shipping or not. The reverse assignment does not make sense because it is not interesting to predict whether an auction has free shipping based on its selling price.

Now imagine we are studying a possible association between scores on the final exam and midterm exam. The logical question is: "Does a student's score on the midterm help to predict his or her score on the final?" Midterm exam score would play the role of x and final exam score would play the role of y. The reverse assignment does not make logical sense because the midterm comes before the final.

In the hair and eye color example, either assignment makes sense. Asking "Can hair color (x) predict eye color (y)?" or "Can eye color (y) predict hair color (x)?" are both logical and interesting questions. Likewise, either assignment works for the Blu-ray and DVD example. "Can the amount consumers spend on Blu-rays predict the amount they spend on DVDs?" and "Can the amount consumers spend on DVDs predict the amount they spend on Blu-rays?" are both questions that make sense.

> Often, logic alone suggests how to cast the variables into the roles of x and y. In general, the correct assignment is made by considering the question being asked and the context of the problem.

Once x and y have been assigned, the analysis first proceeds by finding the marginal distribution of y, i.e., the possible values of y and their frequencies over all individuals in the data. Then, the conditional distribution of y for individuals with some common value of x is found. The conditional distribution is found for each unique value of x in the data. If any of the conditional distributions of y differ from the marginal distribution of y, then x and y have an association—knowing an individual's x value provides additional information about (i.e., narrows down) its possible values of y.

At its core, the analysis of an association is the same thing as asking "Does the distribution of possible y values depend on an individual's x-value?" If yes, then x and y have an association.

2.3 Associations when *y* and *x* are categorical variables

An association exists between two categorical variables if knowledge of the level of x for an individual provides additional information about the possible values for that individual's level of y. Example questions of interest that involve two categorical variables include:

- Is there a relationship between buying on `amazon.com` and gender? If yes, knowing the level of the variable Gender (male vs. female) tells you something about the variable Purchase (buy vs. not buy). The percentages of men and women who buy from `amazon.com` may be different.
- Is there an association between political affiliation and income? If yes, knowing the level of the variable Income (encoded as a categorical variable with levels low/middle/high) tells you something about the variable Affiliation (Republican, Democrat, Independent).

The stereotype is that low-income households tend to lean Democrat, while high-income households tend to lean Republican.

- Does personality change during college? Consider the variables Personality (introvert/extrovert) and Class (freshman, sophomore, etc.). If there is an association, then knowing the level of the variable Class tells us something about the variable Personality. Typically, freshmen have the highest percentage of introverts.

The first step in the analysis is to cast the two variables into the roles of x and y. In this case, the distinction is purely to aid in visualization. The statistical analysis of the association is the same regardless of the assignment. Recall that y is the quantity we want to predict and x is the quantity used to make the prediction. When both variables are categorical, let us think about the assignment in a slightly different manner:

> Let y be the "response" or "variable of interest" (what we're really studying) and let x be the "grouping" variable. To help identify which is which, ask the question: "Is the distribution of y the same for each level of x?"

In the first of the motivating examples, the grouping variable x is Gender while y is Purchase. An association exists between the two if the distribution of y depends on x (i.e., whether a customer buys or not depends on gender). In the second example, the grouping variable x is Affiliation while y is Income. An association exists if the distribution of income varies between affiliations.

When y is a categorical variable, the marginal distribution of y refers to the proportion (or percentage) of all individuals in the data with each level of y. For example, if y is car color, then the marginal distribution of y could be:

Color	Proportion
Red	0.07
Black	0.31
Other	0.62

The conditional distribution of y for some level of x refers to the proportions of each level of y among only those individuals with that common level of x. For example, if x is gender, then the conditional distributions of y could be:

Color	Marginal (Overall)	Conditional (Women)	Conditional (Men)
Red	0.07	0.03	0.10
Black	0.31	0.31	0.31
Other	0.62	0.66	0.59

In this example, the marginal (overall) distribution of car color is 7% red, 31% black, and 62% other. The conditional distribution of car color for women is 3% red, 31% black, and 66% other. For men, it is 10% red, 31% black, and 59% other. Knowing the gender of the individual provides additional information about the distribution of car color (it's not the same between genders), so we say there is an association.

Note: the proportions of *each* level of y (here: red, black, other) do not have to be different for there to be an association. As long as there is at least one difference, we say that an association exists.

2.3.1 Visualizing the association with mosaic plots

The **mosaic plot** allows us to visualize the conditional distribution of y for each level of x. The plot aids in judging the strength of an association, while the χ^2 (pronounced "chi-squared") test is useful for gauging the statistical significance of the relationship.

A mosaic plot is a set of side-by-side segmented bar charts (one for each level of x). These segmented bar charts graphically represent the conditional distributions of y for each level of x. We compare them to a segmented bar chart representing the overall marginal distribution of y. If we see any differences, then an association exists between x and y (knowing the level of x gives additional information about the distribution of y). Bigger discrepancies between the conditional distributions of y indicate a stronger association.

In R `plot(y~x)` can produce a mosaic plot. A more effective display can be made by using `associate()` in package `regclass` since it also gives a segmented bar chart for the marginal distribution of y.

An association between x and y is suspected when there are noticeable differences between the side-by-side segmented bar charts in a mosaic plot. A big discrepancy indicates a strong association. Note: the widths of the bars represent the relative frequencies of each level of x and do not reveal whether x and y have an association.

For example, consider a survey of 579 students in Knoxville, TN, during a 2009 introductory statistics class (the `CALL` data of package `regclass`). These students reported their cell-phone provider (`Provider`) and perceived frequency of dropped calls (`DropCallFreq`). Figure 2.6 shows a mosaic plot of the relationship.

The logical question to ask is: "Can we predict dropped-call frequency from the provider?" (rather than vice versa). The grouping variable x is thus the cell-phone provider. The levels of `Provider` are `ATT`, `Sprint`, `USCellular`, `Verizon`. The response variable y is self-reported frequency of dropped calls. The levels of `DropCallFreq` are `Rarely`, `Occasionally`, `Often`. Each bar in the mosaic plot gives the conditional distribution of perceived dropped-call frequency for that provider.

The widths of the bars in the mosaic plot are proportional to the relative frequencies of the levels of `Provider`. We see that `Verizon` is the thickest since over 50% of students have that carrier. Only about 10% of students have `Sprint` or `USCellular`, so their bars are relatively skinny. The level `Rarely` is found most often for `Verizon` (about 90%) and least often for `ATT` (about 50%).

No statistical analysis is complete without acknowledging its limitations. For this study, the analysis is limited to Knoxville in 2009 (even more specifically, to areas in which students reside and travel). The results may not generalize to other locations or even to the current time period, so it would be misleading to use this data to advertise that Verizon (the provider with the highest chance of rarely having dropped calls) gives superior service.

The data suggests that a strong association exists between `DropCallFreq` and `Provider`. The conditional distributions of dropped-call frequency (the segmented bar charts in the mosaic plot) look substantially different from each other and from the marginal distribution (the separated segmented bar chart on the right). Knowing the student's provider tells us a good deal about the chance that he or she will report often, occasionally, or rarely having dropped calls.

Figure 2.6 — Mosaic plot for cell-phone provider and dropped-call frequency. In a mosaic plot, each level of x gets a bar (the width of a bar corresponds to the relative frequency of that level). Each bar is shaded according to the distribution of y for that level of x and represents the conditional distribution of y for that level. The separated bar on the far right shows the marginal distribution of y, i.e., the overall relative frequencies of each level of y.

In this example, each bar represents a different cell-phone provider (x). The shaded areas within a bar equal the relative frequencies that customers report dropped calls (rarely, occasionally, or often) for that provider (y).

We see that the distribution of dropped-call frequency varies quite a bit between providers. For instance, customers are much more likely to report rarely having dropped calls if they have `Verizon` than if they have `ATT`. Relative to the marginal distribution of dropped-call frequency, a caller that uses AT&T has a much lower chance of reporting `Rarely` and a much higher chance of reporting `Occasionally`.

Knowing the provider substantially narrows down the possible values for dropped-call frequency for at least one of the carriers, indicating the presence of a strong association.

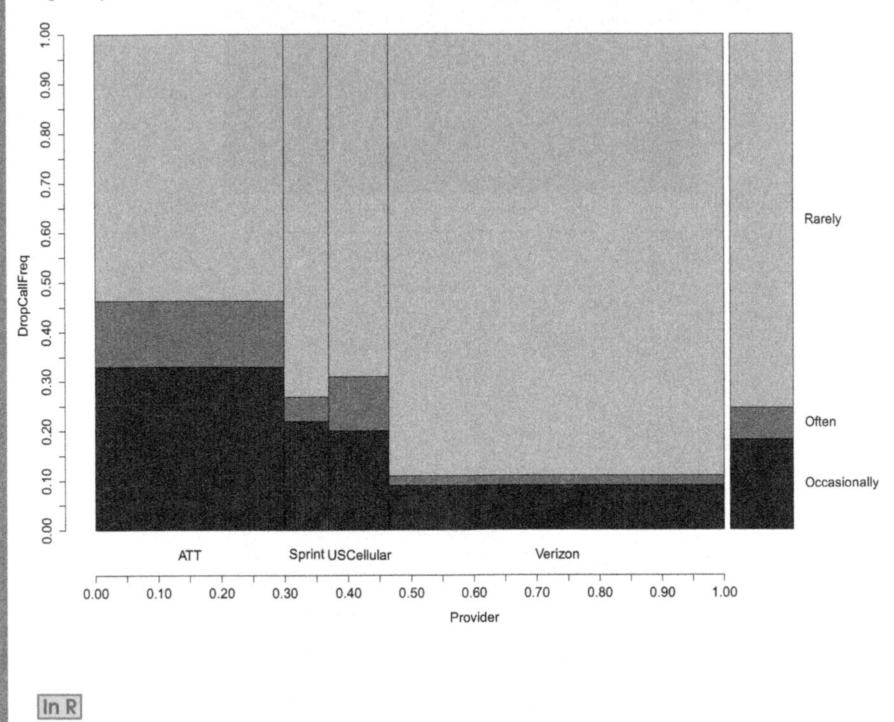

In R

```
data(CALLS)
associate(DropCallFreq~Provider,data=CALLS) #shown
plot(DropCallFreq~Provider,data=CALLS) #alternative
```

Figure 2.7 — Mosaic plots for gender and dating habits. The top plot examines a potential relationship between gender and relationship status, while the bottom plot examines a relationship between gender and how someone attracts a mate in the SURVEY11 data.

The conditional distributions of someone's main weapon to attract a mate look about the same between genders and are nearly identical to the marginal distribution. In this case, knowing the gender of the person does not really narrow down the weapon they use to attract a mate, so we do not suspect an association.

The conditional distributions of relationship status look slightly different from each other and from the overall marginal distribution, so we suspect a weak association. Interestingly, more women than men consider themselves "dating."

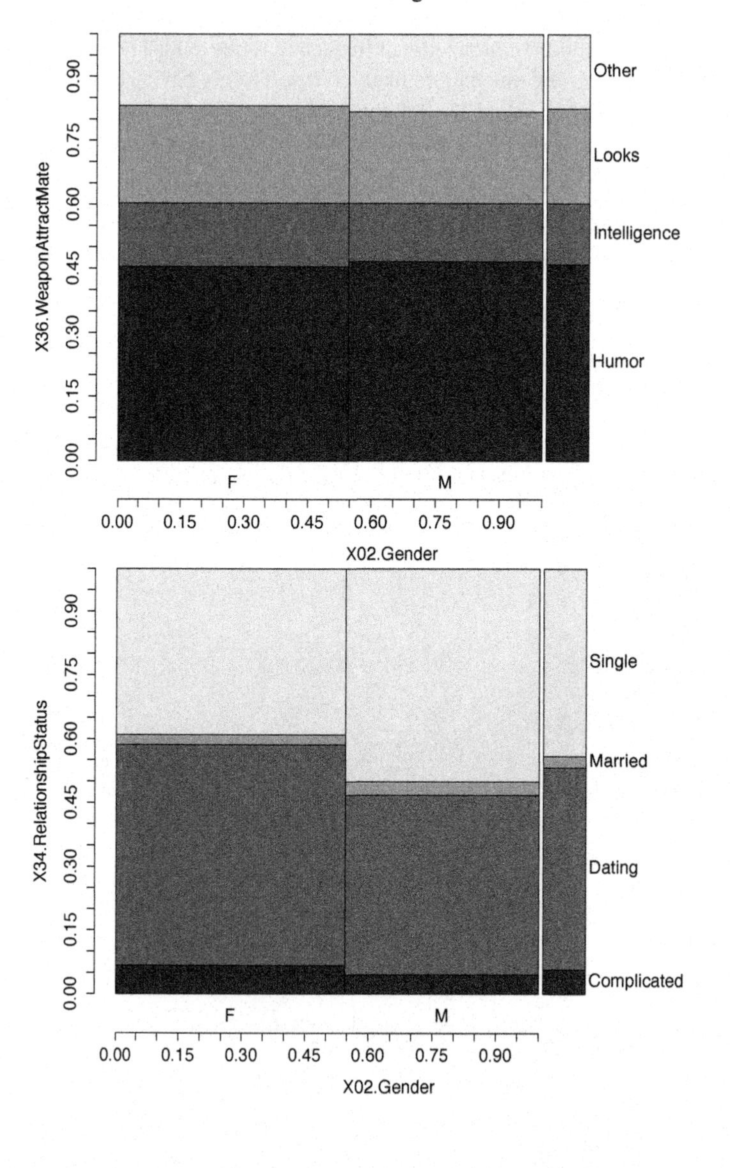

In R

```
associate(X36.WeaponAttractMate~X02.Gender,data=SURVEY11)
associate(X34.RelationshipStatus~X02.Gender,data=SURVEY11)
```

Figure 2.8 — Mosaic plot for gender and computer choice. Let us examine a potential relationship between a person's gender and his or her choice of personal computer (Mac vs. a Windows-based PC).

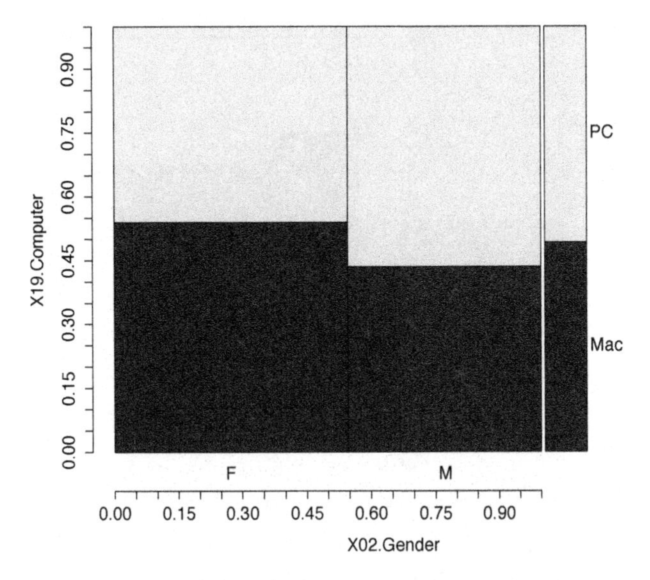

To gauge the strength of an association, we compare the segmented bar charts to each other and to the marginal distribution of y. If the segmented bar charts look about the same, the relationship is weak or perhaps non-existent (the distribution of levels of y does not seem to depend on x). Bigger differences indicate progressively stronger relationships (i.e., the distribution varies more and more between groups).

The marginal distribution of computer choice (separated bar chart on the right) shows almost a 50-50 split between PC and Mac (`SURVEY11` data). The conditional distribution of computer choice for women shows a small majority for Mac, and the conditional distribution for men shows a small majority for PC. Since the conditional distributions look different from each other and from the marginal distribution, we suspect an association: knowing a person's gender provides additional information about his or her likely computer choice. However, because the differences are relatively small, the association is weak.

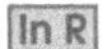

```
associate(X19.Computer~X02.Gender,data=SURVEY11)
```

Additional examples are worthwhile and illuminating. Let us continue to study students with the `SURVEY11` dataset. Consider the relationships between gender and various other variables: relationship status, weapon one uses to attract a mate, and computer of choice. Figures 2.7 and 2.8 show the relevant mosaic plots, and Figure 2.9 investigates whether joining a fraternity or sorority is associated with someone's political beliefs.

There is little to no association between gender and the weapon used to attract a mate (the conditional distributions for men and women as well as the overall marginal distribution look nearly the same). What one uses to attract a mate is quite similar between genders.

Figure 2.9 — Mosaic plot for going Greek and political beliefs. Let us examine a potential relationship between a person's choice to go Greek and his or her political beliefs (SURVEY11 data).

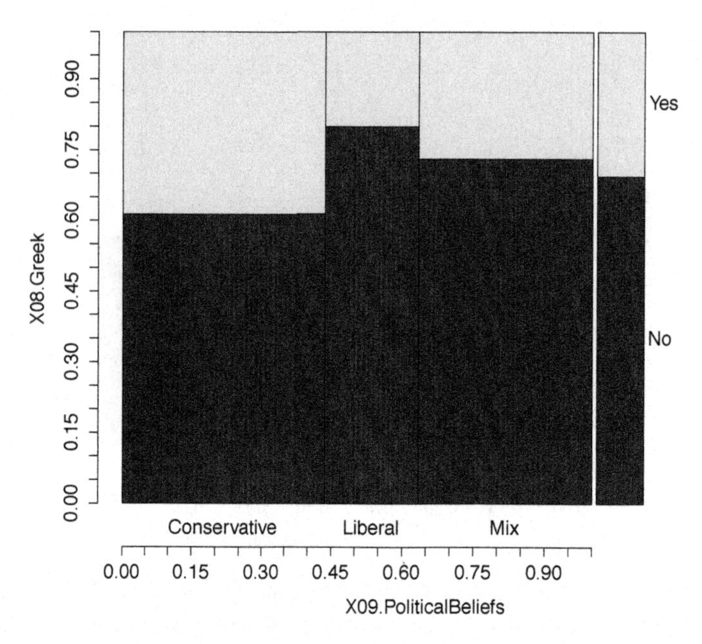

The marginal distribution of going Greek shows that about 30% of students overall join fraternities or sororities. However, based on the conditional distributions of going Greek, about 40%, 20%, and 30% of students with conservative, liberal, or a mix of beliefs join Greek societies. Since the conditional distributions look different from each other and from the marginal distribution, we suspect an association: knowing the beliefs of a person provides additional information about whether he or she may have gone Greek. The differences are rather pronounced, so the association has moderate strength.

In R

```
associate(X08.Greek~X09.PoliticalBeliefs,data=SURVEY11)
```

However, there does look to be an association between relationship status and gender. While the percentages of men and women who responded "It's Complicated" and "Married" are nearly identical, there does look to be a difference between "Single" and "Dating." Specifically, a higher percentage of women responded "Dating" than men, while a higher percentage of men responded "Single" than women. The implications are interesting and open to interpretation.

Further, there looks to be a weak relationship between computer preference and gender (a small majority of women use a Mac, while a small majority of men use a PC) and a moderate relationship between political beliefs and going Greek (it appears that the fraction of people going Greek gets progressively higher for more conservative beliefs).

2.3.2 Contingency table

A **contingency table** provides a numerical summary of the relationship. The entries in the table are the observed frequencies of each combination of y and x. The rows of the table are labeled by the levels of x. The columns of the table are labeled by the levels of y.

The margins of the table give the row and column totals, and the lower right number gives the sample size n (total number of cases) in the data. The row and column totals are the marginal distributions of each variable, i.e., the overall frequency distribution of the levels of y and the overall frequency distribution of the levels of x.

Table 2.2 shows the contingency table for the dropped call data. Since x is `Provider`, each row represents a different cell-phone carrier. Each column represents one of the levels of y: `Occasionally`, `Often`, and `Rarely`.

Table 2.2 — Contingency table example. A contingency table breaks down each variable into its levels and tabulates how often each combination of levels is observed. Here, there are 2 Sprint customers who reported `Often` for dropped calls, etc. The margins of the table (labeled `Sum`) give the *marginal* distributions of `DropCallFreq` and `Provider`, and the bottom right corner gives the number of cases (n) in the data. In this survey, there are 579 individuals. Of these individuals, 173 have AT&T, 41 have Sprint, 55 have US Cellular, and 310 have Verizon (these numbers form the marginal distribution of phone carrier).

	Occasionally	Often	Rarely	Sum
ATT	57	23	93	173
Sprint	9	2	30	41
USCellular	11	6	38	55
Verizon	28	6	276	310
Sum	105	37	437	579

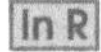

```
data(CALLS)
table(CALLS$Provider,CALLS$DropCallFreq)
associate(DropCallFreq~Provider,data=CALLS)
```

The contingency table can be used to summarize various aspects of the data.

- How many people in the survey use AT&T? 173 (row total of `ATT`)
- How many AT&T customers report they rarely have dropped calls? 93
- Overall, how many people in the survey report they rarely have dropped calls? 437 (column total of `Rarely`)

The (marginal) distribution of cell-phone provider is given by the column of row totals: 173 `ATT`, 41 Sprint, etc. The (marginal) distribution of dropped-call frequency is given by the row of column totals: 105 report occasional dropped calls, 37 report often dropped calls, etc.

The contingency table provides little insight into whether an association exists because different levels of x may have different numbers of individuals. For example, the 57 (the number of AT&T

customers who report `Occasionally`) can't immediately be compared to the 11 (the number of US Cellular customers who reported the same) since the total number of AT&T and US Cellular customers is very different (173 vs. 55).

To take away this dependency on the group sizes, the conditional distribution of y for each level of x is tabulated. The conditional distribution of y for some level of x is simply the fraction of all individuals with that level of x who have each level of y. These fractions can be easily found by dividing the number in each cell of the table by its corresponding row total. In fact, the conditional distributions of y for each level of x are what is represented by the segmented bar charts in the mosaic plot.

For example, the conditional distributions of dropped-call frequency for AT&T and Verizon customers are (after rounding):

Provider	Occasionally	Often	Rarely
ATT	57/173 = 0.33	23/173 = 0.13	93/173 = 0.54
Verizon	28/310 = 0.09	6/310 = 0.02	276/310 = 0.89

Noticeable differences between the conditional and marginal distributions of y indicate an association between x and y. See Table 2.3 for an example.

Table 2.3 — Conditional and marginal distributions of dropped-call frequencies. By dividing the number in each cell of the contingency table by its row total, the conditional distribution of y can be tabulated for each level of x along with the marginal (overall) distribution of y. For example, in Table 2.2, we see 30 of the 41 Sprint customers report rarely having dropped calls. The fraction works out to be $30/41 = 0.732$.

An association between x and y exists when knowing the x-level of an individual tells us something about the value of its y-level. This occurs when the distribution of y is somehow different between at least two levels of x, i.e., if the percentages when scanning down a column don't quite match up.

For `Occasionally`, the marginal frequency is 0.181. For AT&T and Verizon customers, the conditional frequencies are 0.329 and 0.09, respectively. If there was no association, these percentages should be much closer to each other and to the overall marginal percentage.

Overall, 18.1% of customers occasionally have dropped calls. If we know the customer uses AT&T, the chance of him or her occasionally having dropped calls is much higher. If we know the customer uses Verizon, the chance of him or her occasionally having dropped calls is much lower. We suspect a strong association since knowing the provider gives us significant additional information about the dropped-call frequency.

```
           Occasionally      Often    Rarely
ATT          0.32947977 0.13294798 0.5375723
Sprint       0.21951220 0.04878049 0.7317073
USCellular   0.20000000 0.10909091 0.6909091
Verizon      0.09032258 0.01935484 0.8903226
Marginal     0.18134715 0.06390328 0.7547496
```

In R

```
associate(DropCallFreq~Provider,data=CALLS)
```

2.3.3 Statistical test for association (χ^2 test)

Unfortunately, even when two categorical variables are unrelated, the segmented bar charts in the mosaic plot will never appear identical. The conditional distributions of y and the marginal distribution of y will almost always show *some* (usually small) discrepancy when real data is used. A statistical test is required to determine whether the discrepancies are indicative of an underlying association or whether they could have easily resulted from natural chance variation.

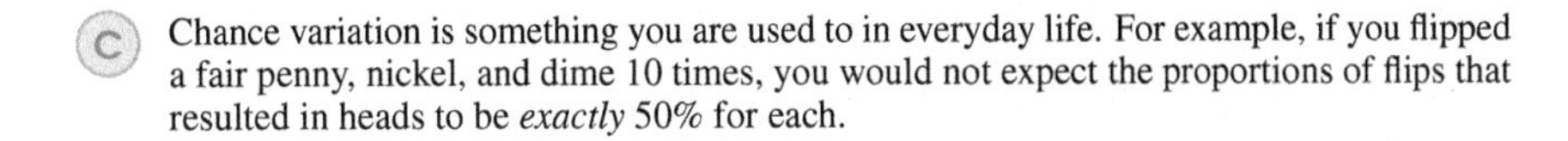

Chance variation is something you are used to in everyday life. For example, if you flipped a fair penny, nickel, and dime 10 times, you would not expect the proportions of flips that resulted in heads to be *exactly* 50% for each.

We must determine if the association is **statistically significant** or if chance alone can explain the observed differences between the conditional and marginal distributions of y.

> An association is statistically significant if it is unlikely (by convention, a probability less than 5%) to have been produced "by chance," i.e., by independent, unrelated quantities.

To gauge the statistical significance of an association, we must first figure out a formal way to measure the difference between the conditional distributions of y across the levels of x and the overall marginal distribution of y. Once this is established, we must then determine the sizes of these differences that do indeed occur by chance when x and y are unrelated. If, by chance, a difference at least as large as the one observed occurs less than 5% of the time, we claim the association is statistically significant.

The convention of claiming statistical significance based on the 5% figure is due to historical reasons. Fisher's book *Statistical Methods for Research Workers* seems to be the first specific mention of the 5% number, but this was likely based on even earlier conventions. Look up the article "On the Origins of the .05 Level of Statistical Significance" in *American Psychologist* from May 1982 for an interesting read.

There are many ways to quantify the difference between the conditional and marginal distributions of y. Our strategy will be to compare the observed counts in the contingency table to the counts we would have *expected* had x and y been independent. If the observed and expected counts are very different, there is strong evidence of an association.

Formally, the statistic used to quantify the difference in conditional and marginal distributions is called the **discrepancy** D:

$$D = \text{sum over every cell of } \frac{(O-E)^2}{E} \tag{2.1}$$

where O is the observed value (not percent) in a cell of the contingency table (e.g., the entries in Table 2.2) and E is the expected count had x and y been independent. The expected count E can be calculated by finding the row and column totals of the cell in question and calculating:

$$E = \frac{\text{Row Total} \times \text{Column Total}}{n} \tag{2.2}$$

For example, to calculate the expected number of AT&T customers who report `Occasionally`, we use Table 2.2. The row total for this cell is 173 (173 customers have `ATT`) and the column total is 105 (105 report `Occasionally`). We multiply these and divide by the sample size (579) to get $173 \times 105/579 = 31.4$.

Mathematically, the formula for E makes sense. Let us illustrate by deriving the expected count in the cell for AT&T customers who report `Occasionally`. If the two variables do not have an association, then the conditional distribution of dropped-call frequency for AT&T customers should be the same as the overall, marginal distribution of dropped-call frequency. Overall, 105 out of the 579 customers report `Occasionally`, which works out to be 18.1%. Note: the 105 is the row total for the `ATT/Occasionally` cell, and the 579 is the number of individuals in the data, n.

If there were no association, then all carriers would have the same dropped-call frequencies. Thus, 18.1% of AT&T customers should report `Occasionally`. Since there are 173 AT&T customers, this works out to be $0.181 \times 173 = 31.4$. Notice the 173 is the column total for the cell in question. Backtracking through our work, we see the expected count is indeed $173 \times 105/79$ or (Row Total/n) $\times$ (Column Total).

To measure D, we need to calculate the expected values for *each* (all 12 in this case) of the entries in the contingency table, calculate $(O-E)^2/E$ for each, and take the sum. For the dropped call data, it can be shown that $D = 78.7$.

	Observed			Expected		
Observed	Occasionally	Often	Rarely	Occasionally	Often	Rarely
AT&T	57	23	93	31.4	11.1	130.6
Sprint	9	2	30	7.4	2.6	30.9
US Cellular	11	6	38	10.0	3.5	41.5
Verizon	28	6	276	56.2	19.8	234.0

$$D = \frac{(57-31.4)^2}{31.4} + \frac{(23-11.1)^2}{11.1} + \ldots + \frac{(6-19.8)^2}{19.8} + \frac{(276-234)^2}{234} = 78.7$$

The next question to ask is whether this discrepancy is "large" or whether we could have found this value "by chance" when the variables are not associated. We will answer this question by using the **permutation procedure**. In the permutation procedure, we create artificial data where, by design, y and x are independent. This is accomplished by shuffling up the observed values of y and randomly assigning them to individuals in the data. In effect, the column of y-values is randomly reordered. The value of D for this "permutation" dataset is computed and recorded, and the process repeats a large number of times.

It is easiest to introduce the permutation procedure when x and y are both quantitative variables. Table 2.4 illustrates the approach.

Table 2.4 — Illustration of permutation procedure. In the permutation procedure, the observed values of y are shuffled up and randomly assigned to each individual. This way, the numerical value for the association is one that has indeed happened "by chance" when x and y are independent. Note: in these permutation datasets, sometimes an individual ends up with its original value of y, but most of the time it does not.

Individual	Observed Data		Permutation 1		Permutation 2		Permutation 3	
	x	y	x	y	x	y	x	y
1	2.2	0.2	2.2	3.4	2.2	5.6	2.2	3.4
2	2.7	3.4	2.7	6.0	2.7	3.4	2.7	0.2
3	2.8	3.4	2.8	5.6	2.8	6.0	2.8	5.6
4	4.9	5.6	4.9	3.4	4.9	3.4	4.9	3.4
5	7.2	6.0	7.2	0.2	7.2	0.2	7.2	6.0

By assigning each individual a random value for y, we guarantee that there is no association between x and y in the permutation dataset. Thus, the value for D (or however we measure the discrepancy) is one that has indeed arisen by chance. After a few hundred rounds of this procedure, we have a very good idea of what values of D can occur when x and y are independent.

The distribution of values of D that arise "by chance" is known as the **sampling distribution** of D under the assumption of no association. The sampling distribution of various statistics forms the underpinning of most statistical tests that are performed. In general, the sampling distribution of a statistic is just the distribution of possible values that the statistic can achieve when data is collected in a certain manner.

Once the permutation procedure has been performed, the statistical significance of the observed association can be judged by calculating the ***p*-value** of the value of D observed in our data.

The p-value of D is the probability of measuring at least as large a discrepancy between observed and expected counts (or between conditional and marginal distributions) by chance alone. In other words, it is the fraction of artificial samples (generated by the permutation procedure, where x and y are not associated) that have a discrepancy at least as large as the observed value of D. By convention, if the p-value is less than 5%, we say that the association is statistically significant since it is unlikely (i.e., the probability is less than 5%) to be observed by chance.

The p-value of the association is being *estimated* using the permutation procedure. The estimated p-value is the fraction of artificial samples whose values of D are at least as large as the observed value for the discrepancy. You can imagine that had you generated a different set of permutation datasets, this fraction would be different. Thus, there is some uncertainty regarding the "actual" p-value. The output of `associate()` gives a 95% confidence interval for the p-value. If 5% is inside the interval, the test is inconclusive and the number of rounds in the permutation procedure should be increased.

Although we say an association is statistically significant if its p-value is less than 5%, this does not mean that the association is "real." There is always *some* probability (perhaps small) of observing a discrepancy at least as large as the one measured in the data by chance. Thus, our analysis cannot *prove* the existence of an association. Likewise, a p-value of 5% or larger is not *proof* that no association exists—the association may have just been too weak to be detected.

> A statistical analysis can never prove that an association exists between x and y, nor can it prove that x and y are independent. The analysis does, however, allow us to take a position on whether we think an association does or does not exist.

Let us illustrate the test with the dropped call data. See Table 2.5 for partial examples of the artificial datasets created with the permutation procedure. After 10,000 rounds, we have a very good idea what values of D occur "by chance." Figure 2.10 shows the values of D from the simulation.

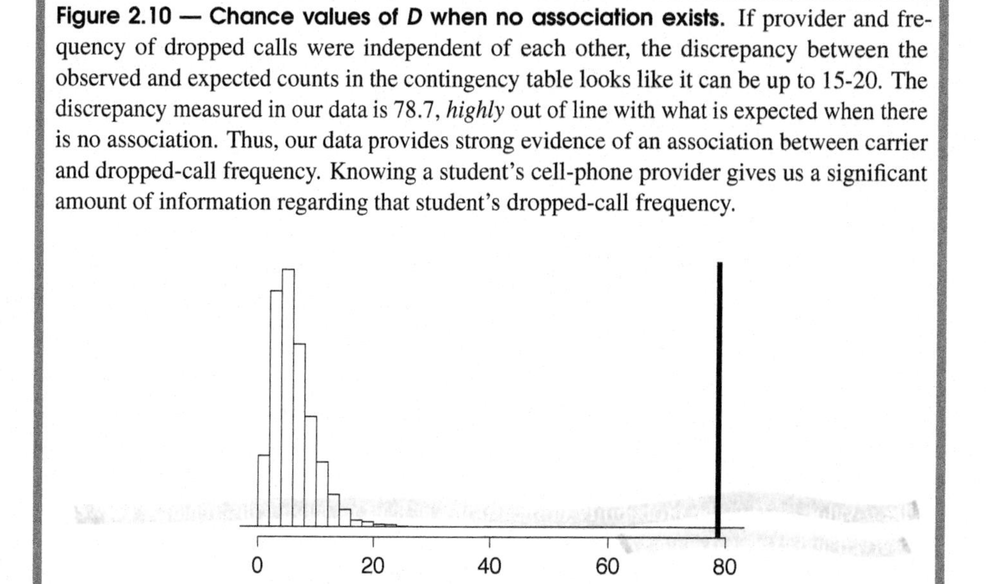

Figure 2.10 — Chance values of *D* when no association exists. If provider and frequency of dropped calls were independent of each other, the discrepancy between the observed and expected counts in the contingency table looks like it can be up to 15-20. The discrepancy measured in our data is 78.7, *highly* out of line with what is expected when there is no association. Thus, our data provides strong evidence of an association between carrier and dropped-call frequency. Knowing a student's cell-phone provider gives us a significant amount of information regarding that student's dropped-call frequency.

In R

```
associate(DropCallFreq~Provider,data=CALLS,permutations=10000)
```

The discrepancy of $D = 78.7$ measured from our data is highly "out of line" with the values that are expected to occur when carrier and dropped-call frequency are independent. Thus, the differences in the conditional distributions of dropped calls in Figure 2.6 are highly unlikely to have arisen "by chance."

The p-value of the observed association between `Provider` and `DropCallFreq` is the fraction of artificial samples (generated using the permutation procedure) whose values of D are at least 78.7. Since the largest value of D observed in our simulation of 10,000 artificial samples is about 30, the p-value is less than 1 in 10,000.

Table 2.5 — Permuting the Dropped Call data. The first six rows of the `CALL` data are shown (`Sprint` does not happen to appear) in the Observed Data column. Two artificial datasets created with the permutation procedure are displayed. These are generated by shuffling up the observed dropped-call frequencies and assigning them to students at random. Note: in the original illustration (Table 2.4), you could easily see how the collection of y values had randomly been reordered for the permutation datasets since there were only 5 individuals. The presented table here only has six of the 579 rows in the data, so some of the original y values appear missing in the permutation datasets. They would be present if the list continued.

	Observed Data		Permutation 1		Permutation 2	
Student	`Provider`	`DropCallFreq`	`Provider`	`DropCallFreq`	`Provider`	`DropCallFreq`
1	`ATT`	`Occasionally`	`ATT`	`Often`	`ATT`	`Rarely`
2	`USCellular`	`Rarely`	`USCellular`	`Rarely`	`USCellular`	`Rarely`
3	`Verizon`	`Occasionally`	`Verizon`	`Rarely`	`Verizon`	`Rarely`
4	`ATT`	`Often`	`ATT`	`Rarely`	`ATT`	`Occasionally`
5	`USCellular`	`Rarely`	`USCellular`	`Rarely`	`USCellular`	`Rarely`
6	`Verizon`	`Occasionally`	`Verizon`	`Rarely`	`Verizon`	`Rarely`
...	...	...	...	...	...	...
	$D = 78.7$		$D = 3.4$		$D = 9.1$	

This implies that there is less than a 0.01% chance of observing our data (and a corresponding association at least as strong) had a student's provider and dropped-call frequency been unrelated. Since this is less than 5%, we conclude the association is statistically significant, i.e., unlikely to have arisen by chance. However, remember that while we have strong evidence of an association, we have not *proven* that an association exists. There is always *some* chance, however small, of observing at least as large a value of D "by chance."

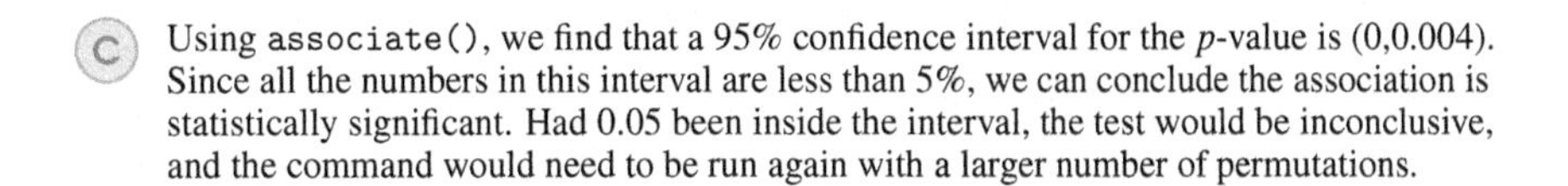

Ⓒ Using `associate()`, we find that a 95% confidence interval for the p-value is (0,0.004). Since all the numbers in this interval are less than 5%, we can conclude the association is statistically significant. Had 0.05 been inside the interval, the test would be inconclusive, and the command would need to be run again with a larger number of permutations.

Since the differences in the conditional distribution are large visually, we conclude that there is a strong, statistically significant association between provider and service, at least among college students in Knoxville, TN, from which the data was collected.

Ⓒ The method for simulating the p-value is computationally burdensome (but for modern computers, still quite quick), but there is a streamlined approach that yields an *approximate* p-value without the need to run simulations. If the dataset is so large that running the simulation would take too long, you can see this approximate p-value by adding the argument `classic=TRUE` to `associate()`.

2.4 Associations when y is quantitative and x is categorical

If y is a quantitative variable like income and x is a categorical variable like profession, we say that an association exists if the distribution of y differs in some way between the levels of x.

Aside 2.1 — *p*-values and statistical significance. The ***p*-value** of a statistic is a fundamental quantity in statistics and is used to gauge statistical significance. The following general definition will suffice for the study of any association.

The p-value is the probability that a random, independent set of quantities would produce an association at least as strong as the one observed from your data.

If the p-value of the association is small, it is unlikely (though not impossible) that independent quantities could have produced the data you collected. Either there is an association between the variables (for whatever reason) and knowing one gives you information about the possible values of the other, or the variables are actually independent and you happened to collect a highly unusual sample. The standard cutoff for a "small" p-value is 5%.

- If the p-value of the association is $< 5\%$, you have strong (though not conclusive) evidence of an association between the two quantities (it is theoretically possible for independent quantities to produce p-values arbitrarily close to 0 by chance).
- If the p-value of the association is $\geq 5\%$, you lack sufficient evidence to establish an association (though it may be the case the association is so weak you were unable to detect it).

When the p-value is less than 5%, we say that the association is **statistically significant**, i.e., unlikely to have been produced by "chance." When the p-value is 5% or greater, the association is not statistically significant. Note: a statistically significant relationship may still be quite weak. Always look at the appropriate visualization of the data and/or the value measuring the association to determine strength.

In other words, knowing an individual's level of x provides additional information regarding his or her possible values of y. Questions that involve this type of association include:

- Is there a relationship between the amounts people spend at Walmart (quantitative) and gender (categorical)? Do men and women spend the same amount on average at Walmart?
- Is there an association between religious conviction (categorical) and college GPA (quantitative)? Are the average GPAs for churchgoers and non-churchgoers the same?
- Are guys who wear glasses (categorical) perceived to be less attractive (quantitative, assuming attractiveness is measured as a score)? Is the average score for guys with glasses lower than the average for guys without glasses?

Formally, if the marginal distribution of y (over all individuals in the dataset) is different from at least one of the conditional distributions of y (for all individuals who are a common level for x), then we say that an association exists between x and y. However, determining whether there is such a difference in distributions turns out to be a rather hard problem. Rather, our strategy will be to assess whether there are any significant differences in the *average* or *median* value of y between levels of x.

Most of the time, it's the difference in averages or medians that is interesting rather than the distribution as a whole. For example, a merchant is often only concerned whether the typical sales to women and men are the same. If there is a difference (e.g., if men spend more than women), this suggests that more efforts could be made to bring women into the store so that overall sales are increased. Now imagine men and women spend the same amount on average, but the range of amounts for women is larger than for men. The existence of such an association does not suggest an obvious strategy to increase sales.

By focusing on the "typical value" of y, we will be unable to detect certain types of associations (see Figure 2.11 for examples). However, looking for differences in averages is by far one of the most common tasks in analytics, so the loss is not great. As you learn how to perform this analysis, do keep in mind this limitation!

Two showers may have the same pleasant temperature on average, but one shower's temperature could be a lot more variable (and a lot more unpleasant). An association exists between shower and temperature, but our chosen line of analysis will not be able to detect it.

Figure 2.11 — Equal averages but different distributions. An association exists between x and y when there are differences in the conditional distributions of y between the levels of x. The plots below show that the distribution of y is different for groups A and B, so there is an association between y and $x = Group$. On the left, groups A and B have the same average value of y, but the standard deviation of values for group B is larger. On the right, groups A and B have the same average value *and* standard deviation of y (but the distributions still look quite different).

Unfortunately, determining whether there is a difference between the marginal and conditional distributions of y as a whole is hard. Typically, the question we *really* want to answer is whether there is any difference in averages or medians between levels of x. This is an easier question. However, by restricting ourselves to this particular line of inquiry, we limit ourselves in the kinds of associations we can detect. In both examples below, x and y have obvious associations, but the *average* values of y are identical. Our analysis will miss this type of association!

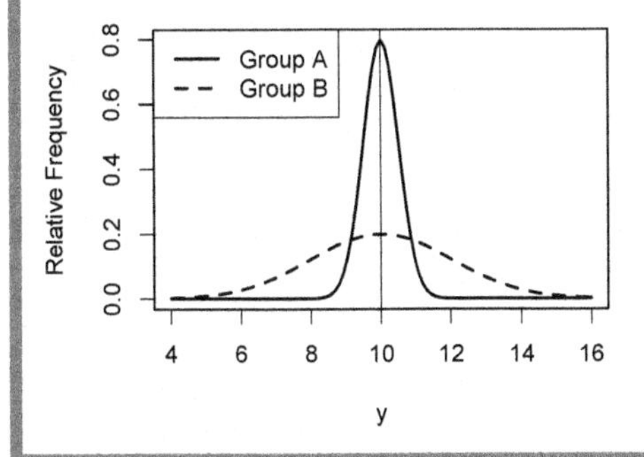

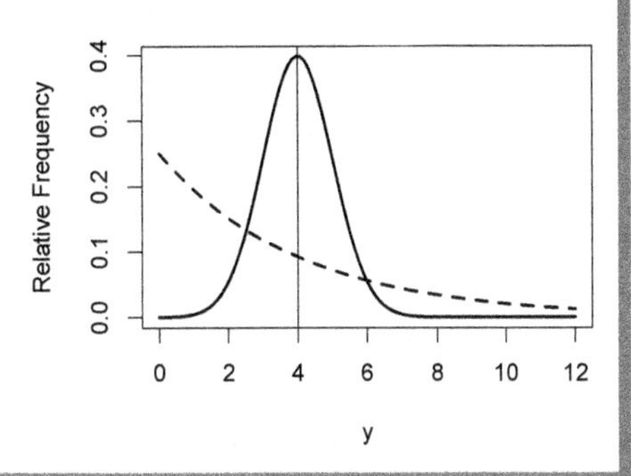

To motivate this line of analysis, let us consider data on people's appearance and attractiveness. Students in six statistics classes rated the attractiveness of men and women who had posted pictures of themselves on an online dating site. The average rating over all students in the class was designated to be the "attractiveness score" of the person in the picture. `ATTRACTF` and `ATTRACTM` contain the scores and various other characteristics of 70 men and women.

Students were instructed to rate the gender to which they were most attracted, and no distinction was made between opposite-sex and same-sex ratings.

Is there an association between attractiveness score and smiling? Wearing glasses? Hair color? Do people who smile have a higher average attractiveness than people who do not smile, etc.?

2.4.1 Visualizations with side-by-side box plots

The first step in analyzing the association is to visualize the conditional distributions of y for each level of x. An association exists if there are differences, i.e., not all box plots look "about the same"—knowing the level of x provides information about the possible values of y. Larger differences indicate stronger associations.

> Since looking "about the same" is hard to describe statistically, we will instead keep things simple and say that an association exists if the *average* or *median* value of y is not the same between levels of x. In other words, their "typical values" are different.

When visually assessing the existence or strength of an association, we first look at the box plots and histograms of the conditional distributions of y for each level of x. To determine what (means vs. medians) we are comparing, we note the shape of the distributions.

> If the distributions of y are roughly symmetric with no extreme outliers (i.e., roughly Normal), we will compare the average values of y between levels of x. Otherwise, we will compare the median values of y between the levels of x.

In R Making side-by-side box plots in R can be accomplished by `plot(y~x)`, though these box plots will not display the averages. Making histograms for each level of x is more involved. Running `associate()` from the `regclass` package shows side-by-side box plots (including averages), all histograms, and Q-Q plots to gauge whether the distributions are "close" to a Normal distribution.

If the averages/medians in each box plot are about equal, then we will say the association between y and x is weak or perhaps non-existent. If the averages/medians look noticeably different, there may be a significant association, and a formal statistical test is required.

Figure 2.12 shows side-by-side box plots of the attractiveness scores for women with certain characteristics in the `ATTRACTF` dataset. It looks like wearing glasses, hair color, and apparent race have a strong and meaningful association with attractiveness (the averages look very different), while smiling does not (the averages are about the same).

When there are only two groups (x has two levels), we say an association exists if the averages or medians are different. When there are three or more levels of x, we say an association exists if not all levels have identical averages or medians (i.e., two or more levels may have the same average, but at least one level is different than the others). If the association looks strong enough to be of any practical significance, we can run a formal test to see if such a difference is statistically significant or could have just happened "by chance."

Figure 2.12 — Visualizing associations involving attractiveness. To check for an association and to gauge its strength, we compare the averages/medians of the box plots. The magnitude of the difference reveals the strength of the association. In these examples, the distribution of attractiveness score is roughly symmetric with no extreme outliers, so we will compare averages.

The average score for girls wearing glasses is much lower than for girls with no glasses—attractiveness and eyewear have an association. The same goes for hair color (lighter-haired girls have a higher average score). However, there does not seem to be much of an association between score and smiling (the averages are nearly identical). Apparent race may be associated with score due to noticeably differing averages.

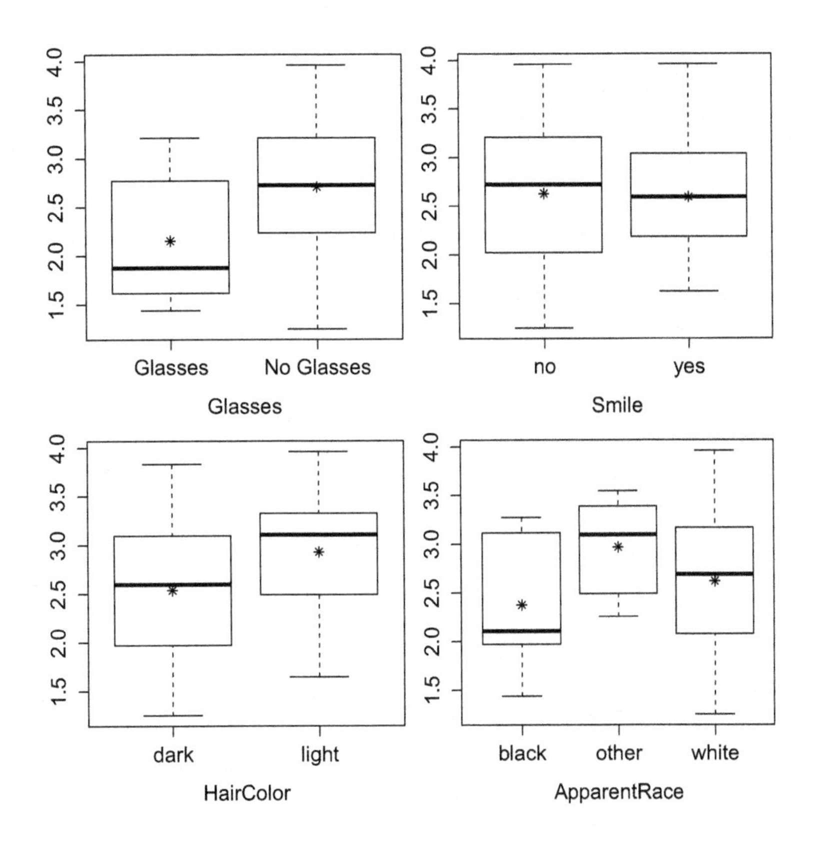

In R

```
data(ATTRACT)
associate(Score~Glasses,data=ATTRACTF)
associate(Score~HairColor,data=ATTRACTF)
associate(Score~ApparentRace,data=ATTRACTF)
```

2.4.2 Tests for association

The test of statistical significance depends on the shapes of the conditional distributions of y for each level of x.

- If all distributions are roughly symmetric, have about the same spread, and have no extreme outliers (i.e., well-described by Normal distributions), the analysis of variance (**ANOVA**) test is used, and the average values of y are compared across the levels of x.
- If all distributions are roughly symmetric and have about the same spread, but one or more contain extreme outliers, the **Kruskal-Wallis test** should be used instead of the ANOVA.
- Otherwise, the **median test** is used, and the median values of y are compared across the levels of x.

ANOVA (averages)

When it makes sense to compare the average value of y between the levels of x (distributions are well-described by a Normal curve, i.e., roughly symmetric, approximately equal spread, with no extreme outliers), the analysis of variance (**ANOVA**) test is used to determine if the association is statistically significant.

While the mechanics are relatively complex, the test essentially compares the observed variability in the averages across the levels of x to the expected variability in averages had there been no association (i.e., the conditional distribution of y for each level of x is identical to the marginal, overall distribution of y).

The difference between the observed and expected variability in averages is measured by the F statistic.

$$F = \frac{\text{Observed variability of group averages}}{\text{Expected variability of group averages}} \tag{2.3}$$

A value of F of 3.2 means that the observed variability in group averages is 3.2 times higher than the variability we would expect by chance (if there was no association). Values of the F statistic much greater than 1.0 are evidence that y and x have an association (at least two of the levels of x have different average values for y) since the differences in averages is much higher than what would be expected "by chance." A value of F close to 1.0 is consistent with the groups having the same fundamental underlying average. Figure 2.13 provides a visual justification for this reasoning.

To determine whether the association (i.e., difference in averages) is statistically significant, we need to find the probability of measuring a difference at least as large as the observed value of F "by chance." The p-value of the test provides us with the answer.

> The p-value of the ANOVA tells us the probability of finding at least as big a discrepancy in averages (i.e., at least as large a value for F) "by chance" when x and y are independent (i.e., all levels of x have the same distribution of y).
>
> If the p-value is $< 5\%$, the association is statistically significant. There is strong (though not conclusive) evidence that at least two levels of x have different average values of y.
>
> If the p-value is $\geq 5\%$, the association is not statistically significant. If a difference in averages exists at all, it is too small to be detected with the data.

Figure 2.13 — Motivation behind ANOVA. An ANOVA compares the observed variability in the average values of y across levels of x (here, given by the three dotted horizontal lines) to the variability we would expect if there were no association.

On the left, each of the three levels of x (by design) have the same distribution of y (i.e., y and x have no association). The observed variability in averages is about what we'd expect, and the F statistic is about 1.0.

On the right, each of the three levels of x (by design) have very different distributions of y (i.e., y and x have a strong association). Knowing an individual's level of x tells us a good deal about his or her possible values of y—individuals in A have relatively small values while individuals in C have relatively large values. The F statistic is much greater than 1.0, indicating that the observed variability in the averages is much larger than what would have been expected by chance.

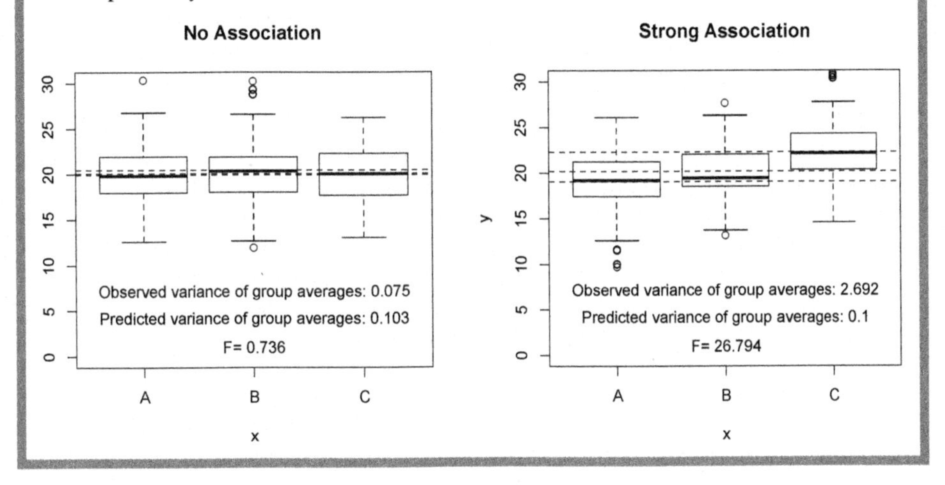

To find the p-value, we need to know what values of F are likely to appear "by chance." We can once again use the permutation procedure to gain this insight.

1. Create an artificial dataset by shuffling up the observed values of y and randomly assigning them to individuals. See the table below. Calculate the value of F. By design, this procedure guarantees that there is no underlying relationship between x and y so that the measured value of F is one that can occur "by chance."

Individual	Observed Data		Permutation 1		Permutation 2		Permutation 3	
	x	y	x	y	x	y	x	y
1	A	0.2	A	3.4	A	5.6	A	3.4
2	B	3.4	B	6.0	B	3.4	B	0.2
3	B	3.4	B	5.6	B	6.0	B	5.6
4	B	5.6	B	3.4	B	3.4	B	3.4
5	A	6.0	A	0.2	A	0.2	A	6.0
	$F = 0.19$		$F = 4.08$		$F = 0.35$		$F = 0.53$	

2. Repeat this procedure many times to build up a distribution of values of F that occur by chance.
3. The (estimated) p-value of the association is the fraction of these artificial datasets whose values of F are at least as large as the value measured on the original data.

4. If the p-value is less than 5%, the observed variation in averages (and thus association between y and x) is statistically significant—it is unlikely (probability less than 0.05) for the levels of x to exhibit the observed differences in averages by chance.
5. Note: always check the 95% confidence interval for the p-value. If 0.05 is inside this interval, the test is inconclusive, and the number of permutations must be increased.

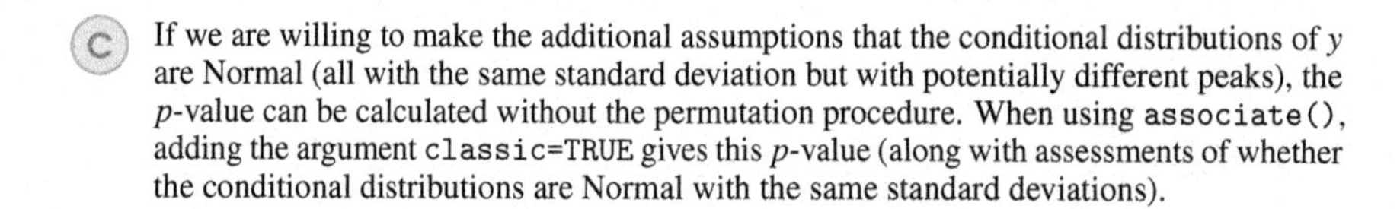

If we are willing to make the additional assumptions that the conditional distributions of y are Normal (all with the same standard deviation but with potentially different peaks), the p-value can be calculated without the permutation procedure. When using `associate()`, adding the argument `classic=TRUE` gives this p-value (along with assessments of whether the conditional distributions are Normal with the same standard deviations).

Regarding the attractiveness scores of women in the `ATTRACTF` dataset, it is found that the estimated p-values (after 50,000 permutations) of the associations between score and wearing glasses, smile, hair color, and apparent race are 1.5%, 84.4%, 5.4%, and 19.3%, respectively. Thus, the only feature that has a statistically significant association with attractiveness score is wearing glasses. See Figure 2.14.

Figure 2.14 — Finding *p*-values for associations involving Attraction Score. The possible values of F (a measure of the discrepancy in averages between levels) when all levels have the same underlying average can be simulated to find the p-value of the association. These plots show the distribution of F when attractiveness score (`Score`) does *not* have associations with smiling (`Smile`) or apparent race (`ApparentRace`). The vertical line represents the observed value of F from the `ATTRACTF` data.

Regarding `Smile`, it is clear that our value of F is out of line with what we expect when there is no association. In fact, the p-value is about 1.5% (only 1.5% of artificial samples produce F values at least as large "by chance"), implying that the association is statistically significant—the average attractiveness score depends on whether or not the girl is smiling.

Regarding `ApparentRace`, we see the observed value of F is pretty typical of what is found when there is no association. Since the p-value is about 20% (much greater than the cutoff of 5%), the association is not statistically significant. It looks like the average attractiveness score is the same regardless of the girl's perceived race.

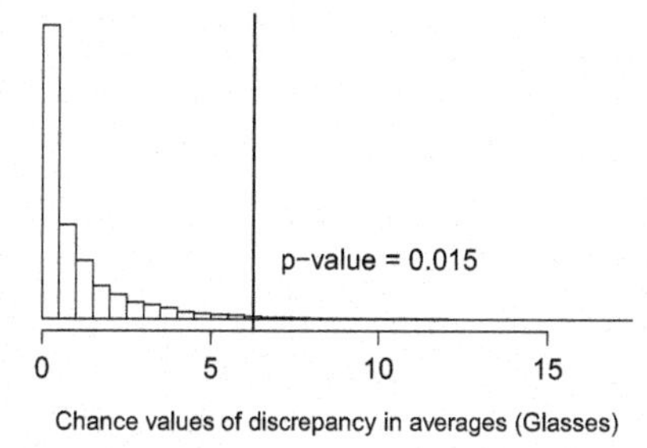

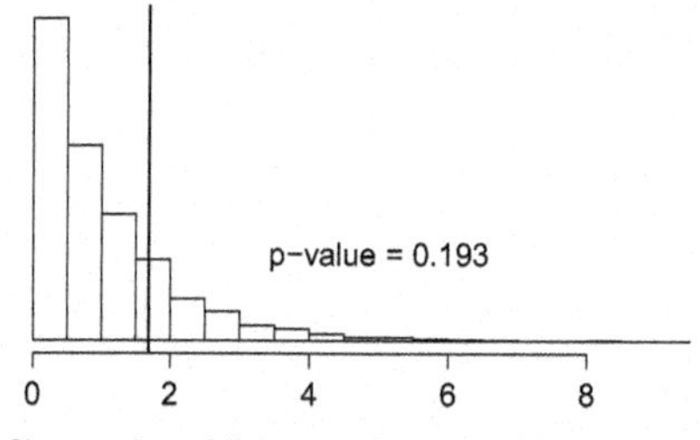

In R

```
associate(Score~Smile,data=ATTRACTF)
associate(Score~ApparentRace,data=ATTRACTF)
```

While we are not surprised to find that the association between attractiveness and smile is not significant (their averages are about the same in Figure 2.12), we may be somewhat surprised to find that the associations between attractiveness and hair color or apparent race (which did look to have reasonably large differences in averages) are not significant either. Thus, it is necessary to perform the statistical test when the association looks to be strong. A "strong" looking association may *not* be statistically significant!

If the association is statistically significant, we have evidence that at least two levels of x have different average values of y. Unfortunately, the ANOVA does not tell us *which* levels have different average values. This requires what is known as a post-hoc test and is beyond the scope of this text. An Internet search (or Wikipedia) for the Least Significant Difference (LSD) test, Tukey's Honest Significant Difference (HSD), or Scheffe's test will fill you in on the details.

Median test

If a distribution has noticeable skewness or extreme outliers, the Normal curve does not provide a good approximation to its shape, and the average may not represent a "typical" value. Rather, the median provides a more useful summary (see Figure 2.15). If the conditional distribution of y for at least one of the levels of x has these properties, then the median values of y should be compared across levels. The median test should be used to evaluate statistical significance.

Figure 2.15 — Failure of average to capture the "typical" value. When the distribution is skewed (left panel), the average gets pulled out from the peak of the distribution toward the tail. The average value is no longer representative of a typical value (in this case the average is 4.5, which is larger than 70% of the values).

When the distribution has outliers (right panel), the average gets dragged toward them. The average value may no longer represent a typical value from the distribution (in this case, values are tightly clustered around a central peak, but the outlier has shifted the average up above the peak entirely).

The median is much less sensitive to the shape of the distribution or to outliers and better represents a typical value (closer to the peak) in these cases.

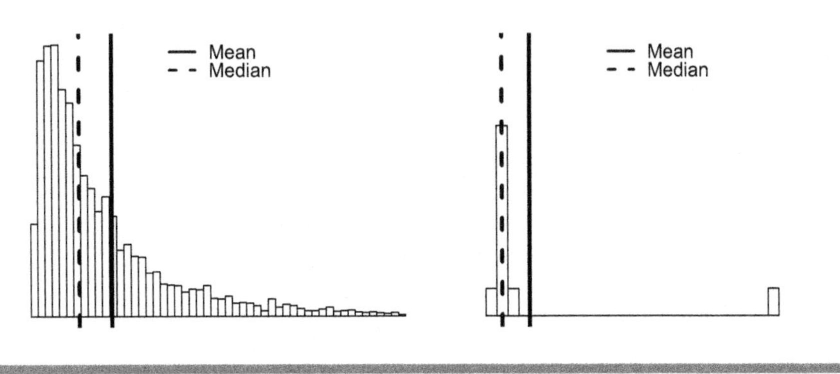

The test proceeds by reasoning that if the median values of y for each level of x were the same (i.e., no association exists between x and y), then about half of the values of y for each level of x should be less than this common median and the other half should be larger. If a noticeable majority of y values for one level of x is below the common median, then that level of x typically has smaller values of y than the other levels. In that case, knowing x provides additional information about the typical value of y, so there is indeed an association.

The "common" median is estimated by finding the median of the marginal distribution of y, i.e., the collection of y values over all individuals in the data.

To illustrate, consider the potential existence of an association between the rating of a new product and the rater's apparent race. The common median (of all ratings) is 3.1. We may suspect an association since all scores for "Black" are above the median, while all but one for "White" is below.

	Values							Larger than median (of 3.1)						
White	3.1	2.1	3.7	1.8	2.3	1.9		no	no	yes	no	no	no	
Black	3.7	3.3	4.1	3.4				yes	yes	yes	yes			
Other	4.1	1.9	3.0	1.7	4.2	3.6	1.6	yes	no	no	no	yes	yes	no

The median test is conducted by converting the original data into a contingency table and performing the χ^2 test for association between the (now) two categorical variables x and y (Yes/No, depending on if the value is larger than the median).

	Larger than median	
Race	Yes	No
White	1	5
Black	4	0
Other	3	4

In this example, the p-value of the median test is 4.4%. Since it is less than 5%, we say that there is evidence of an association between rating and race—the median ratings between at least two levels of race are different. As with the ANOVA, the test does not tell us *which* levels of x have different medians.

Kruskal-Wallis test for symmetric distributions with outliers

When the distributions of y for each level of x are roughly symmetric and have about the same spread but contain extreme outliers, the average may not necessarily represent the "typical" value, as seen in Figure 2.15. While the median test can be conducted to determine if x and y have an association, an alternative (more specialized) analysis called the Kruskal-Wallis test can be used instead.

The Kruskal-Wallis test replaces the original values in the data with their relative *ranks*, then essentially conducts the ANOVA on the dataset of ranks. For example, consider two samples (men vs. women) of times spent on a website. Let us recode the observed values into relative ranks and then calculate the average rank for each sample.

	Time on Website					Relative Ranks					Average Rank
Men	1.2	3.4	3.6	5.0	12.5	1	3	4	5	9	4.4
Women	3.3	5.1	5.3	8.8	20.5	2	6	7	8	10	6.6

If there was no association (men and women have the same typical value for time on the website), then we would expect each sample to have a mix of high and low ranks. If one sample typically has larger values than the other, then the ranks of this sample will be larger as well. If the observed variability in the average ranks between levels of x is much larger than the variability we would expect by chance, then there is evidence for an association.

The p-value can be calculated using the permutation procedure, and as with other tests, if the p-value is less than 5%, then the association is statistically significant (at least two levels have different typical values). If the p-value is 5% or larger, then the association is not significant since the variability in average ranks could have "easily" occurred by chance.

In the example above, we see that women's times are larger (as well as the average rank of the values), so there is some evidence for an association. However, the p-value turns out to be about 31%, indicating that there is no association between someone's gender and the time he or she spends on a website (the difference in average ranks is not statistically significant) in this study.

Choosing the correct test

The median test can always be used to test for an association between a quantitative y (amount spent, height, income, etc.) and a categorical x (gender, race, homeowner/renter), so why don't we always just use it? The median test has the lowest **power** of the tests we have discussed, meaning that it has the smallest chance of detecting an association when it exists (weak associations often go undetected when using the median test). When other tests are appropriate, we should use them since they are more likely to discover the association when it is present.

- If the distributions of y for each level of x are roughly symmetric, have about the same spread, lack extreme outliers, and are well-described by a Normal distribution, the average provides a useful summary of the "typical" value of y. Use the ANOVA.
- If all distributions are roughly symmetric, but one or more have extreme outliers, use the rank-based test (Kruskal-Wallis) since the average may not represent the typical value.
- If one or more of the distributions of y are quite skewed (potentially with extreme outliers), the median best represents a typical value. Use the median test.

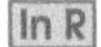

As with any analysis of associations, `associate()` in package `regclass` will provide the relevant graphical and statistical analysis. Specifically, side-by-side box plots and histograms are provided, as well as the distribution of "chance" values for the difference in averages, mean ranks, and medians found via the permutation procedure. The p-values (and associated 95% confidence intervals) of the ANOVA, Kruskal-Wallis, and median tests are provided. Adding the argument `classic=TRUE` also gives Q-Q plots for each level of x and the p-value from the classic ANOVA test (which assumes that each conditional distribution is Normal with the same standard deviation).

2.5 Associations when y is categorical and x is quantitative

If y is a categorical variable like buy vs. not buy and x is a quantitative variable like income, we say that an association exists if the distribution of the levels of y changes with x. In other words, if we look at the segmented bar charts for the distribution of y for individuals who share some common value of x, their appearance will depend on the exact value of x we have selected. Questions that involve this type of association include:

- Is there an association between being hired (yes/no; categorical) and college GPA (quantitative)? Does the probability of being hired steadily increase with GPA?

- Is there a relationship between the probability a customer shops at Target (yes/no; categorical) and the distance the customer lives from the nearest store (quantitative)?

This particular type of association can be difficult to analyze since it is quite possible that each individual in the data has a unique value for x. Previously, we could graphically examine and statistically compare the conditional distributions of y (either categorical or quantitative) for each level of a categorical x. When x is quantitative, it is impossible to glimpse the conditional distribution of y for all possible values of x because many values of x may have only been recorded once and many values of x may not have been recorded at all. See Table 2.6.

Table 2.6 — Difficulty assessing conditional distributions of y when x is quantitative. Imagine our data consists solely of the following nine individuals (these happen to be the first nine individuals in the STUDENT data).

Churchgoer (y)	HSGPA (x)
No	3.18
No	3.20
Yes	3.40
Yes	3.14
Yes	4.00
Yes	3.85
Yes	3.60
No	3.25
No	3.60

An association exists between someone's high school GPA (x) and whether he or she is a churchgoer (y) if the fraction of people who regularly go to church is higher for some values of GPA and lower for others. Unfortunately, only a single GPA occurs twice (3.60) and many GPAs are absent (e.g., 3.90), making estimating the fraction of churchgoers at each possible value of GPA impossible.

One strategy to analyze the association is to group individuals with similar values of x together, e.g., 0-5, 5-10, 10-15, and to treat these groups as levels of a categorical variable. A mosaic plot and χ^2 test can be used to study the association.

Figure 2.16 shows such an analysis of a potential association between someone's high school GPA and whether he or she regularly attended church. The possible values of GPA have been split into six categories with about 100 students each.

Overall, the marginal distribution shows that slightly fewer than half of the students are regular churchgoers. Knowing the student's GPA appears to add additional information about going go church. Among students with very low GPAs (2.34 to 3.33), the proportion of churchgoers is noticeably lower. Among students with high GPAs (3.9 to 4), the proportion of students is noticeably higher. Because we see *some* differences in the conditional distributions of going to church, we have evidence of an association.

Indeed, the p-value of the association (as estimated by the permutation procedure) is only 0.4%, so the association is statistically significant.

Figure 2.16 — Association between going to church and high school GPA. For this problem, we are interested in predicting whether someone regularly goes to church (y) based on his or her GPA in high school (x). Since GPA is a quantitative variable, it is not possible to estimate the conditional distribution of going to church for all allowable GPAs because not all values were observed and some were observed only once. Thus, high school GPA is converted into a categorical variable with 6 levels (with about 100 students in each): 2.34-3.34, 3.34-3.54, etc. The analysis proceeds as if we were studying an association between two categorical variables.

Because the conditional distributions of y (going to church) do look different from each other and from the marginal distribution, we say that there is visual evidence for an association. In fact, the analysis shows that, among these students, the probability of being a churchgoer appears to be higher for students with higher GPAs.

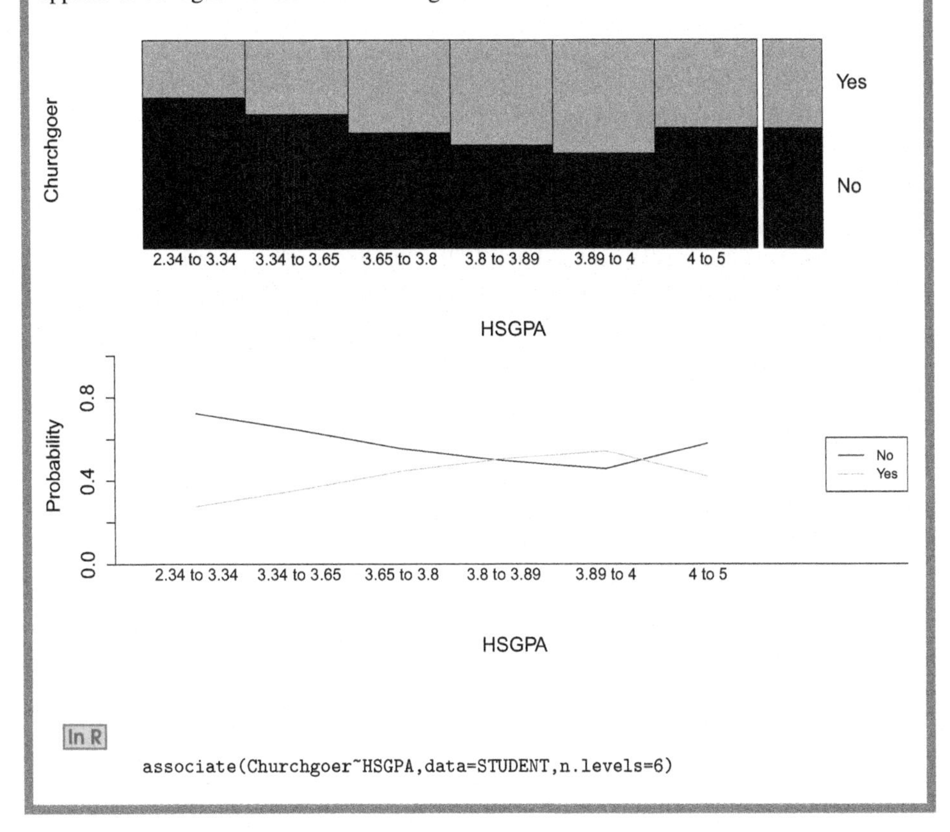

In R

```
associate(Churchgoer~HSGPA,data=STUDENT,n.levels=6)
```

In R

`associate()` in package `regclass` will perform the relevant analysis when y is categorical and x is quantitative. In this case, the default number of levels when converting x into a categorical variable is about $n/10$, where n is the sample size (this way, about 10 individuals have each level of x). If you want a different number of levels (e.g., 6 as in the church and GPA example), add the additional argument `n.levels=6`.

2.6 Associations when y and x are quantitative variables

An association exists between two quantitative variables when knowing the value of one provides additional information about the possible values for the other. Questions that involve this type of association include:

- Is there a relationship between your final exam score and number of hours that you study?
- Is there an association between the amount of money people spend at grocery stores and at fast-food restaurants?
- Is the first week's sales of a new product indicative of sales 10 weeks after launch?
- Do SAT/ACT scores really indicate future success in college (higher college GPA)?

When an association exists, information can potentially be exploited. For instance, admissions counselors only want to let students into college who will be successful. Since they cannot peer into the future, they seek to find quantities that are associated with college GPA (one measure of success). By identifying such a quantity, like the number of high school clubs or the household income of the parents, they can focus on acquiring students similar to those who have succeeded in the past. If the association indeed generalizes to new students, the counselors will improve the student body.

To analyze an association, the first step is to cast the variables into the roles of x and y. In this case, the distinction only affects the visualization of the relationship and not the statistical analysis. Based on the question at hand, recall the convention for assignment. Let y be the quantity you wish to predict and x be the quantity used to make predictions.

In other words, assign x and y so that the following question makes sense: "Can x help to predict y?" We treat x as the "predictor variable" and y as the "response" (or variable of interest). For example:

- If we are analyzing the association between ACT score and college GPA, then y will be GPA and x will be ACT score. We want to predict college GPAs from ACT scores.
- If we analyze the association between the amount of sales in the first and tenth weeks after launch, then y will be sales in the tenth week and x will be sales in the first week (we want to predict tenth week from first week sales).

The association is visualized using a **scatterplot**, where x and y values of individuals are plotted in pairs. We refer to the shape of the cloud of points as the "stream of points." If the stream of points looks like a flat, featureless, rectangular band, then no association exists (the conditional distributions of y for each x look about the same). If the stream exhibits a pattern, then the conditional distribution of y for at least one value of x is different. In that case, x and y have an association since knowing an individual's x value provides additional information about his or her possible y-values.

The only "pattern" that is not indicative of an association is when there are horizontal "gaps" in the stream of points. This is an artifact of the data collection procedure and indicates that x values in the gaps are relatively rare. The presence of these gaps make no comment on whether x and y have an association.

Figure 2.17 shows examples of scatterplots where associations do and do not exist.

Figure 2.17 — Appearance of scatterplots when associations do and do not exist. The top three plots show examples where x and y do not have an association. Knowing the x-value of an individual does not give any additional information about that individual's y value since it appears that the distribution of y is roughly the same everywhere. For example, in the first plot, values are centered around 10, give or take 2.5 or so. In the third plot, there are gaps around $x = 3$ and $x = 6$ to 8. This is a relic of how data was collected (or indicates that individuals with these x values are very rare). Horizontal gaps do not contain any information about whether x and y have an association.

The bottom three plots show examples where x and y have an association. On the left, the typical value of y is larger for individuals with larger values of x. In the middle, the typical value of y is always about 100, but the spread of possible y values is larger for individuals with larger values of x. On the right, individuals who have x values close to 0 have y values close to ± 1. When individuals have x values close to ± 1, they have y values close to 0. In all three cases, the distribution of possible values of y changes with x. Thus, knowing an individual's value of x yields additional insight about the individual's possible values of y.

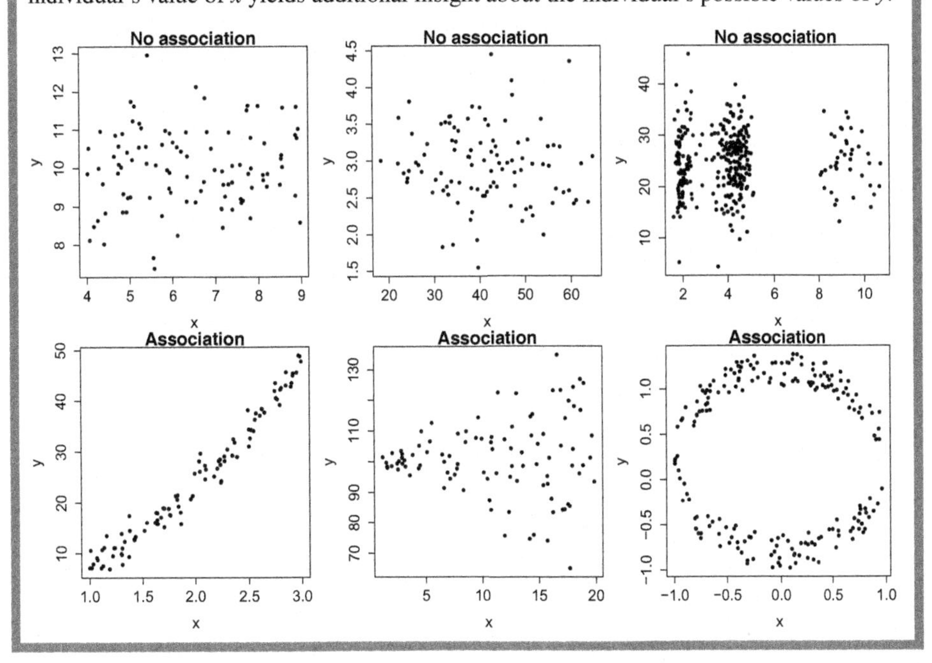

The strength of the association is gauged by the amount of (vertical) scatter in the stream of points and, more formally, by either Pearson's correlation coefficient r or Spearman's rank correlation. Formal tests can be conducted to determine whether the association is statistically significant, but the value of the correlation itself is the final judge of whether the association is of any practical importance.

2.6.1 Visualizing the association with scatterplots

A scatterplot shows how values of x and y vary together. By convention, y has values along the vertical (up/down) axis and x has values along the horizontal (left/right) axis. To describe the association, we note features of the stream of points, specifically its **direction** and **form**. The direction may be positive, negative, or a bit of both (**non-monotonic**), and the form may be linear or nonlinear. See Figure 2.18 for examples.

Direction

The direction of a relationship refers to the trajectory of the stream of points and describes how the variables change together. There are three kinds of directions: positive, negative, or non-monotonic (a mixture of positive and negative).

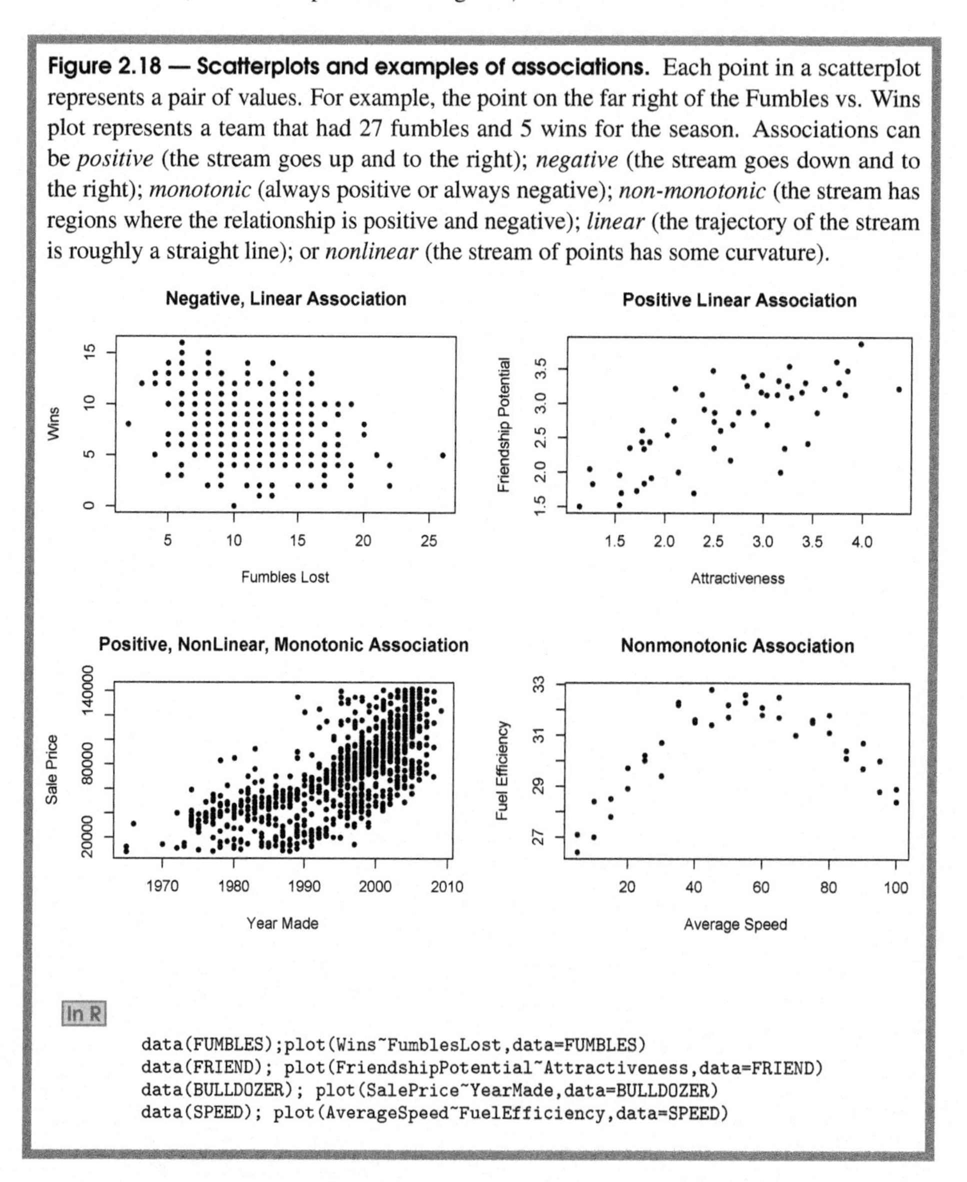

Figure 2.18 — Scatterplots and examples of associations. Each point in a scatterplot represents a pair of values. For example, the point on the far right of the Fumbles vs. Wins plot represents a team that had 27 fumbles and 5 wins for the season. Associations can be *positive* (the stream goes up and to the right); *negative* (the stream goes down and to the right); *monotonic* (always positive or always negative); *non-monotonic* (the stream has regions where the relationship is positive and negative); *linear* (the trajectory of the stream is roughly a straight line); or *nonlinear* (the stream of points has some curvature).

```
data(FUMBLES);plot(Wins~FumblesLost,data=FUMBLES)
data(FRIEND); plot(FriendshipPotential~Attractiveness,data=FRIEND)
data(BULLDOZER); plot(SalePrice~YearMade,data=BULLDOZER)
data(SPEED); plot(AverageSpeed~FuelEfficiency,data=SPEED)
```

Positive association

Two variables have a positive association when above-average values of y are typically found with above-average values of x (the same goes for below-average values). The trajectory of the stream of points heads up and to the right of the plot.

The upper-right scatterplot in Figure 2.18 shows the relationship between the attractiveness score of a woman (as gauged by straight males rating a picture) and her "friendship potential" (a rating of how likely female students said they would be friends with the woman after viewing the same picture). Interestingly, the association is noticeably positive. Women who are above average in terms of attractiveness also have above-average scores for friendship potential. Women of below-average attractiveness typically have below-average friendship scores.

The lower-left scatterplot shows a positive association between the selling price of bulldozers at auctions and the year that the bulldozer was made. Typically, newer bulldozers (above average values for Year Made) are found with above average values of Sale Price.

Negative association

Two variables have a negative association when above-average values of y are typically found with below-average values of x (and vice versa). The stream of points heads down and to the right of the plot. The upper-left scatterplot in Figure 2.18 shows a negative association between the number of wins per season of an NFL team and the number of lost fumbles. Typically, teams with an above-average number of wins had a below-average number of lost fumbles and vice versa.

Non-monotonic vs. monotonic associations

Two variables have a monotonic relationship when the direction is either all positive or all negative. Most relationships are monotonic. Non-monotonic associations occur when the direction of the relationship changes, i.e., has a mix of positive and negative parts. The lower-right scatterplot in Figure 2.18 shows the relationship between the fuel efficiency and speeds of cars. The relationship is non-monotonic because the trajectory is positive for low speeds and negative for high speeds. The optimal fuel efficiency is reached at about 58 miles per hour.

In 1974, then-president Nixon signed a law that made the national speed limit 55 mph. The goal was to force people to drive at more fuel-efficient speeds and to decrease the demand for foreign oil. It wasn't until 1995 that Congress finally repealed the law. Some interstates still have the default 55 mph speed posted.

Form - Linear vs. Nonlinear

The form of a relationship refers to the shape of the trajectory of the stream of points. A **linear** relationship is when the trajectory is well-described by a straight line. The term **nonlinear** is used otherwise (noticeable curvature, discontinuities, etc.). In Figure 2.18, the relationships between the number of wins and number of lost fumbles as well as between the attractiveness scores and friendship potentials of women look quite linear. The relationships between a bulldozer's selling price and its model year as well as between the fuel efficiency and speed of cars look nonlinear.

Strength

The strength of an association between two categorical variables is assessed by comparing the segmented bar charts for each level of x. Larger discrepancies indicate stronger associations. The strength of an association between a categorical and quantitative variable is assessed by comparing the average or median values of y between levels of x. Bigger differences imply stronger associations.

The strength of an association between two quantitative variables is related to how much vertical scatter is present in the stream of points and to its tilt.

> Among streams with the same amount of tilt, less vertical scatter implies a stronger association. Among streams with equal amounts of scatter, more tilt implies a stronger relationship.

There is an intuitive justification for this rule. When two streams have the same amount of tilt, knowing the value of x narrows down the range of possible values of y more for the stream with less scatter. When two streams have the same amount of scatter, knowing the value of x narrows down the typical value of y more for the stream with larger tilt. For example, consider Figure 2.19.

Figure 2.19 — Gauging the strength of associations with scatterplots. In these three plots, y ranges between 1 and 2. On the left, this variation is the same regardless of x, so knowing x doesn't narrow down the possible values of y: x and y do not have an association. In the middle, we see a distinct tilt to the stream of points and less scatter. When $x = 2.8$, y varies between 1.15 and 1.55, while when $x = 6$, y varies between 1.38 and 1.78. Knowing x somewhat narrows down the possible values of y, so there is a moderate association. On the right, there is very little scatter in the stream. When $x = 2.8$, y ranges between 1.025 and 1.1, while when $x = 6$, y ranges between 1.57 and 1.65. Knowing x greatly narrows down the possible values of y, and there is a strong association.

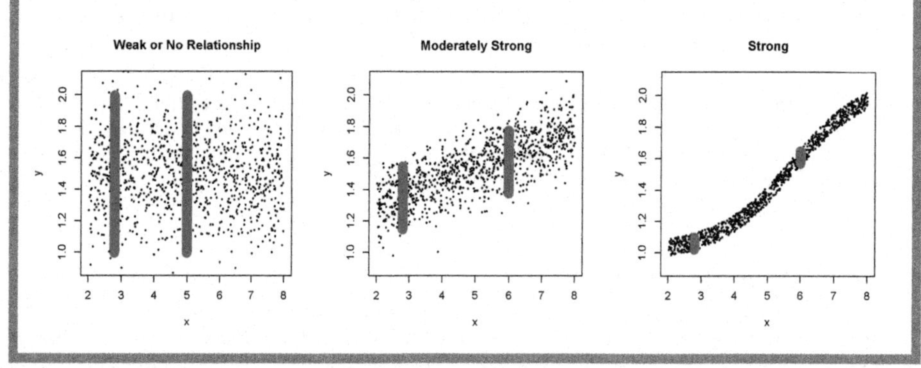

Let us now turn to numerically measuring the strength of the relationship. Based on our reasoning so far, it makes sense to compare the *overall* variability of y to the variability of y *once we know* x.

2.6.2 Pearson's correlation *r* for linear relationships

When the trajectory of the stream of points is *linear*, **Pearson's correlation** coefficient r is used to describe the strength of the association between x and y. Further, we use the word **correlation** rather than *association*. Key properties of r are:

- $-1 \leq r \leq 1$: A correlation of 0 means there is no linear component to the relationship between x and y while a correlation of ± 1 means that the stream of points is *exactly* a straight line (no vertical scatter).
- Values of r farther from 0 (either more positive or more negative) indicate progressively stronger relationships.
- A positive correlation indicates the direction of the relationship is positive. A negative correlation indicates the direction is negative.
- Having $r = 0$ does *not* mean that there is no association between x and y, just that there is no *linear* relationship.
- Do not use r to describe a relationship that is not linear.

(C) The formula that gives r is involved enough that a detailed discussion is omitted. What is important to know is that the formula uses information about how far individuals' x- and y-values are from their respective averages, as well as about the standard deviations of x and y. Since averages and standard deviations are sensitive to outliers, the value of r is also sensitive to outliers.

Graphical illustrations of what various correlations look like (as well as cases where $r = 0$) can be found in Figure 2.20.

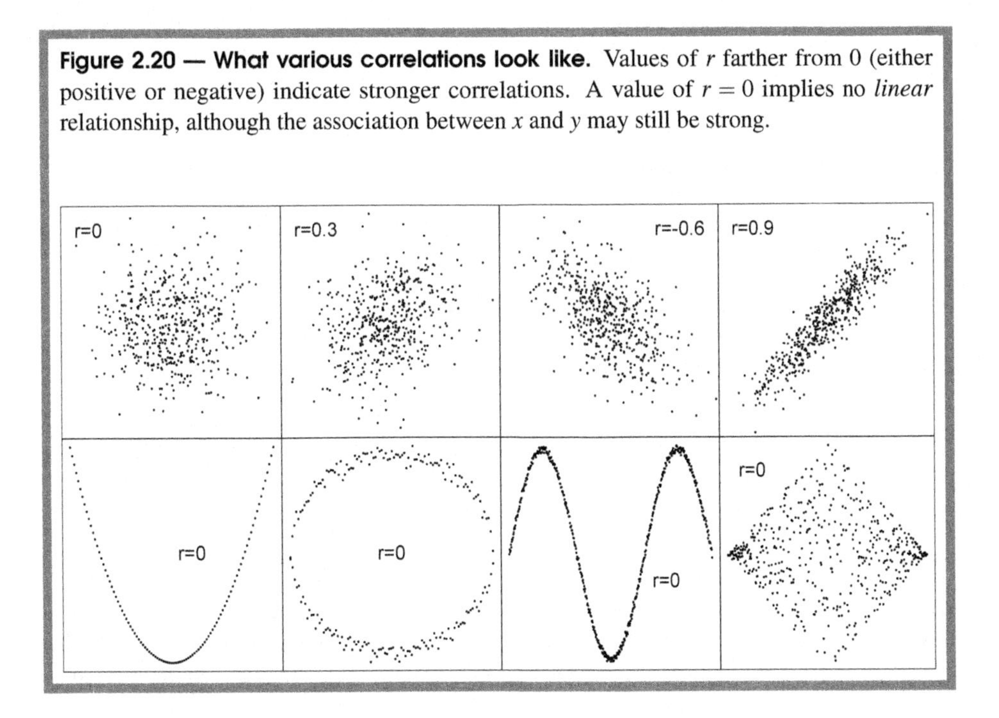

Figure 2.20 — What various correlations look like. Values of r farther from 0 (either positive or negative) indicate stronger correlations. A value of $r = 0$ implies no *linear* relationship, although the association between x and y may still be strong.

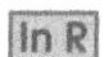

`cor.demo()` from package `regclass` is an interactive demo designed to show you what different correlations look like and to show the effect of outliers on the correlation. When you run it, click the scatterplot to add points and watch the value of r update. Note: be sure to click the red END button when you are done adding points.

Interpretation of r

A value of r close to zero indicates a relationship with a weak linear component (the association may still be nonlinear and strong). Values of r far from 0 (either positive or negative) imply the relationship has a strong linear component. To interpret the value of r, we first square it.

> The quantity r^2 tells us the percentage of the overall variation in y that can be "attributed" to (or "explained" by) knowledge of x. Informally, "knowing x gets us $100r^2\%$ of the way to knowing y." We will call r^2 the **coefficient of determination**. r^2 is only appropriate for linear relationships.

Let us revisit the relationship between attractiveness score and friendship potential (Figure 2.18), which has a moderately strong, positive, linear relationship. Attractiveness scores vary between about 1.5 and 4.0, but this variation is reduced once we focus on a specific value of friendship potential. It turns out that $r = 0.75$ and $r^2 = 56.25\%$. Knowing how females would rate the friendship potential of a woman gets you about 56% of the way to knowing how males would rate this woman's attractiveness.

For the NFL dataset in Figure 2.18, the correlation between Wins and Fumbles Lost is about -0.34, so $r^2 = 12\%$. About 12% of the variation in the number of wins among NFL teams can be "explained" once the number of lost fumbles for the season is known. The remainder of the variation must be due to other factors.

Requirements for using Pearson's correlation r

While a numerical value for r can be computed for any pair of quantitative variables, the number is only meaningful under certain conditions.

1. The trajectory of the stream of points is linear.
2. The shape of the stream of points is well-described by an ellipse.
3. The stream should not have extreme outliers (points that are "far" from the stream).

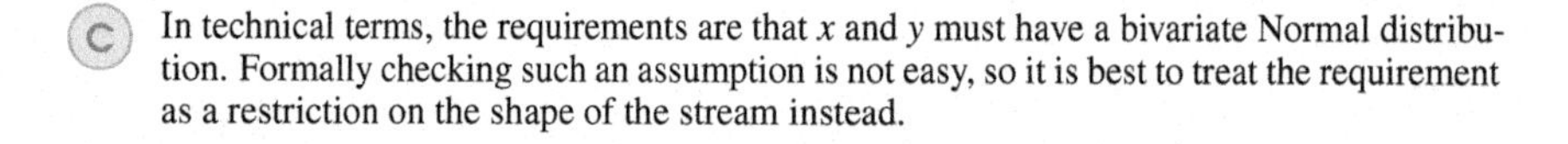

In technical terms, the requirements are that x and y must have a bivariate Normal distribution. Formally checking such an assumption is not easy, so it is best to treat the requirement as a restriction on the shape of the stream instead.

Always check the scatterplot to make sure that measuring Pearson's correlation makes sense—the value of r alone without context is not informative. Figure 2.21 shows three scatterplots where $r = 0$ but obvious (nonlinear) relationships between x and y exist (see also Figure 2.20). The relationship between a bulldozer's selling price and the year that it is made as well as the relationship between the fuel efficiency and speed of a car (Figure 2.18) would not be well-summarized by r due to nonlinearities.

Figure 2.21 — Examples where x and y are associated but r=0. Pearson's correlation r only measures the strength of linear relationships where the stream of points is elliptical with no outliers. In the left panel, y has a nonlinear relationship with x (a violation of the first assumption) since y (by design) exactly equals $7+0.1(x-15)^2$. Since y is completely determined by x, a value of $r=0$ gives the most misleading indication of the strength possible.

In the middle panel, the trajectory is linear, but the stream is not elliptical and the variation of y depends on x (for small x there is very little variation in y, for large x there is large variation in y). While x and y have a clear association (knowing x narrows down the possible values for y), the correlation is measured to be $r=0$.

The right panel shows the effect of an outlier. Without the outlier, the correlation is $r=0.96$. With the outlier, the correlation is $r=0$.

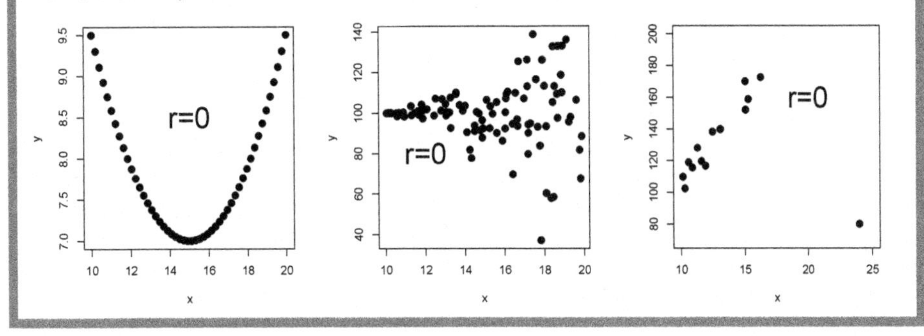

2.6.3 Statistical significance of linear associations

Even when x and y are completely unrelated, the measured value of r in a sample will rarely equal exactly zero. For the association to be statistically significant, r must be far enough from zero that it is unlikely that an unrelated set of quantities could have produced at least as strong a correlation "by chance."

The p-value in a test for correlation tells us the probability that a random, unrelated set of points could have produced a correlation at least as strong (i.e., as far from 0, either positive or negative) as the observed value of r.

If the p-value is $< 5\%$, the correlation is statistically significant.

If the p-value is $\geq 5\%$, the correlation is not statistically significant (if there is a correlation between x and y, it is too weak to be detected with your data).

To find the p-value, we need to determine what values of r are possible "by chance" when x and y are unrelated. The permutation procedure can once again help us approximate the p-value.

1. Create an artificial dataset by shuffling up the observed values of y and randomly assigning them to individuals. Refer to the example in Table 2.4. Calculate the value of r. By design, this procedure guarantees there is no underlying relationship between individuals' x and y values, so this value of r is one that can occur "by chance."

2. Repeat this procedure many times to build up a distribution of values of r that occur by chance.
3. The (estimated) p-value of the observed correlation is the fraction of these artificial datasets whose values of r are at least as far from zero as the correlation measured on the original data. See Figure 2.22.
4. If the p-value is less than 5%, the observed correlation is statistically significant—it is unlikely that a random pairing of points would produce such a strong correlation by chance.
5. Note: always check the 95% confidence interval for the p-value. If 0.05 is inside the interval, the test is inconclusive, and the number of permutations must be increased.

With modern computers, it is easy to find the p-value of a correlation with the permutation procedure. We can also find an approximate p-value with a formula if we assume x and y have a bivariate Normal distribution (a very specific way of having an elliptical stream of points). Using `cor.test()` in R or `associate()` from package `regclass` (adding the additional argument `classic=TRUE`) will show this p-value.

For example, consider whether the attractiveness score of a male (as rated by mostly straight females) is related with how fashionable he is (fashionableness "scores" are the number of seven people, men and women, who agreed the man was fashionable). The `ATTRACTM` dataset contains these quantities. The scatterplot (Figure 2.22) shows vague hints of a positive association. The stream looks linear and elliptical enough that the correlation should be a good measure of its strength. The correlation turns out to be $r = 0.28$, so only about $r^2 = 8\%$ of the variation in attractiveness scores can be attributed to a guy's fashionableness. Is such a small value statistically significant?

After 50,000 rounds of the permutation procedure, it is found that 979 (2%) have values of r that are at least as strong as $r = 0.28$ (i.e., larger than 0.28 or smaller than -0.28). The p-value is thus 2%. Since this is smaller than 5%, we conclude that the correlation is statistically significant. However, it is by no means strong since $r^2 = 8\%$.

2.6.4 Effect of outliers on correlation

It is critical that the "no extreme outliers" assumption is met for the value of r to accurately reflect the strength of the relationship. A *single* outlying point can greatly affect the value of the correlation. Figure 2.23 shows examples of how an outlier can induce a strong correlation when otherwise there is none, how an outlier can destroy an otherwise strong correlation, and how an outlier can strengthen an already moderately strong relationship.

The key point is that outliers do not affect the correlation in a consistent manner: sometimes adding an outlier makes the correlation stronger and other times it makes the correlation weaker. You must *always* check the scatterplot to make sure extreme outliers do not exist before using r to measure the strength of a relationship or to comment on its statistical significance.

In R

Use `cor.demo()` to explore the effect of outliers on the correlation. Click on the blank plot to add points. The correlations with and without the most recently-added point will be displayed. Can you make an example where an outlier destroys an otherwise strong relationship? Can you make an example of where an outlier induces an apparently strong relationship when there really is none? Note: be sure to press the red END button to stop adding points.

Figure 2.22 — Assessing the statistical significance of a correlation. The correlation between the attractiveness scores and fashion scores of males in the ATTRACTM data is only $r = 0.28$. We need the p-value to assess whether the correlation is statistically significant. The p-value is the probability of observing a correlation at least as strong as what was measured in the data when x and y are unrelated (i.e., a correlation less than -0.28 or larger than 0.28). The right plot shows values of r from artificial samples made with the permutation procedure where x- and y-values are paired together randomly. Only 2% of such artificial samples have correlations at least as strong as the original sample, so the p-value of the correlation is 2%. The correlation is statistically significant.

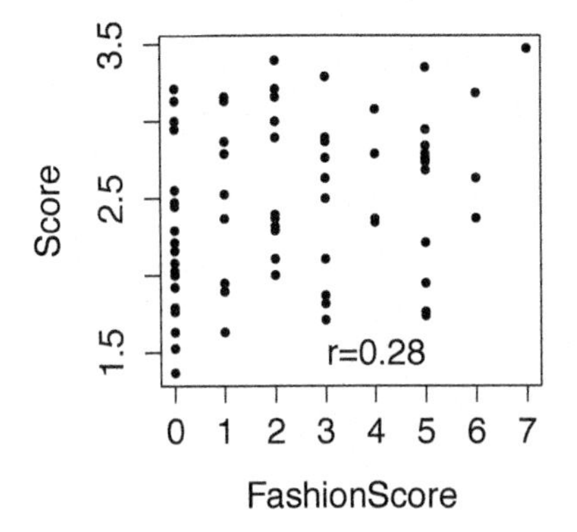

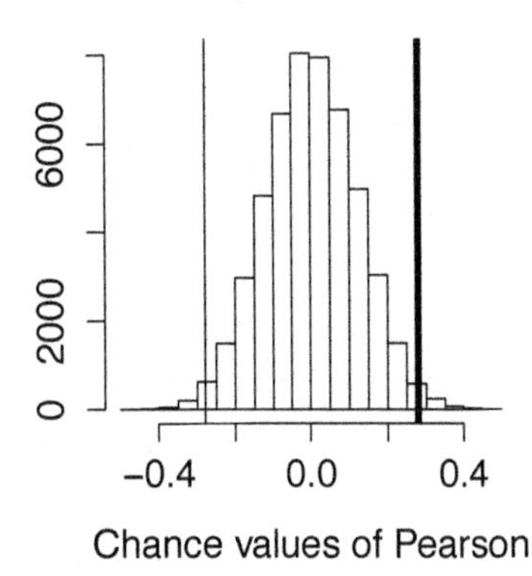

In R

```
data(ATTRACTM)
associate(Score~FashionScore,data=ATTRACTM,permutations=50000)
```

Figure 2.23 — Illustrating the effect of an outlier on the correlation. In the left panel, the relationship between the black points is nonexistent ($r = 0$). Adding in the red dot makes $r = 0.87$, thus giving the impression that a strong relationship exists. In the middle panel, the correlation between the black points is very strong ($r = -0.91$). Adding in the red dot makes $r = 0.1$, thus giving the impression that x and y are weakly (positively!) correlated. In the right panel, the correlation between the black points is strong ($r = 0.74$). Adding in the red dot makes $r = 0.98$, thus giving the impression that the relationship is stronger than what it "really" is.

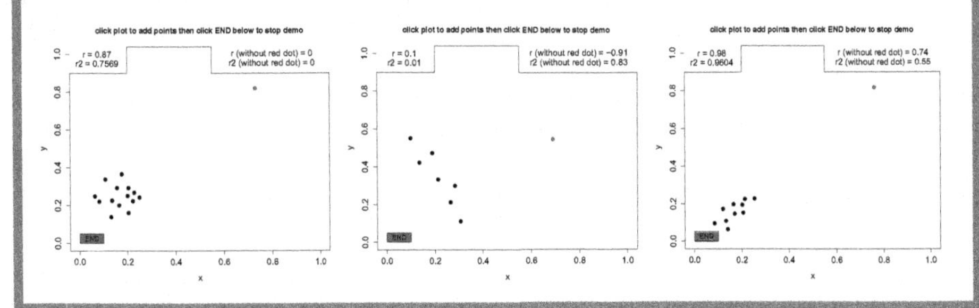

2.6.5 Spearman's rank correlation

When the stream of points is nonlinear and/or non-elliptical, or when outliers exist, Pearson's correlation r may not be effective at measuring the strength of the association. As long as the relationship is monotonic, **Spearman's rank correlation** is used instead.

The strength of a non-monotonic relationship is notoriously difficult to measure. In Chapter 4.5.1, we will discuss fitting a polynomial curve to a stream of points. A value called the adjusted R^2 will be calculated and used to quantify the strength of the relationship.

Similar to the Kruskal-Wallis test for comparing the typical value of y between levels of x, Spearman's method uses the *ranks* of the values instead of the actual values themselves. Calculation of Spearman's rank correlation is straightforward: replace the original values with their ranks and find the (Pearson) *correlation between the ranks*. See Table 2.7.

Table 2.7 — Spearman's method. Spearman's method replaces the original values in the dataset by their ranks, then finds Pearson's correlation between the ranks.

Original x	Original y	Rank x	Rank y
4.2	12.1	1	1
7.8	22.0	2	3
8.8	16.3	3	2
11.1	26.2	5	4
10.2	28.5	4	5
$r = 0.865$		Spearman = 0.8	

The statistical significance of the association is determined from its p-value: the probability that two unrelated quantities would produce an association at least as strong (measured by Spearman) "by chance." As with Pearson's correlation r, the p-value of Spearman's rank correlation can be estimated via the permutation procedure. The association is statistically significant if the p-value is less than 5%.

Figure 2.24 shows three associations whose strengths must be measured using Spearman's rank correlation. Though the relationships are statistically significant regardless of which measure is used, Pearson's r gives an inferior way to measure the strength.

The `DONOR` dataset provides an example where the choice of Pearson vs. Spearman is critical. In this data, information about nearly 20,000 donors to a charity has been recorded. We may be curious to know if there is an association between the amount people have donated to this charity (`LIFETIME_GIFT_AMOUNT`) and their income (which the charity does not know, but rather estimates with the typical household income of the donor's neighborhood, `MEDIAN_HOUSEHOLD_INCOME`). Figure 2.25 shows the relevant graphics. It is clear that Spearman's measure must be used since there are outliers and the stream of points is not elliptical (the histograms and Q-Q plots show the distributions of each variable individually is far from Normal).

Pearson's r equals 0.02 and has a p-value of 0.01. Spearman's rank correlation equals -0.002 and has a p-value of 0.80. Although both measures show that any association is weak, using Pearson's measure makes us mistakenly conclude that the association is statistically significant.

Figure 2.24 — Examples where Spearman must be used to gauge strength. The left panel displays the relationship between the body fat percentages and heights of 252 people. It requires Spearman because of the extreme outlier. The middle panel shows the relationship between the horsepower of a car and its fuel efficiency (km per liter). It requires Spearman because of nonlinearity. The right panel shows the relationship between the number of minutes students spend on Facebook and the number of texts they send each day. It requires Spearman because the stream of points is not elliptical. In all cases, Spearman's measure gives a better idea of the strength of the relationship than Pearson's r (though sometimes the values are similar, and the relationships in this case are statistically significant regardless of the way the strength is measured).

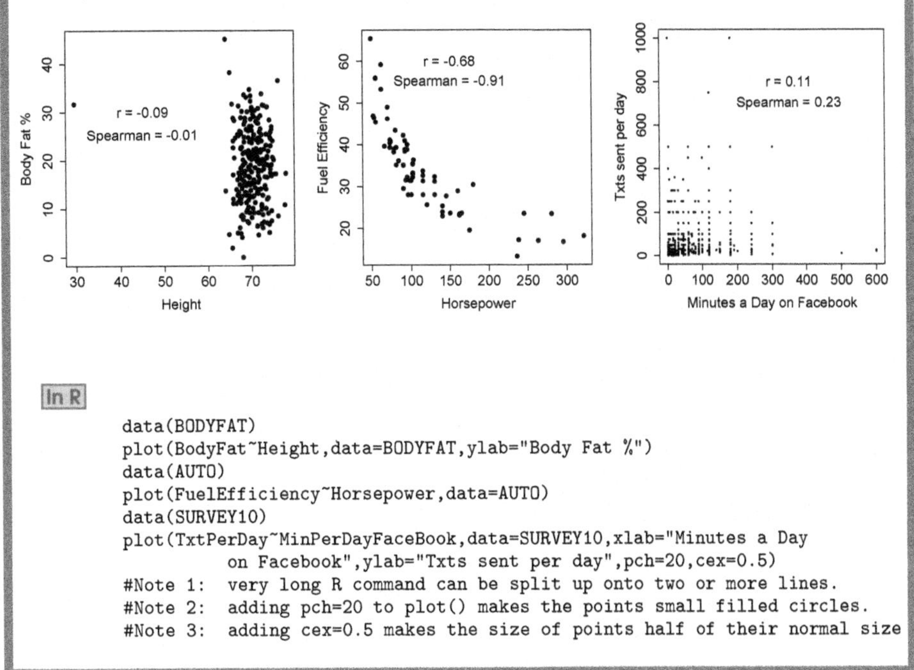

In R

```
data(BODYFAT)
plot(BodyFat~Height,data=BODYFAT,ylab="Body Fat %")
data(AUTO)
plot(FuelEfficiency~Horsepower,data=AUTO)
data(SURVEY10)
plot(TxtPerDay~MinPerDayFaceBook,data=SURVEY10,xlab="Minutes a Day
         on Facebook",ylab="Txts sent per day",pch=20,cex=0.5)
#Note 1:  very long R command can be split up onto two or more lines.
#Note 2:  adding pch=20 to plot() makes the points small filled circles.
#Note 3:  adding cex=0.5 makes the size of points half of their normal size
```

2.7 Causality and lurking variables

Regardless of the types of variables involved in the analysis, when an association is found to be statistically significant, great care must be taken not to *overinterpret* the result. The existence of an association (even with a p-value less than one in a trillion) *never* implies that there is an underlying cause and effect connection between the two variables (i.e., that changing an individual's x value will cause his or her y variable to change). Rather, establishing cause and effect requires a scientific theory and even a bit of philosophy.

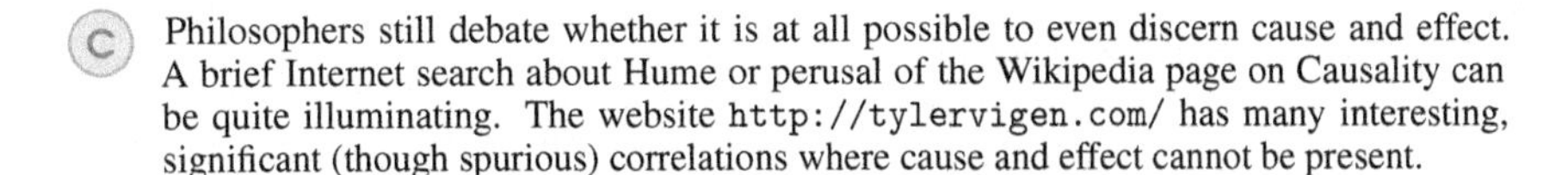

Philosophers still debate whether it is at all possible to even discern cause and effect. A brief Internet search about Hume or perusal of the Wikipedia page on Causality can be quite illuminating. The website `http://tylervigen.com/` has many interesting, significant (though spurious) correlations where cause and effect cannot be present.

Figure 2.25 — Pearson vs. Spearman choice importance. The stream of points describing the relationship between individuals' lifetime gift amounts and their (estimated) household income is non-elliptical (the histograms and Q-Q plots show the distributions of both variables are not Normal). Thus, Spearman's rank correlation must be used to describe the relationship. Its value is -0.002 with a p-value of 0.80, so we would conclude that there is no association between these variables.

Pearson's correlation is $r = 0.02$ with a p-value of 0.01. Incorrectly using this measure would lead you to believe the relationship is statistically significant.

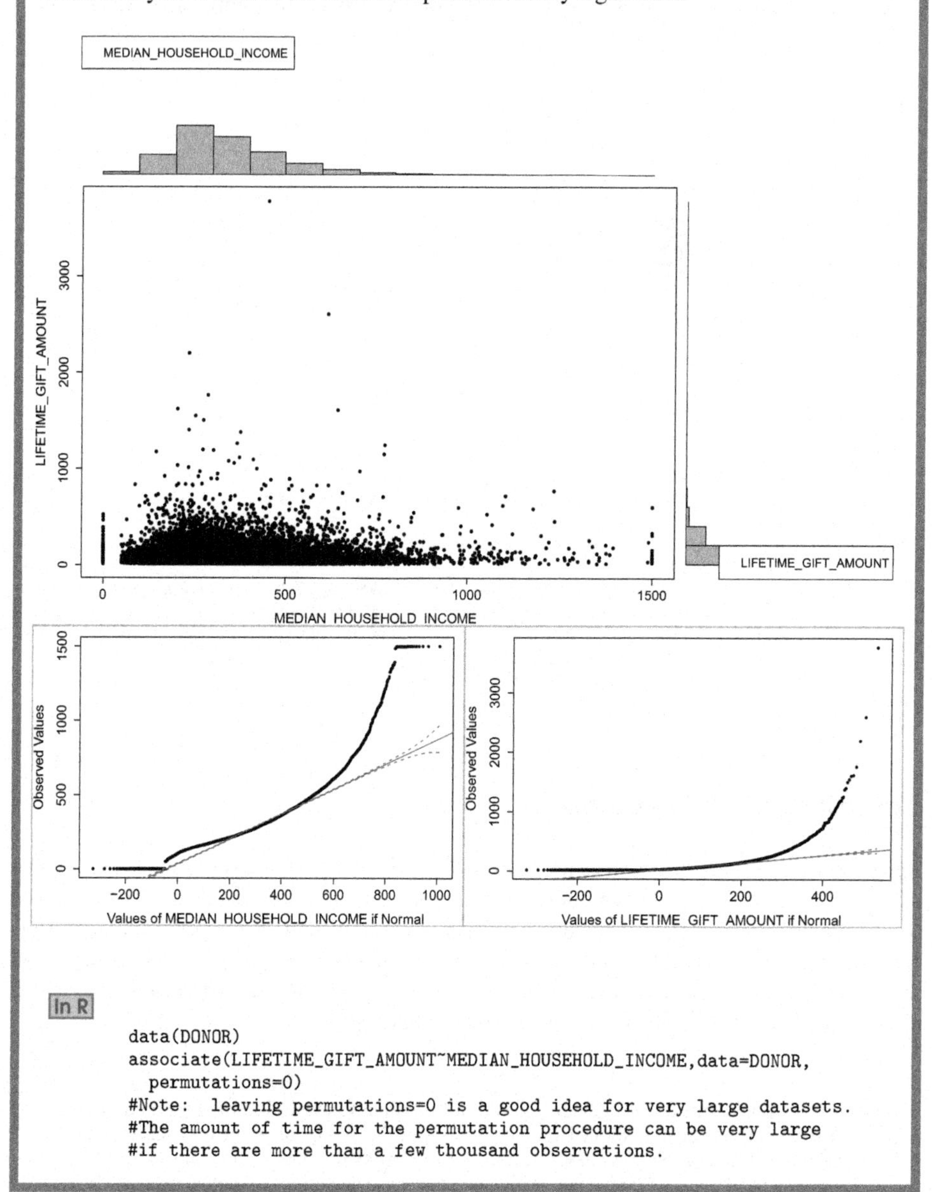

In R

```
data(DONOR)
associate(LIFETIME_GIFT_AMOUNT~MEDIAN_HOUSEHOLD_INCOME,data=DONOR,
  permutations=0)
#Note:  leaving permutations=0 is a good idea for very large datasets.
#The amount of time for the permutation procedure can be very large
#if there are more than a few thousand observations.
```

Causation can *never* be established solely with statistical analysis for two reasons:

1. Using the tests we have discussed, it is impossible for the p-value to equal zero. There is *always* some chance (however remote) that a set of random, unrelated quantities could have produced the association observed in the data because a random shuffling of y-values *could* in theory produce the exact sequence of observed y-values. Since we can never rule out chance, we cannot prove causality.
2. There may be a **lurking variable** (a common cause) that is inducing the association. For example, ice cream consumption and the number of drowning deaths are positively associated. However, banning ice cream sales won't decrease the number of drownings because there is no causal link. Rather, the observed association is induced by the time of year and temperature. In hot summer months, ice cream sales are larger than they are in winter months. Drowning deaths are also higher in summer months than winter months because more people are swimming.

When you find a statistically significant association, you should always ask yourself "Why?" What other reasons, besides cause and effect, may explain the relationship? In Chapter 4 (multiple regression), we will learn about techniques that allow us to account for lurking variables. Doing so will make the relationship between two variables clearer, but the question will always remain whether we have identified *every* important lurking variable. Even when all lurking variables have been accounted for, independent quantities always have *some* chance of producing the associations we observe. Thus, even a precise statistical analysis can never establish cause and effect.

That being said, if there is an underlying cause and effect relationship (e.g., the force applied to an object and its resulting acceleration), an association analysis should pick up on it.

> A *better* interpretation of r^2 would be: "For *whatever* reason, $100r^2$% of the variation in y can be attributed to x." A better statement when commenting on significance would be: "For whatever reason, x and y have a statistically significant association."

For example, consider the association between the number of piercings on someone's body and his or her height (Figure 2.26) in the `SURVEY10` dataset (699 students in a statistics class in 2010). The correlation is fairly strong ($r = -0.58$), implying that about 33% of the variation in people's heights can be "explained" (for whatever reason) by the number of piercings they have. The p-value is less than 1 in a billion, so the correlation is highly statistically significant. However, it would be absurd to suggest that getting an additional piercing will cause someone to shrink. The lurking variable, or common cause, in this example is gender. Women are typically shorter than men and typically have more piercings, making it look like there's a negative relationship between height and piercings.

Another example involves the relationship between the weight and top speeds of cars in a study of European models in the `AUTO` dataset (Figure 2.27). Based on the left plot, the relationship between weight and top speed of a car is positive and quite strong. At first, this may seem counterintuitive—you may know from personal experience that your car slows down when you load it up with more stuff.

While this is true for a *particular* vehicle, our data consists of many *different* cars. When we compare two points in the plot, these cars not only differ in weight, but also (behind the scenes) cab volume, horsepower, and fuel efficiency.

Figure 2.26 — Gender as a Lurking Variable. The negative relationship ($r = -0.58$) between height and number of piercings is highly statistically significant. Obviously, there is no causal connection (putting an additional piercing in a person's ear will not make him or her shrink). The lurking variable (common cause) is gender. Points are coded by gender (women are red, men are blue). When the association analysis is done separately for men and women, we find that $r_{women} = -0.10$ and $r_{men} = -0.06$. Thus, the correlation "disappears" once we account for gender. Gender induces the correlation here because women are in the upper left of the plot (shorter, more piercings) and guys are clumped in the bottom right (taller, fewer piercings).

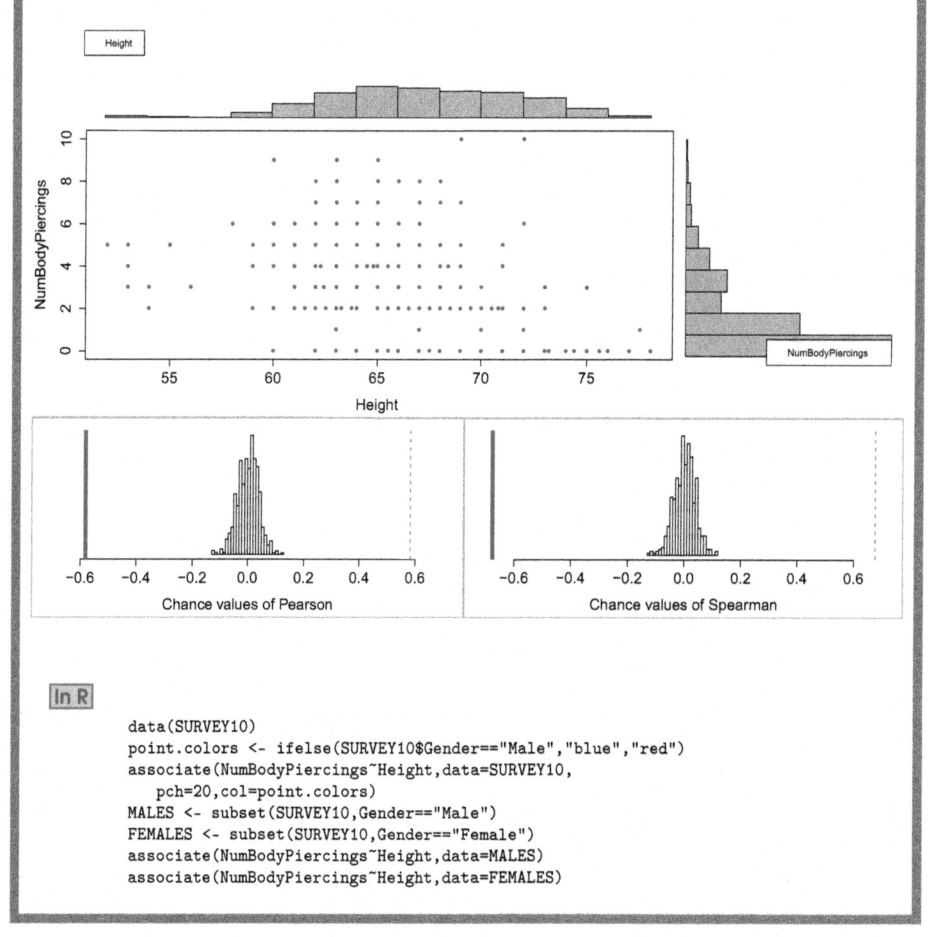

In R

```
data(SURVEY10)
point.colors <- ifelse(SURVEY10$Gender=="Male","blue","red")
associate(NumBodyPiercings~Height,data=SURVEY10,
   pch=20,col=point.colors)
MALES <- subset(SURVEY10,Gender=="Male")
FEMALES <- subset(SURVEY10,Gender=="Female")
associate(NumBodyPiercings~Height,data=MALES)
associate(NumBodyPiercings~Height,data=FEMALES)
```

The correlation is induced by the horsepower of the car. The middle panel shows that heavier vehicles tend to have engines with higher horsepowers. The third panel shows that cars with higher horsepower engines achieve higher top speeds. Thus, the positive relationship between the top speed and the weight of a car exists by the virtue of heavier cars having engines with more horsepower, and engines with more horsepower allowing a higher speed.

If all cars in the data had the same horsepower, cab volume, etc., and *only* differed in weight, we would see that heavier cars have lower top speeds due to the laws of physics.

Figure 2.27 — Counterintuitive relationship due to lurking variable. Common sense and physics tell us that a car achieves a lower top speed when it is weighed down. However, in the AUTO dataset, the relationship between weight and top speed is positive and strong. The reason is due to the lurking variable "horsepower." Heavier cars in this dataset are built with higher horsepower engines (middle panel), and higher horsepower engines lead to higher top speeds (right panel). The net result is a positive relationship between weight and top speed of cars in the data when we know cause and effect works differently for a particular car.

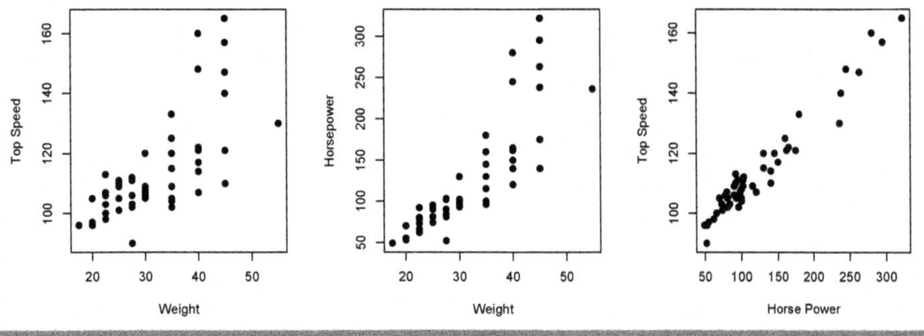

2.8 Practical significance versus statistical significance

An association has **practical significance** if it is both statistically significant and strong enough to be interesting or useful. Practical significance is subjective and depends on the context of the problem.

On one hand, if the correlation between amounts shoppers spend at Walmart and the amounts shoppers spend at The Home Depot is $r = 0.02$, very few people (if any) would be excited. The association is so weak that knowing the amount spent at one store gets you only $0.02^2 = 0.0004 = 0.04\%$ of the way to knowing the amount spent at the other.

On the other hand, if the correlation between today's closing price of Disney and Cola-Cola's closing price one week ago had a correlation of $r = 0.02$, traders would take notice. If the correlation was reflective of a real, causal relationship between the stocks, then even the smallest ability to predict a closing price can make a lot of money.

The result of a test for an association is a p-value and a comment about its *statistical* significance, i.e., whether it is likely that the association in the data could have been produced "by chance." Unfortunately, a p-value reveals *nothing* about the strength of an association or whether it is large enough to be useful.

The p-value of a test for significance does *not* indicate whether the association is strong, interesting, or of any practical value. The magnitude and utility of an association must be judged separately using the mosaic plot, side-by-side box plots, scatterplot, or r^2 (depending on the types of variables). For datasets with many observations, extremely small and inconsequential associations can be statistically significant.

For example, imagine a marketer needs to decide whether a new type of frequent flyer program should be mostly marketed to men or to women (or if gender matters at all). The question becomes: "Is there an association between interest in the program and gender?"

Imagine that a survey of 50 men and 50 women finds that 35 men (70%) are interested in the program compared to 34 women (68%). Figure 2.28 shows the mosaic plot. Right away, we see that any association is weak at best. The conditional distribution of "Interest" (segmented bar charts) is nearly identical for both genders.

Indeed, a statistical test measures a discrepancy of $D = 0.0468$ and a p-value much larger than 5%, so the association is not statistically significant. However, now imagine that the same proportion of men and women are interested (70% vs. 68%), but the total number of men and women in the survey is 50,000 each. The mosaic plot will look the same (it plots percentages, not counts), but now the test measures a discrepancy of $D = 46.75$ and a p-value of 0.0001, implying the association is highly statistically significant! Thus, *always* be sure to take statistical significance with a grain of salt. Even the weakest association will be statistically significant if the sample size is large enough.

Figure 2.28 — Mosaic plots for frequent flier program. The mosaic plot reveals that the association between interest in a new program and gender is weak (if it exists at all) since the segmented bar charts look nearly identical. However, depending on the sample size, a statistical test may or may not claim the association is statistically significant. The plot below was constructed using a sample of 50 men and women (35 men and 34 women had Interest=Yes). However, the plot will look identical for a sample of 50,000 men and women (with 35,000 and 34,000 women having Interest=Yes)! The test for the smaller sample has a p-value of about 1.0 (no statistically significant association), while the test for the larger sample has a p-value of 0.0001 (highly statistically significant association). In both cases, the association is so weak that it lacks practical significance and importance. Thus, the p-value alone never tells you the strength of an association.

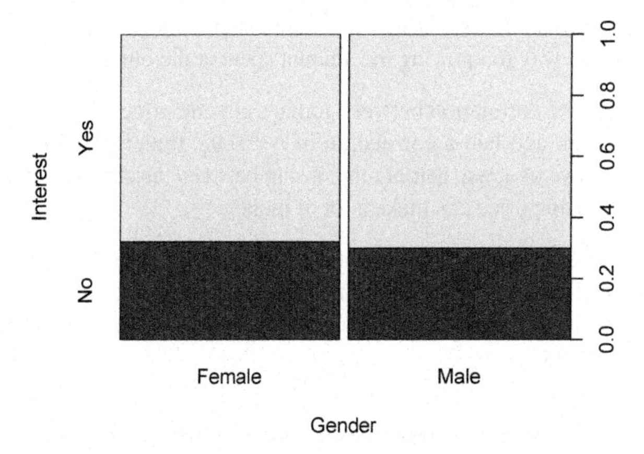

In R

```
data(SMALLFLYER); data(LARGEFLYER)
associate(Interest~Gender,data=SMALLFLYER,permutations=0,classic=TRUE)
associate(Interest~Gender,data=LARGEFLYER,permutations=0,classic=TRUE)
```

A statistically significant association may be extremely weak and may not carry any practical significance or value to your problem. Always visually assess the strength of an association with the relevant plots to decide whether the association (if statistically significant) has any practical consequence or value to you and the question at hand.

2.9 Summary

Gauging whether two quantities have a statistically significant association is a fundamental question in every line of research. When an association exists, knowing the value of one variable provides additional information and narrows the value of the other, for whatever reason.

Knowing that the probability of buying a product is associated with owning a pet, driving a red car, etc., may allow advertisers to execute campaigns more efficiently. Knowing that college GPA is associated with playing a musical instrument or having done volunteer work in high school may allow colleges to make smarter admission decisions.

An association analysis begins with a visual display. Graphics allow us to check whether the association is strong or of any practical importance. The marginal (overall) distribution of y in the data is examined, and then the conditional distributions of y for individuals who have some common characteristic (same value of x) are considered. If some of the conditional distributions are different from each other and from the marginal distribution, then knowing an individual's x-value can provide additional information about his or her possible y-values.

If the association would have practical significance to you, the next step is to conduct a test and examine the p-value. The p-value of an association is the probability that two random, unrelated quantities would produce an association at least as strong as what was measured in the data "by chance." This p-value can be estimated via the permutation procedure, where artificial samples are generated by shuffling up the values of y and randomly assigning them to individuals. Associations measured on these artificial datasets give an idea of what values occur "by chance," and the p-value is estimated to be the fraction of these samples whose associations at are least as strong as the association in the original data.

By convention, if the p-value is less than 5%, the association is statistically significant. The implication is that the probability that chance alone could produce the association measured in the data is less than 5%, but it is still possible. If the p-value is 5% or larger, the association is not statistically significant. If this is the case, either x and y do not have an association, or it is so weak that it remained undetected by the analysis.

Remember that the p-value is not quite the end of the story. If an association is statistically significant, an assessment of whether it holds any *practical* value or importance needs to occur. Practical significance is subjective. For example, if the amount of money people donate to charity has a highly significant association with gender, but if the difference in average amounts for men vs. women is one cent, the association is meaningless for all intents and purposes.

Finally, you must always be careful not to overinterpret a statistically significant association. A statistically significant association is never proof of a causal connection between x and y due to the possibility of a lurking variable (and there is always a possibility that unrelated variables could produce an association as strong by chance).

The remainder of this book will move forward from asking "Do x and y have an association?" to asking deeper, more specific questions about the association. What equation best relates y to x, and how can we *predict* the value of y once we know an individual's value of x?

Analysis of associations summary

	y categorical x categorical	y quantitative x categorical	y quantitative x quantitative
Visualize	Mosaic plot	Side-by-side box plots	Scatterplots
What to look for	Differences in side-by-side segmented bar charts	Differences in averages or medians	Scatter and tilt in stream of points
Test	**Chi-squared χ^2 test**	**ANOVA** (roughly Normal) **Kruskal-Wallis** (symmetric with outliers) **median** (any distribution)	**Pearson's r** (linear, elliptical) **Spearman** (nonlinear, outliers, non-elliptical, monotonic)

2.10 Exercises

1: Assigning the variables to the roles of x and y is critical for making visualizations (though the statistical test comes out the same). For the following examples, which variable should be x and which should be y (use common sense)?

a) Color of background vs. Time spent on website
b) Waiting time in line vs. Number of open cashiers
c) Price of item vs. Probability of purchasing
d) Weather vs. Demand
e) Click on ad vs. Mobile device type

2: Below is a contingency table that studies the association between where people sit (Location) and their gender (Gender).

	Location				
Gender	Back	Front	Middle	Varies	Total
Female	62	127	126	14	329
Male	45	89	106	10	250
Total	107	216	232	24	579

a) How many students are in the survey? In other words, what is the sample size?
b) How many males sit in the front?
c) Report the marginal distribution of Location. Give the numbers as percentages instead of counts. Round to the nearest percent.
d) Report the conditional distribution of Location for Females. Give the numbers as percentages instead of counts. Round to the nearest percent. Comparing the conditional distribution to the marginal distribution from the previous question, would you say that there is significant evidence of an association? Why or why not?

e) Calculate the expected count of Females who sit in the Middle if there was no association between Location and Gender. Round to one decimal place.

f) The value of the discrepancy between all expected and observed counts turns out to be 1.017. Below is the simulated sampling distribution of D for 5000 samples with no association. Is the association between Location and Gender statistically significant? Why or why not?

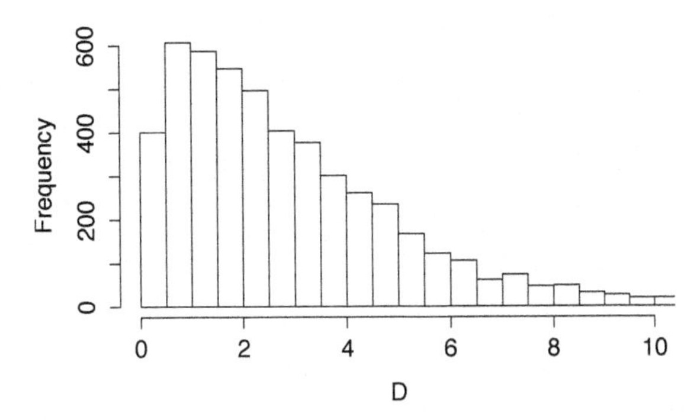

3: Consider the daily demand for bicycles at kiosks in DC. Below are side-by-side box plots of the distributions of demand for each day of the week.

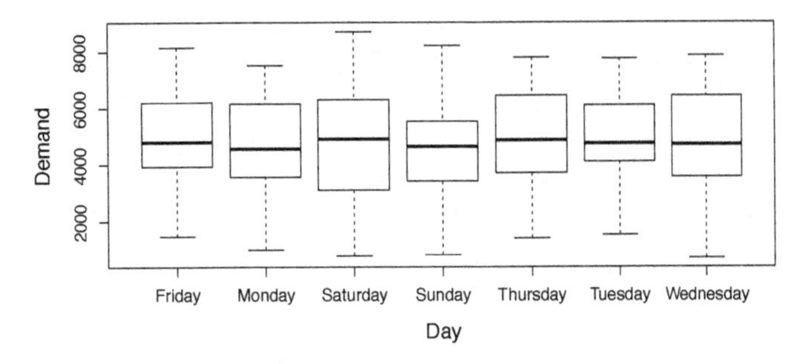

a) What about this plot suggests that there may be an association between Day and Demand?

b) The F statistic has been calculated for this data, and it turns out it is 4.7. What is the practical interpretation of this number?

c) Below is the sampling distribution of F for 5000 samples when no association exists between Day and Demand. Is the observed association statistically significant?

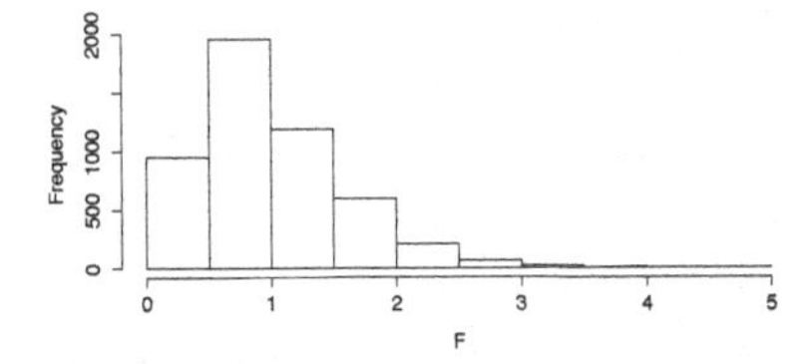

d) Management only cares whether the demands vary from day to day by about 1000. Thus, does the association carry any practical significance?

4: True or False. Imagine the sample size is at least a dozen.

a) A test for an association comes back with a p-value of 0.003

1) The association must be statistically significant.

2) The association must have practical significance.
3) The association must be strong.

b) A test for an association comes back with a p-value of 0.32
1) The association must be statistically significant.
2) The association has practical significance.
3) The association must be weak, if it exists at all.

5: The government conducts the census every 10 years, but not everyone responds. Follow-up workers interview the people who don't mail back their form. To intelligently allocate workers, we need to figure out which quantities are associated with the response rate. Use `EX2.CENSUS`. Most columns give the percentages of each neighborhood with a certain property, e.g., `Suburban` gives the percentage of that neighborhood that is considered "suburban", `Hispanics` gives the percentage of individuals that identify as Hispanic, `Age45to65` gives the percentage of the individuals within that age range. Other columns like `VacantUnits` and `RentingHH` give the fraction of housing units or households with that quality.

a) We want to predict `ResponseRate`. What five variables are most strongly correlated (may be positive or negative) with `ResponseRate`. Hint: use `all.correlations()`.
b) The variable most correlated with the response rate is `HomewownerHH`, the fraction of households that own their home. Calculate r^2 and interpret its value.
c) Is the association between `HomewownerHH` and `ResponseRate` statistically significant? Explain. Do you think it holds practical significance? Explain.
d) Explore the association between `logMedianHouseValue` (the logarithm of the median home value) and `MedianHHIncomeCity` (the median income of households in the city). Use `associate()` (let x be `MedianHHIncomeCity`) and describe the direction and form of the stream of points. Does the stream have "unusual features"? Which measure (Pearson vs. Spearman) should be used to measure the strength of the association and why?

6: Use `EX2.TIPS`. This dataset records the bill and tip amounts (along with tip percentage) as well as the party size, who was at the table, whether they smoked, and the time of visit.

a) We are curious whether there is an association between the size of the party and whether they smoke. Party sizes range between 1 and 6, so in this case, it is appropriate to compare the average between groups (when y only takes on a few different values, using the average is typically the best way to go regardless of what the distribution looks like). Run `associate()` to perform a test of significance using the default number of permutations. Why is the test inconclusive?
b) Change the number of permutations to 5000. The test should now be conclusive. Is there a statistically significant difference in average party size between smokers/non-smokers? Would you say this difference carries any practical significance?
c) Examine the association between the bill and tip amounts with the graphical and statistical output of `associate()`. Which measure (Pearson vs. Spearman) is appropriate for measuring the strength of the relationship? Is the relationship statistically significant? Does the choice of Pearson vs. Spearman affect this conclusion?
d) Examine the association between $y =$ `Day_Night` (whether the table was seated for lunch vs. dinner) and $x =$ `Smoker`. Examine graphical output and the result of the statistical test. Is the fraction of non-smokers who dine at lunch larger or smaller than for smokers? Is the association statistically significant? Explain.

7: Draw four scatterplots (label them A, B, C, D) and put in a stream of points with the following properties.

a) Positive, linear, heteroscedastic
b) Negative, nonlinear
c) Non-monotonic
d) A relationship whose strength would be well-modeled by Pearson's r

8: Visit `www.tylervigen.com` and click "Discover a new correlation" at the top. Choose one of the variable types (Interesting variables, Marriage rates, etc.). Scan through the list of variables, choose one, and click Correlate. Scan through the list of possible correlations and choose one with a "large" correlation.

a) Report the two variables you selected and include the plot the website provides.
b) Report the value of r and calculate r^2. Interpret this value.
c) These variables have a statistically significant correlation (or association) that also has practical significance (since it's so strong). However, is there a cause and effect link between them? Explain.

9: Run the function `cor.demo()`

a) Generate a scatterplot that has a correlation of about -0.80 (give or take ± 0.02). Have this be the correlation displayed in the upper right.
b) Generate a scatterplot that has a stream of points with an extreme outlier. Without the outlier (red dot), the stream should have a correlation of around $|r| = 0.7$. With the outlier (red dot), the stream should have a correlation near 0.
c) Generate a scatterplot that has a stream of points with an extreme outlier. Without the outlier (red dot), the stream should have a correlation of around $r = 0$ (say, within 0.2). With the outlier (red dot), the stream should have a correlation near 1 (say, within 0.2).

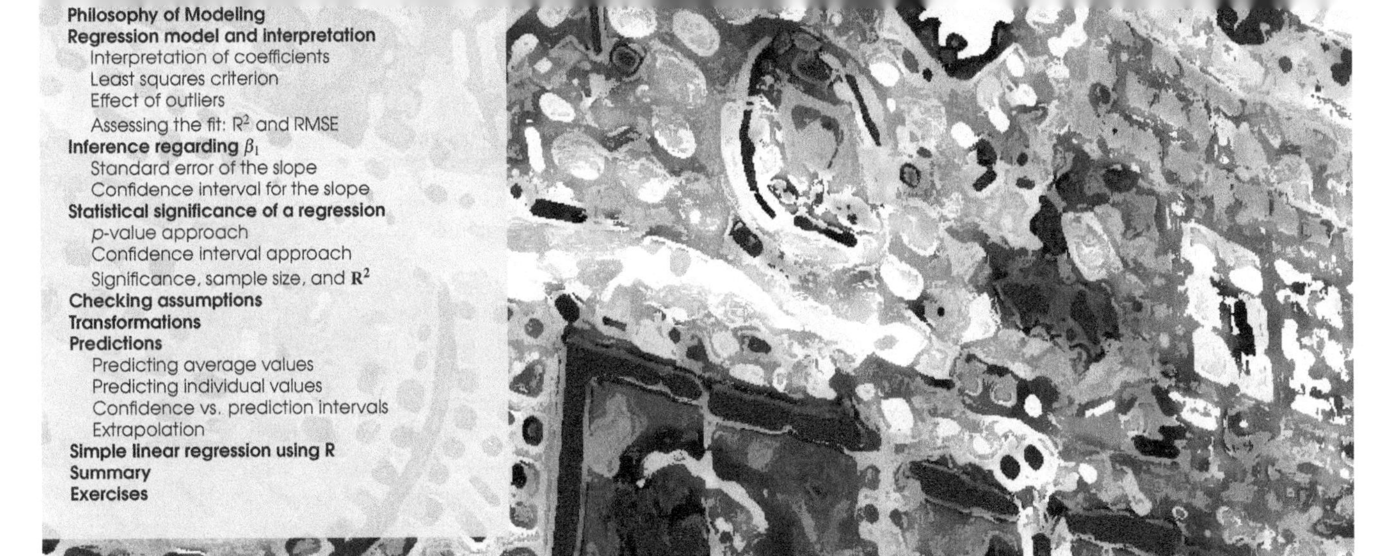

Philosophy of Modeling
Regression model and interpretation
- Interpretation of coefficients
- Least squares criterion
- Effect of outliers
- Assessing the fit: R^2 and RMSE

Inference regarding β_1
- Standard error of the slope
- Confidence interval for the slope

Statistical significance of a regression
- p-value approach
- Confidence interval approach
- Significance, sample size, and R^2

Checking assumptions
Transformations
Predictions
- Predicting average values
- Predicting individual values
- Confidence vs. prediction intervals
- Extrapolation

Simple linear regression using R
Summary
Exercises

3. Simple Linear Regression

The world is full of associations. The number of wins of an NFL team (and the chance that a team will win any particular game) is associated with the number of times the team fumbles. An individual's perceived attractiveness is associated with whether he or she wears glasses and whether he or she is in shape. The sales of a newly released product are associated with the amount spent on TV advertising.

The last chapter was concerned with measuring the strength and statistical significance of an association. An association exists between two quantities when knowing the value of one narrows down the possible values of the other. Such an analysis can be useful for determining what appears to be connected (for whatever reason) to the variable of interest. However, we often want to take the analysis a step further and come up with an equation that relates both variables and/or makes predictions.

For example, consider a sample of employee salaries at a large company. Hiring and retention rules dictate that an individual's monthly pay depends on that individual's job position, time with the company, years of prior work experience, years of education, etc. We already know "what matters" when determining salary (each of these variables probably have highly statistically significant relationships with pay), so an analysis of associations is not interesting.

Rather, we may want to know the impact of each variable on pay. How much higher is the expected salary for each additional year of work experience, etc.? Perhaps you are considering applying to a job at the company and you would like to know which is more valuable: an additional year of work experience or an additional year of being with that company.

- Is it best to stay employed at your current job for an additional year (and enjoy the salary bump that comes with an additional year's work experience)?
- Is it best to be hired now (at a lower salary, but with a raise after a year)?

Such questions can be answered by fitting a **simple linear regression**. In effect, a simple linear regression is just an equation that relates the average value of some quantity y (salary) to some predictor variable x (e.g., years work experience):

$$\text{Average value of } y = \mu_y = \beta_0 + \beta_1 x \qquad (3.1)$$

The equation is "simple" because only one predictor variable x is included; we will see in later chapters how to extend the framework to *multiple* regression, where multiple predictors are used simultaneously to predict y.

However, before delving into the details and methods of the procedure, it is worth discussing the philosophy of regression modeling. The linear regression equation is not an equation that captures a physical law (such as $E = mc^2$) because it is not a statement of cause and effect. Rather, a regression deals with how the y values of two individuals are expected to differ from each other. We will begin the chapter with an overview of modeling philosophy, then discuss how to make and interpret simple linear regressions. As with all analyses in statistics, a linear regression requires a special set of assumptions to be valid, and it is always important to check them.

3.1 Philosophy of Modeling

The reality in which we live is hopelessly complex and cannot be *fully* described using any tools known today. In fact, even predicting simple quantities like the exact time it takes a ball to fall to the ground is impossible. To calculate this time, you would need to know to infinite precision:

- The shape of the ball
- The current atmospheric conditions (to take into account air resistance)
- The composition of the Earth's interior since the force of gravity varies slightly depending on where you are on Earth and what is beneath you.

In fact, it is *still* unclear whether gravity itself is the result of one mass "tugging" on another (via the interaction of fundamental particles known as gravitons), the consequence of objects moving through curved space-time as explained in Einstein's general relativity, or due to some other mechanism.

Rather, we make *approximations* to reality that make describing some behavior of interest tractable. This set of approximations consist of our *model* for reality. For example, in an introductory physics class, to calculate the time it takes a ball to fall to the ground, the following approximations are made:

- the ball is a point mass with zero volume (obviously wrong since no such things exist)
- there is no air and thus no air resistance (obviously wrong since the drop is occurring on Earth)
- there is known, constant force g from gravity (wrong because the exact value of the force is unknown and the force varies slightly as the ball moves closer to the ground)

When these approximations are made, and if the ball is dropped with no initial speed from a known distance above the ground d, the time it will take to fall to the ground is $t = \sqrt{2d/g}$. If someone actually performs the experiment in the real world and compares the measured falling time to this prediction, the two times will not be equal. However, they will be pretty close. In other words, even though the model was fundamentally wrong, it proves to be fairly accurate and rather useful.

Likewise, the Mercator projection is a rectangular map of the spherical Earth. It heavily distorts the area near the polar regions but gives a good approximation of the layout of the rest of the landmasses. We have all used and seen this (obviously wrong) map before, and we have all found it informative.

In general, all models are an *approximate* description of how reality works. The late George Box coined what will be the mantra of this book:

All models are *wrong* but some are *useful.*

The quality of the model depends on the accuracy of its assumptions about reality. One can make models increasingly more complex (and accurate) to mimic progressively more subtle effects, but this is often quite difficult.

NASA has used Newton's law of universal gravitation and Einstein's general relativity to successfully land people on the moon, land a probe on a comet, and fly spaceprobes past every planet, including Pluto. Even though the equations behind these two theories are incomplete and "wrong," they provide good enough descriptions of the universe to be immensely useful.

The simple linear regression model ($\mu_y = \beta_0 + \beta_1 x$) is an equation for a straight line. The model assumes that the average value of y (among all individuals with a common value of x) has a perfectly linear relationship with x. Do we think this is the way reality works? Of course not! We understand that the real world is more complex.

Imagine we were omnipotent and possessed data on every potential individual in existence (i.e., we possessed a **census**). We could then find the actual average value of y for each unique value of x. These averages would most definitely *not* fall exactly on a line. Thus, our model is wrong *a priori*, but it may still be quite useful in describing, at least *approximately*, how x and y vary together. Of course, the utility and accuracy of our model depends on the reasonableness of this linearity assumption.

From here on out, we will assume that the equation $\mu_y = \beta_0 + \beta_1 x$ holds *exactly* and is "the truth." Our task then becomes estimating β_0 and β_1 from the data we have collected. The downside is that our estimates will never equal the "true" values. The upside (and this is quite remarkable) is that by making a few additional assumptions about how much individuals deviate from the average, we will be able to determine just how far our guesses are likely to be from the truth.

Before beginning, it is worthwhile to split models into two broad categories: descriptive and predictive models.

Descriptive Modeling

The goal of a descriptive model is to describe reality in as much detail as possible, e.g., what is the expected difference in salaries between two people who differ in their education levels by one year? In the context of regression, this means trying to estimate the quantities β_0 and (more importantly) β_1 with as much precision as possible. When we discuss multiple regression and model the average value of y with numerous predictor variables, the focus will also be on determining *which* set of predictors is necessary (typically not all the information available in the dataset is required).

Since a descriptive model attempts to get close to how the real world works, and because "all models are wrong," descriptive modeling is an inherently difficult task. While the model won't be a perfect reflection of reality, it should be, at the very least, somewhat informative. The majority of this book is devoted to building descriptive models because of all of the intricacies involved.

Predictive Modeling

One goal of a predictive model is to predict the average value of y of all individuals who share some common value for x, e.g., what is the average salary among all employees with six years of education and two years of experience? Another goal is to predict the y value of a single individual who happens to have some value of x. What is your anticipated salary if you graduated college but have no work experience?

These types of models are unconcerned with the values of β_0, β_1, or even what variables are being used to make the predictions. The worth of a predictive model is gauged by the typical difference between its predicted values and the actual y values of yet-to-be-observed individuals. As such, a predictive model is allowed to be a "hack job"—it doesn't matter much what the model "looks like"; as long as it works, use it!

In some sense, a predictive model is easier to build than a descriptive model since it can be somewhat detached from reality as long as it makes good predictions. What makes predictive modeling tricky is that there is a much broader assortment of models to choose from, and the time it takes to build one is longer.

3.2 Regression model and interpretation

The simple linear regression equation is:

$$\mu_{y|x} = \beta_0 + \beta_1 x \tag{3.2}$$

Here, $\mu_{y|x}$ (pronounced "mu of y given x") represents the average value of y among all individuals who share some common value of x (e.g., the average pay among all individuals with three years of work experience). β_0 and β_1 are the **coefficients** of the model. The regression equation is that of a straight line, so the model says that the average value of y has a linear relationship with x. The intercept of the line (i.e., where the line crosses the y-axis) is β_0, and the slope of the line (i.e., its steepness) is β_1. See Figure 3.1 for a visual depiction of these two quantities.

3.2.1 Interpretation of coefficients

For descriptive modeling, the interpretation of the coefficients in the regression equation is paramount. Each coefficient tells us something about the average value of y.

- β_0: intercept. This represents the average value of y among all individuals who have $x = 0$ and is where the line crosses the y-axis (if the graph happens to be drawn out that far). Typically, this quantity is no more important than the average value of y among all individuals who have some other common value of x, but a line needs an intercept, so we give it "special" treatment. The value of the intercept will be meaningless if $x = 0$ is not a possible value or if $x = 0$ is far outside the values of x used to build the model.
- β_1: slope. This represents the expected or average difference in y between two individuals who happen to differ in x by one unit. If two individuals differ in x by four units, we would expect them to differ in y by $4\beta_i$ units, etc.

(C) Note: when we compare two individuals that differ in x by one unit, their difference in y values probably will not *exactly* equal β_1, but the difference should be close (this is why we refer to it as the expected or average difference).

Figure 3.1 — Visualizing coefficients of a simple linear regression equation. The intercept β_0 is where the line happens to cross the y-axis. However, scatterplots are usually *not* drawn so that the y-axis corresponds to the left edge of the graph, so do not use the edge as a reference (find the location where $x = 0$; it may not even be on the plot). The slope β_1 measures the "steepness" of the line. It is the ratio between how much y changes for a given change in x and is often referred to as the "rise over the run." The slope is the key quantity of a regression since typically, the value of y when $x = 0$ (i.e., the intercept) is no more special than the value of y for any other value of x.

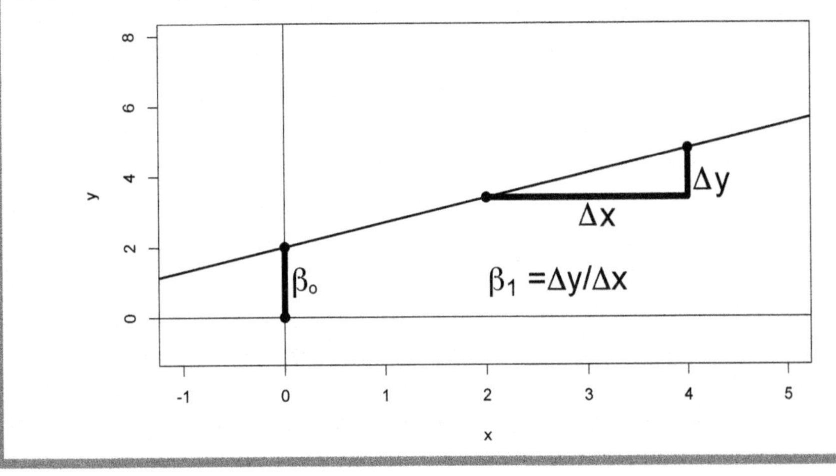

The following boxed expression is the recommended interpretation for the slope. During interpretation, be sure to replace "x" and "y" with their variable names and "units" with the actual units of measurement to give the appropriate context.

> Two entities that differ in x by one unit are expected to differ in y by β_1 units (for whatever reason). If β_1 is positive, the entity with the larger value of x is expected to have the larger value of y (if β_1 is negative, the entity with the larger value of x is expected to have the smaller value of y).

It is critically important not to overextend the interpretation of β_1. The regression describes the average *difference* in individuals' values of y when they differ in x by one unit. It does not describe what *happens* to an individual's value of y when its x-value increases by one unit. The "for whatever reason" is an important part of the interpretation since regression does not assume a cause/effect relationship and is not a physical law.

(C) A regression is not a law of nature like $E = mc^2$, though it can be used to estimate the coefficients of a physical law when one exists. It does not make any attempt to quantify what will happen to an *individual's* value of y when his or her x value changes. Rather, the regression equation describes how the y values of various individuals are expected to differ based on their values of x. To make as bold a statement as how x and y are causally related, or to describe what happens to an individual experiencing change, one needs a scientific theory, a physical mechanism connecting them, and a dataset that has numerous measurements on a single individual instead of a single measurement on many different individuals.

For example, recall the relationships between the number of piercings and height among college students addressed in Figure 2.26. A reasonable model relating the two is:

$$Height = 70 - 1.25Piercings$$

The model implies that, for whatever reason, two people who differ in the number of piercings by one are expected to differ in heights by 1.25 inches (the person with more piercings is expected to be shorter).

Obviously, the model is not a statement on cause and effect and does not reflect any physical law. The "reason" that people differ in height is certainly not the number of piercings they have. Rather, gender is a lurking variable and the "common cause" that induces this relationship (girls tend to have more piercings and tend to be shorter than guys).

Example - Salary data

Consider the SALARY dataset. We are interested in seeing how an employee's salary is related to his or her education and work experience at a particular company. See Figure 3.2 for scatterplots of these relationships.

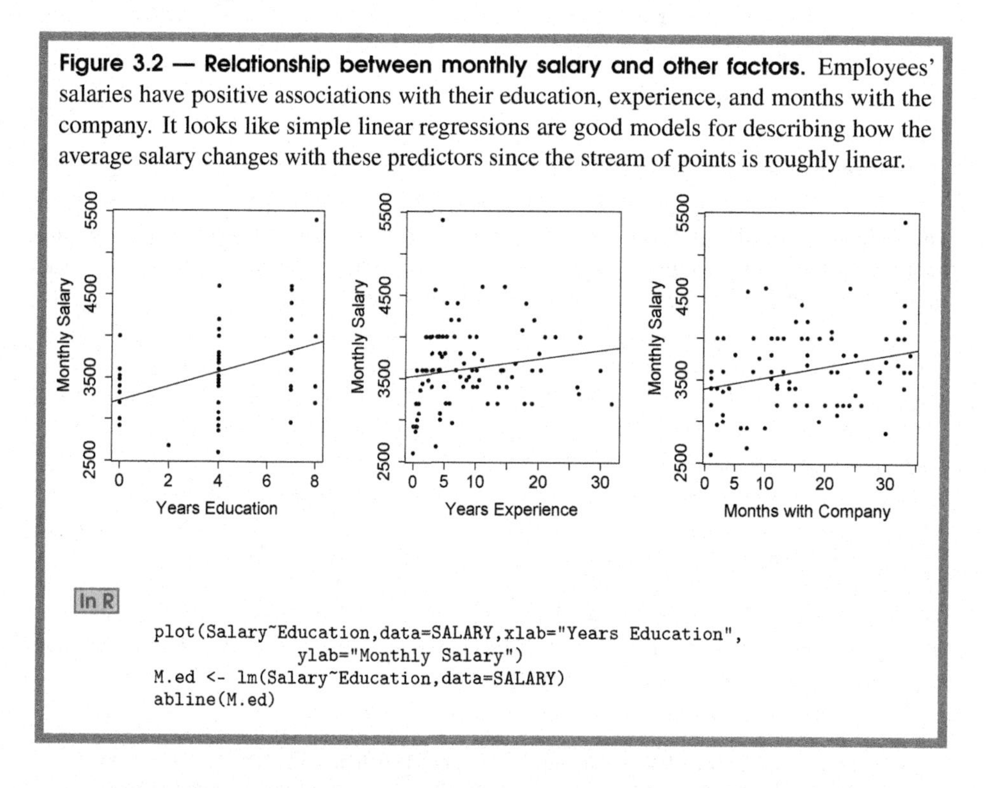

Figure 3.2 — Relationship between monthly salary and other factors. Employees' salaries have positive associations with their education, experience, and months with the company. It looks like simple linear regressions are good models for describing how the average salary changes with these predictors since the stream of points is roughly linear.

```
plot(Salary~Education,data=SALARY,xlab="Years Education",
                  ylab="Monthly Salary")
M.ed <- lm(Salary~Education,data=SALARY)
abline(M.ed)
```

The data records the monthly salaries of 93 individuals along with:

- Education—the number of years of education beyond high school (0 means high school graduate, 4 means college graduate, and numbers higher than 4 represent some sort of graduate school)
- Experience—number of years of prior work experience before joining the company

- `Months`—number of months the employee has worked at the company
- `Gender`—the gender of the individual. Incorporating categorical variables as predictors will be discussed in Chapter 5.

A regression model looks appropriate since the average value of y (`Salary`) does look to vary linearly with each predictor x. Let us propose some regression equations and interpret the coefficients.

Education

The regression equation is $\mu_{Salary} = 3229 + 85.4 Education$.

- The intercept of 3329 implies the average monthly salary among high school graduates (`Education`=0) is $3229.
- The slope of 85.4 implies that two employees who differ in one year of education are expected to differ in monthly salaries by $85.40 (the more educated employee is expected to have the higher salary).
- Note that this interpretation cannot be extended to comment on what would happen to your salary if *you* stayed in school another year and then got hired at this company since the equation is not a physical law. The coefficient talks about differences between individuals in the company, not what happens when an individual experiences change.

Experience

The regression equation is $\mu_{Salary} = 3526 + 10.4 Experience$.

- The intercept of 3526 implies the average monthly salary with no prior work experience (`Experience`=0) is $3526.
- The slope of 10.4 implies that two individuals who differ in work experience by one year are expected to differ in salaries by $10.40 (more experience is associated with higher salary).
- Once again, this does *not* imply that if *you* stayed at your current job another year, and then got hired by this company, that *you* would be paid an additional $10.40 per month (that would be a statement of cause/effect).

Months with company

The regression equation is $\mu_{Salary} = 3393 + 13.2 Months$.

- The intercept of 3393 implies that the average monthly salary for a new employee (`Months`=0) is $3393.
- The slope of 13.2 implies that an individual who has worked at the company for one month longer than another is expected to have a monthly salary that is $13.20 higher.
- Note that this does *not* necessarily imply that the average yearly raise is $12 \times 13.2 =$ $158.40 since the slope refers to differences between individuals, not what happens to a particular individual experiencing change. The only way this is an estimate of the average raise is if there are predetermined rules in place at the company for raises (i.e., an established cause/effect relationship).

Example - Tips data

In the `TIPS` data, a waiter kept track of the bill amounts of each table (`Bill`), the party size at the table (`PartySize`), the tip that was left (`Tip`), etc. Figure 3.3 shows scatterplots of how

`TipPercentage` (tip divided by bill amount written as a percent) is related to the bill amount and number of people at the table. Since the trajectory of the stream of points is linear in both cases, a regression equation should be a reasonable approximation for how the average tip percentage varies with these quantities.

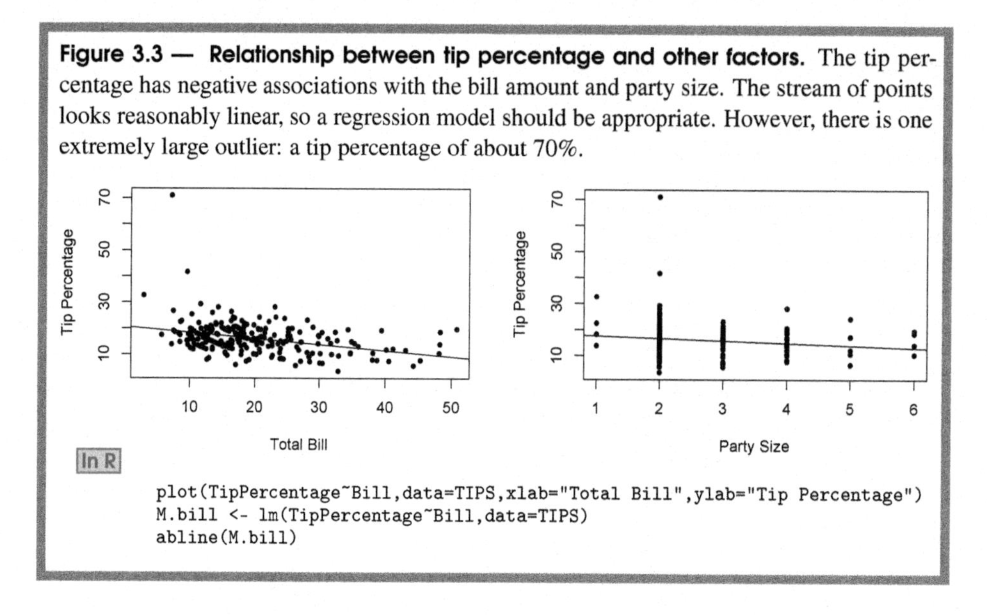

Figure 3.3 — Relationship between tip percentage and other factors. The tip percentage has negative associations with the bill amount and party size. The stream of points looks reasonably linear, so a regression model should be appropriate. However, there is one extremely large outlier: a tip percentage of about 70%.

```
plot(TipPercentage~Bill,data=TIPS,xlab="Total Bill",ylab="Tip Percentage")
M.bill <- lm(TipPercentage~Bill,data=TIPS)
abline(M.bill)
```

Bill

The regression equation is $\mu_{TipPercent} = 20.7 - 0.23Bill$.

- The intercept of 20.7% gives the average tip percentage among bills with `Bill`=0. Obviously, this quantity lacks interpretability since bill amounts are not zero.
- The slope of -0.23 implies that two bills that differ by \$1 are expected to have tip percentages that differ by 0.23% (higher bills are associated with smaller percentages). Note that this does *not* necessarily imply that talking your table into ordering an appetizer is going to decrease your tip percentage. The slope refers to differences in two different bills, not what happens when a certain bill becomes larger (which would be a statement on causality).

Party size

The regression equation is $\mu_{TipPercent} = 18.4 - 0.9PartySize$.

- The intercept of 18.4% gives the average tip percentage among bills coming from parties of size 0. Once again, this quantity lacks interpretability since party sizes have a minimum of one.
- The slope of -0.9 implies that when two bills come from parties that differ in size by one, the one with the larger party is expected to have a tip percentage that is 0.9% lower. Again, this does not necessarily imply that, if an additional person shows up mid-meal to join the party, the tip percentage will decrease. The regression is powerless to comment on what happens to an individual experiencing change.

3.2.2 Least squares criterion

How do we obtain the intercept and slope of the line that best summarizes how the average value of y changes with x? Since we typically don't know $\mu_{y|x}$ (the data collected only yields individual values of y and not the overall average), it makes sense to come up with a line that comes "closest" to the data points as a whole. There are many ways of accomplishing this feat depending on how you define "closest," but the industry standard is to use the **least squares criterion**.

The least squares criterion finds the line that minimizes the sum of the squared errors made by the line. In statistics, the errors are called the **residuals** of the model and are defined as:

$$Residual = Actual - Predicted \tag{3.3}$$

Residuals can be positive (point is above the line) or negative (point is below the line), which is part of the reason we *square* the error (i.e., so they don't cancel each other out when we sum the errors). See Figure 3.4 for a visual illustration.

Figure 3.4 — Residuals. Residuals are the errors made by the regression and represent the distances from the points (observed values of individuals) to the line (values predicted by the model). Residuals are positive when the actual point is above the line and are negative when the actual point is below the line.

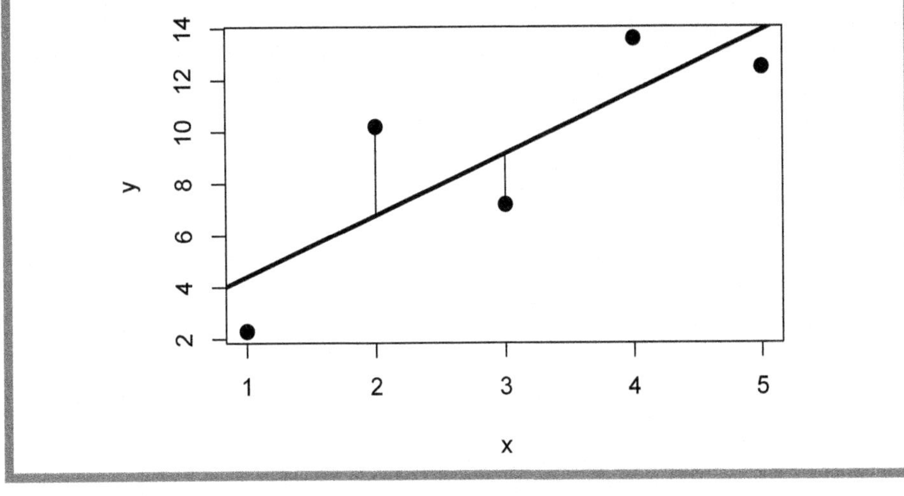

You could find the line that minimizes the sum of the absolute values of the errors, the square root of the absolute values of the errors, etc. The math is easiest when minimizing the sum of the squared errors, and that is the reason the least squares criterion was originally used. Often, there is very little difference between lines found with the different criteria. However, there are better alternatives to least squares that are resistant to outliers and other unusual points. These alternatives were difficult to use in the pre-computer era, but all software packages have some implementation of "robust regression" methods.

Remarkably, there are very simple equations that provide the coefficients of the regression equation that minimizes the sum of the squared errors. If we had a **census**, i.e., data on every possible individual, then the slope and intercept are given by:

$$\beta_1 = r \times \frac{SD_y}{SD_x} \qquad \beta_0 = \bar{y} - b_1\bar{x} \tag{3.4}$$

Here, r is the correlation between x and y, $\bar{x}$ and $\bar{y}$ are the averages, and SD_x and SD_y are the standard deviations. In particular, cast in this form, the slope has a special interpretation. Two individuals who differ in x by one standard deviation (in x) are expected to differ in y by only r standard deviations (in y).

(C) Originally, regression was thought of as "regression to the mean" and was discussed when predicting the height of a son based on the height of his father (Sir Francis Galton in the late 1880s). It was noted that fathers who were extremely tall or short (i.e., had x-values that were many standard deviations away from the average) tended to have sons that were not as unusual in height (i.e., have y-values that were not as many standard deviations from the average). The formula for the slope reaffirms this observation. Values that are one standard deviation from the average in x are expected to be only r standard deviations from the average in y. Since $-1 \leq r \leq 1$, individuals with extreme values of x are not expected to be quite as extreme in y.

Typically, the data that has been collected does not represent a census. When this is the case, the data is referred to as a **sample**, and it is not possible to calculate β_1 and β_0. Instead, the quantities b_1 and b_0 (the sample slope and sample intercept, respectively) are calculated in a similar manner using the observations in the sample and are used to estimate β_1 and β_0. We will return to just how far off b_1 may be from β_1 (i.e., the standard error of the sample slope) shortly.

(C) To determine if your data contains a census or is a sample, ask yourself the question: "Is it theoretically possible to collect more data?" If the answer is no, then you possess a census. If the answer is yes, then you possess a sample. For example, the `NFL` dataset contains information on all teams in the NFL over the course of about a decade. Since it is not possible to collect more data, this represents a census from that time period. The `ATTRACTM` and `ATTRACF` datasets contain information on the physical attractiveness of 70 men and women. Theoretically, it would have been possible to collect more data (by obtaining more pictures or by having students rate them), so the data represents a sample.

3.2.3 Effect of outliers

Since the real world is more complex than our model, there will occasionally be some individuals who just happen to be far from the regression line. These points are called **outliers**. The estimated slope and intercept of the regression line can be very sensitive to outliers. Consider Figure 3.5, which shows two regression lines: one with and one without an outlier.

An outlier "pulls" the regression line toward it since the line tries to minimize the sum of the squared errors. Since an outlier would have a very large residual (with respect to the line constructed without it), the line naturally tries to get as close to the outlier as possible. Just like how an extreme outlier can give a very misleading value for a correlation (Figure 2.23), an extreme outlier can give a very misleading impression of the slope, i.e., the average difference in y among entities that differ in x by one unit. Always check scatterplots to make sure that the regression model looks reasonable.

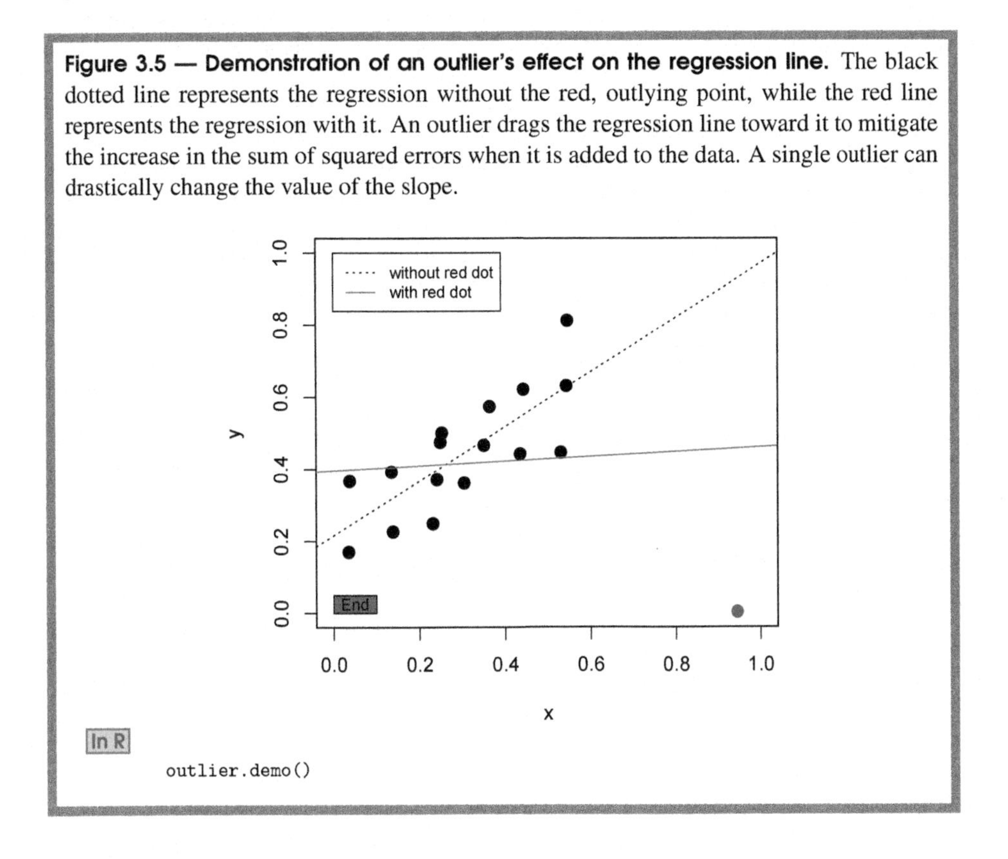

Figure 3.5 — Demonstration of an outlier's effect on the regression line. The black dotted line represents the regression without the red, outlying point, while the red line represents the regression with it. An outlier drags the regression line toward it to mitigate the increase in the sum of squared errors when it is added to the data. A single outlier can drastically change the value of the slope.

```
outlier.demo()
```

3.2.4 Assessing the fit: R^2 and RMSE

The goal of the least squares criterion is to find the line that minimizes the sum of the squared residuals. Once this is completed, we want to know how well the model "fits" the data. There are two main measures for evaluating the fit: $\mathbf{R^2}$ and **RMSE**. R^2 can vary between 0 and 1, with values closer to 1 indicating a better fit. The *RMSE* is the "root mean squared error" and represents the typical size of the residual. Smaller values of *RMSE* are better, but just how small is "good" depends on the context (and units) of the problem.

R^2

In the context of simple linear regression, R^2 equals the square of correlation between x and y, i.e., r^2. As such, it represents the percentage of the variability in y that can be attributed to our model.

R^2 is also used to gauge how well a multiple regression model (predicting y from many different variables) fits the data. When there is more than one predictor in the model, there is no simple relationship between R^2 and the individual Pearson correlations between y and the x's.

Let us interpret R^2 in the context of the errors made by the model. First, we consider the errors made by the **naive model**. This model predicts each individual's value of y to be $\bar{y}$, the overall average value of y in the data (i.e., ignoring any potential information from x). Then, we consider the errors made by the regression model. The decrease in the sum of squared errors when using the model is used to calculate R^2. See Figure 3.6 for a visual illustration.

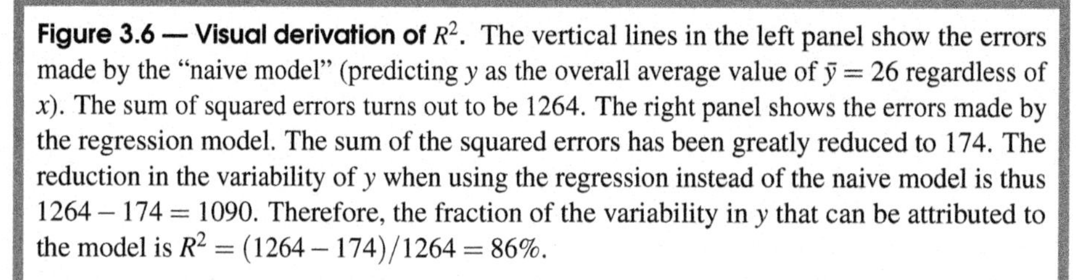

Figure 3.6 — Visual derivation of R^2. The vertical lines in the left panel show the errors made by the "naive model" (predicting y as the overall average value of $\bar{y} = 26$ regardless of x). The sum of squared errors turns out to be 1264. The right panel shows the errors made by the regression model. The sum of the squared errors has been greatly reduced to 174. The reduction in the variability of y when using the regression instead of the naive model is thus $1264 - 174 = 1090$. Therefore, the fraction of the variability in y that can be attributed to the model is $R^2 = (1264 - 174)/1264 = 86\%$.

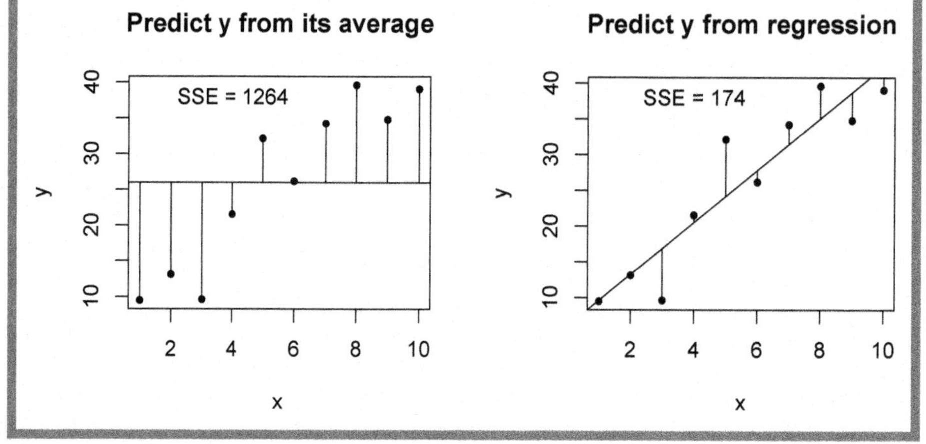

R^2 is the percentage reduction in sum of squared errors when we go from using the naive model (predicting y from $\bar{y}$) to using the regression model (predicting y from x).

Let SSE be the abbreviation for "sum of squared errors." Then we can write the equation for R^2 as:

$$R^2 = \frac{(\text{SSE when using } \bar{y} \text{ to predict } y) - (\text{SSE when using regression to predict } y)}{\text{SSE when using } \bar{y} \text{ to predict } y} \tag{3.5}$$

A model that fits the data extremely well will have an R^2 close to 100%. A model that fits the data poorly will have an R^2 close to 0%. There is no set cutoff for how large R^2 must be for the model to be useful. In business analytics, a "good" R^2 may be as low as 20-40%, and an R^2 of 80% or higher is generally quite impressive. In science, when validating a proposed physical law or equation, it would be disappointing to get an R^2 lower than 90% or so.

Before moving on, it must be noted that just because a model has a large R^2 does *not* mean that it is a "good" model for the data. It is easy for an outlier to induce a large value of R^2, or for a nonlinear relationship to have an R^2 close to 100%. See Figure 3.7. To stress once again, it is *always* necessary to visualize your data before interpreting any number you get from a correlation or regression analysis!

Figure 3.7 — High R^2 doesn't always mean a good model. In the left panel, the extreme outlier gives the impression that a strong relationship exists between x and y. However, looking more closely at the scatterplot, we see x and y have essentially no association and that the large R^2 is induced by the outlier. Even though $R^2 = 97\%$ for the line, it is a very poor model for the data. In the right panel, R^2 for the regression is 99%. However, the line is a poor model for the data since in reality the relationship has obvious curvature.

Do not be fooled into thinking that a large R^2 means the regression line is an appropriate model for the data. A large R^2 just means that the fraction of variability in y that can be explained by the model is large.

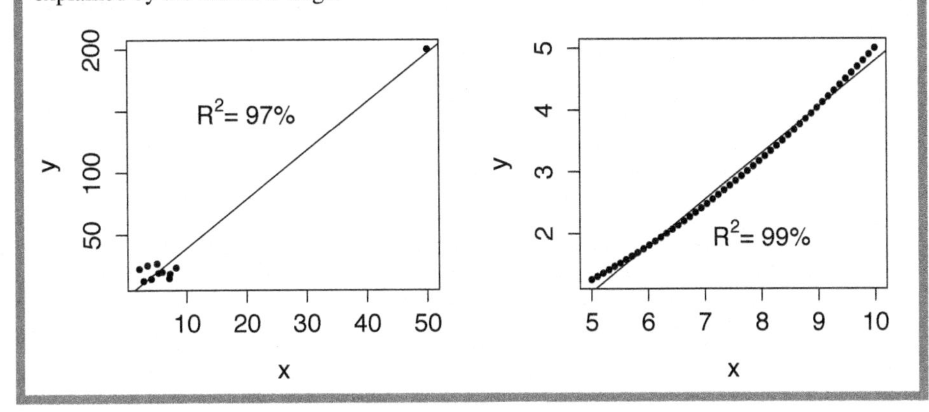

RMSE

The root mean squared error, or RMSE, is the "typical" error made by the regression line. Alternatively, you can think of the RMSE as the typical size of the residual or as the typical distance that points are from the line.

As with R^2, there is no set cutoff for how small the RMSE should be for the model to be useful, but smaller values are better. For some models, it may be an impressive feat if the size of the typical error is $1.00 (e.g., predicting how much money people will spend at Walmart in the next 90 days), while for others, such an error would be disastrous (e.g., predicting the price of a "penny stock" at the end of the trading week).

One thing that can be done is to compare the RMSE to the standard deviation of the y-values in the data. This standard deviation essentially tells you the RMSE of the naive model. If the RMSE of the regression is much smaller than this, your model is much more useful than no model at all.

3.3 Inference regarding β_1

A simple linear regression assumes that the average value of y has a linear relationship with x: $\mu_{y|x} = \beta_0 + \beta_1 x$. Unless we have a census, we estimate β_0 and β_1 with the intercept and slope of the regression line constructed via least squares on our sample. We call these **point estimates** b_0 and b_1, and they serve as our best "guesses" as to what the true values of β_0 and β_1 may be. The followup question is then: how far off might the estimated slope b_1 be from "the truth"?

It turns out it is possible to answer this question *if* we are willing to make additional assumptions about how much individuals' values of y vary about the average, i.e., the distribution of distances of individuals from the regression line. The complete **simple linear regression model** is:

$$y_i = \beta_0 + \beta_1 x_i + \varepsilon_i = \mu_{y|x} + \varepsilon_i \qquad \varepsilon_i \sim N(0, \sigma) \tag{3.6}$$

In this equation, y_i and x_i are the y- and x-values of individual i. The coefficients β_0 and β_1 are still the "true" intercept and slope (the values that would be measured if the data represented a census). The symbol ε_i (pronounced "epsilon") represents the *difference* between the y-value of individual i (who has some value of x) and the average value of y (among all individuals with that value of x). This difference is also the vertical distance of individual i from the line and is often referred to as a **disturbance**.

C Equation 3.2 gives the regression *equation*, i.e., the equation of a line relating the average value of y to x. Equation 3.6 gives the regression *model*, i.e., a full description about how individual values of y are related to x.

Recall the quantity $\beta_0 + \beta_1 x_i$ is the average value of y among all individuals with the common value x_i (Equation 3.2 referred to this as $\mu_{y|x}$, "the average of y given the value of x"). The regression model essentially says: "An individual's value of y is the average value of y among all individuals who share that same common value of x give or take a little, and oh, by the way, the average value of y has a linear relationship with x."

To determine how far the estimated slope b_1 may be from the "truth" β_1, we make very special assumptions regarding the possible values for ε. Specifically:

$$\varepsilon_i \sim N(0, \sigma) \tag{3.7}$$

In other words, the distribution of the possible disturbances is Normal with a mean of zero and a standard deviation of σ. Written this way, this fundamental assumption behind the regression model is rather abstract. Let us recast the assumption as a set of visual constraints about the stream of points. See Figure 3.8. To have $\varepsilon_i \sim N(0, \sigma)$:

- The trajectory of the stream of points must be linear. When the mean of residuals is zero, then the average value of y falls *exactly* on the line (Equation 3.2) as desired.
- The *vertical* spread of points away from the line is the same everywhere. When this is true, the standard deviation of residuals is the number σ (regardless of the characteristics of the individuals) as desired.
- A histogram/QQ-plot of residuals at every value of x (and taken as a whole) looks Normal.
- If x is a variable that measures time either explicitly (days since product was released) or implicitly (items in shopping carts in sequential visits), the residuals of observations that come later in time must be independent of the residuals that came earlier in time.

C It is possible to simultaneously model the correlation in residuals and to fit a linear regression with correlated errors. This type of modeling is called time-series analysis and is beyond the scope of this book.

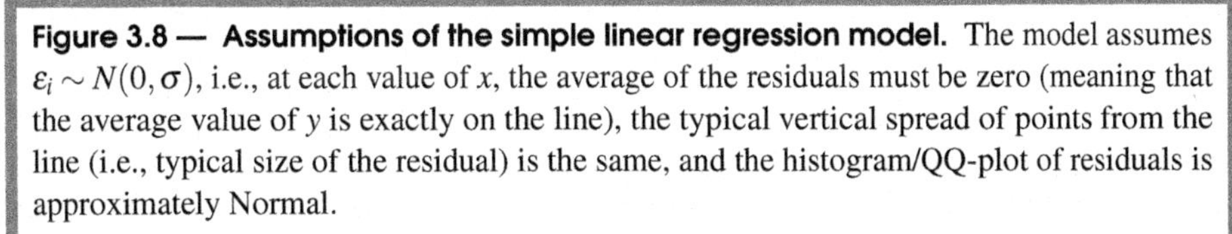

Figure 3.8 — Assumptions of the simple linear regression model. The model assumes $\varepsilon_i \sim N(0, \sigma)$, i.e., at each value of x, the average of the residuals must be zero (meaning that the average value of y is exactly on the line), the typical vertical spread of points from the line (i.e., typical size of the residual) is the same, and the histogram/QQ-plot of residuals is approximately Normal.

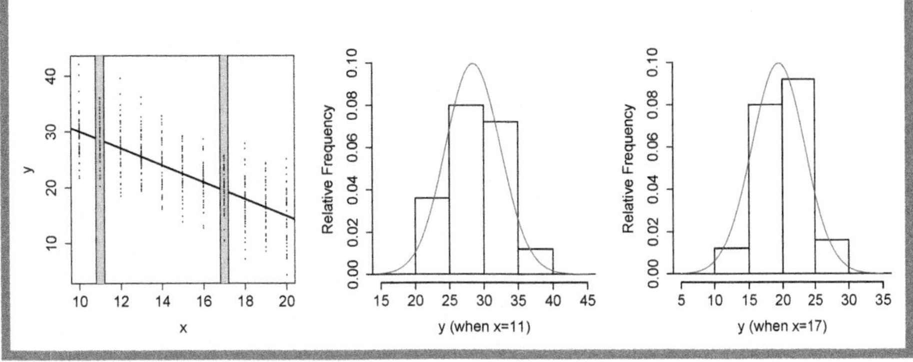

3.3.1 Standard error of the slope

When the simple linear regression model is valid, the slope measured from a sample (b_1) can only be "so far" from the truth (β_1). Consider the following illustrative simulation:

- A random sample of y-values is generated from the model $y_i = 3 + 5x_i + \varepsilon_i$, where $x = 1, 2, \ldots, 10$ and $\varepsilon_i \sim N(0, 2)$.
- The slope is found via least squares and then recorded.
- The first two steps are repeated 10,000 times, and a histogram of the slopes from the 10,000 samples is made.

Figure 3.9 shows the distribution of the measured slopes (b_1) from the simulation. The distribution is centered around $\beta_1 = 5$ (the truth) and looks symmetric. Typically, the measured slopes are about 0.5 or so from the truth (some are closer, some are farther). We can say that in general, the measured slope from a sample is likely to be about 0.5 from $\beta_1 = 5$. In other words, the standard error of b_1 is about 0.5.

The **standard error** of the slope is the typical difference between the measured value from a sample and "the truth" (i.e., $b_1 - \beta_1$).

The standard error is a fundamental, critical quantity that all analysts must understand. When we try to estimate the true value of some parameter θ (e.g., the slope of the "true" regression line) from the statistic $\hat{\theta}$ (e.g., the slope of the sample regression line), then the standard error of $\hat{\theta}$ gives the typical difference between our estimate $\hat{\theta}$ and "the truth" θ. There are often formulas that give this value using only the collected data (without knowing the truth).

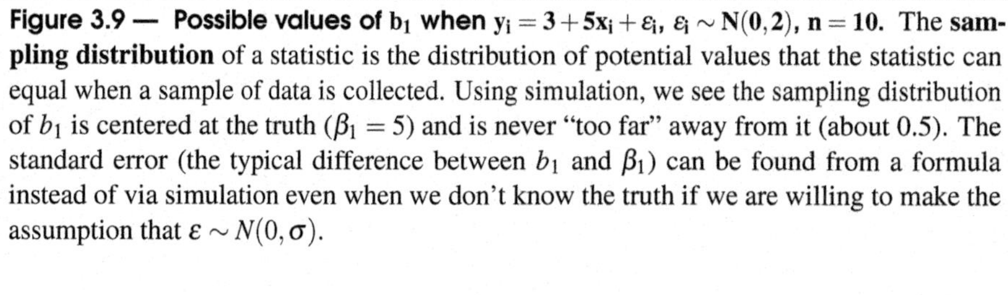

Figure 3.9 — Possible values of b_1 when $y_i = 3 + 5x_i + \varepsilon_i$, $\varepsilon_i \sim N(0,2)$, $n = 10$. The **sampling distribution** of a statistic is the distribution of potential values that the statistic can equal when a sample of data is collected. Using simulation, we see the sampling distribution of b_1 is centered at the truth ($\beta_1 = 5$) and is never "too far" away from it (about 0.5). The standard error (the typical difference between b_1 and β_1) can be found from a formula instead of via simulation even when we don't know the truth if we are willing to make the assumption that $\varepsilon \sim N(0, \sigma)$.

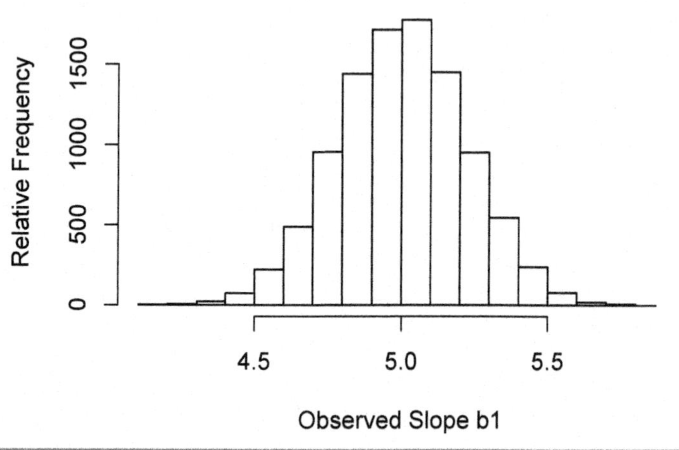

Remarkably, even though we'll *never* know β_1 (unless we possess a census), there is a formula that estimates the value of the standard error of the slope (abbreviated SE_{b_1}) from the data that has been collected.

$$SE_{b_1} = \frac{RMSE}{\sqrt{(n-1) \times SD_x^2}} \tag{3.8}$$

Given the typical size of the residual (RMSE), the sample size (n), and the standard deviation of the predictor variable (x), we can anticipate how far off our measured value of b_1 is likely to be from the truth. The formula for the standard error yields some interesting insights (which can be visualized in Figure 3.10).

- The standard error and RMSE are proportional to each other. When there is more scatter in the stream of points (larger RMSE), the slope of the best-fitting line is more uncertain (many lines "look" like they'd well-summarize the trajectory of the stream).
- The standard error of the slope depends on the spread of the recorded x-values (as measured by the standard deviation). If two experiments are being conducted to estimate β_1, the slope found on the data whose x's are more spread out will probably be closer to the truth.
- With more data (bigger n), your estimated slope will be closer to the truth.

Figure 3.10 — Relationship of standard error of slope with RMSE and SD_x. The left panel serves as a baseline and shows the actual estimated regression equation with a thick solid line along with five "reasonable" regressions (lines that also fit the data well) with dotted lines. There is not much scatter in the stream of points, so nearly all of these lines are on top of each other and all lines have about the same slope. In other words, the standard error of the slope is small.

The middle panel shows the effect of increasing the RMSE. With more scatter in the stream of points, the slopes of five "reasonable" regressions are noticeably different. In other words, as the RMSE increases, the standard error of the slope increases.

The right panel shows what happens when the standard deviation of x's is smaller. The "reasonable" regressions vary quite a bit. The standard error of the slope is larger when the range of x in the collected data is smaller.

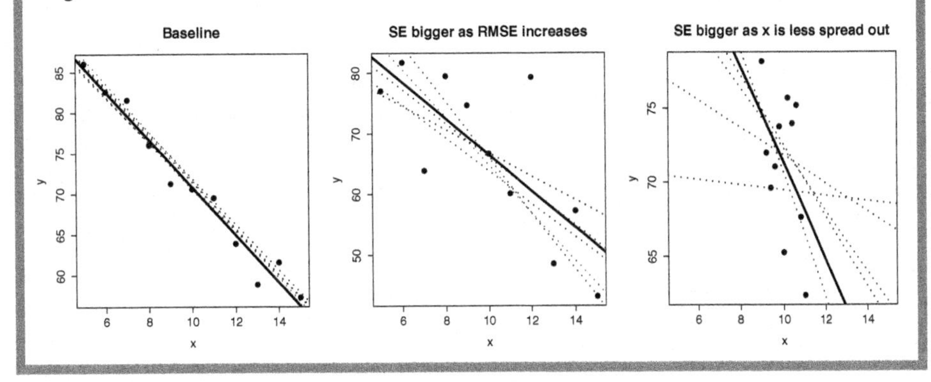

3.3.2 Confidence interval for the slope

Once we have estimated how far the measured slope (b_1) is likely to be from "the truth" (β_1), we can construct a **confidence interval** for the true slope β_1.

In general, a confidence interval is a range of values that has a high probability of covering the true value of the parameter we are trying to estimate. Typically, "high probability" is chosen to be 95%. When the regression assumptions are true, we can derive such an interval by using the following logic:

- When all regression assumptions are true, about 95% of random samples will have their measured slopes b_1 be at most about two standard errors from β_1.
- Thus, if we take our measured slope b_1 and go about ± 2 standard errors from it, the corresponding interval should have about a 95% chance of covering β_1.
- For an interval with a higher level of confidence, we need to go more than two standard errors from b_1, etc.

An approximate 95% confidence interval for β_1 is $b_1 \pm 2SE_{b_1}$. The number in front of SE_{b_1} may be a little larger or smaller than 2 depending on the sample size. Software can be used to calculate an "exact" number. However, since the real world is more complex than our model, using 2 is typically a reasonable shortcut.

A 95% confidence interval gives a range of plausible values for β_1 that are consistent with the collected data. There is always a possibility that the confidence interval is wrong (β_1 is outside its bounds), but the procedure will get it right for about 95% of random samples when the regression model provides a reasonable description of the data.

The term "confidence" may appear confusing at first. The "confidence" in confidence interval refers to the probability that the *procedure* makes an interval that is correct, i.e., includes the truth β_1. You will never know whether *your* confidence interval for a particular dataset is correct, but in the long-run, the procedure makes an interval that will include β_1 about 95% of the time.

To illustrate, consider Figure 3.11. A total of 100 different samples have been generated using the model $y_i = 3 + 5x_i + \varepsilon_i$, $\varepsilon \sim N(0,2)$. The confidence intervals for each sample are displayed by vertical lines. Out of these 100 intervals, four are incorrect (they do not contain the true slope of 5). This demonstration illustrates what "confidence" means. While you will never know whether the confidence interval for *your particular* dataset is correct, in the long-run, about 95% of datasets yield 95% confidence intervals that include β_1.

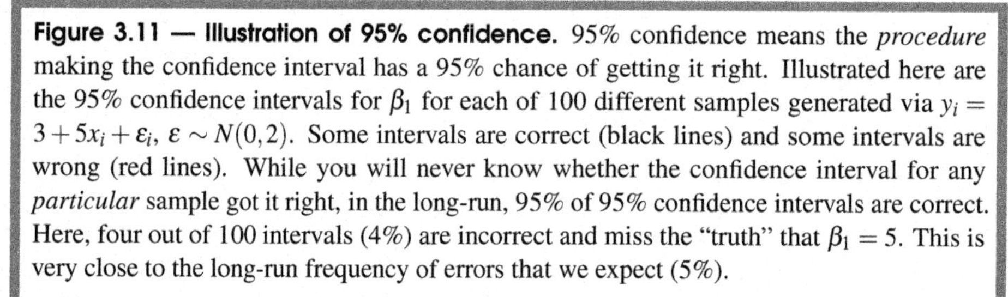

Figure 3.11 — Illustration of 95% confidence. 95% confidence means the *procedure* making the confidence interval has a 95% chance of getting it right. Illustrated here are the 95% confidence intervals for β_1 for each of 100 different samples generated via $y_i = 3 + 5x_i + \varepsilon_i$, $\varepsilon \sim N(0,2)$. Some intervals are correct (black lines) and some intervals are wrong (red lines). While you will never know whether the confidence interval for any *particular* sample got it right, in the long-run, 95% of 95% confidence intervals are correct. Here, four out of 100 intervals (4%) are incorrect and miss the "truth" that $\beta_1 = 5$. This is very close to the long-run frequency of errors that we expect (5%).

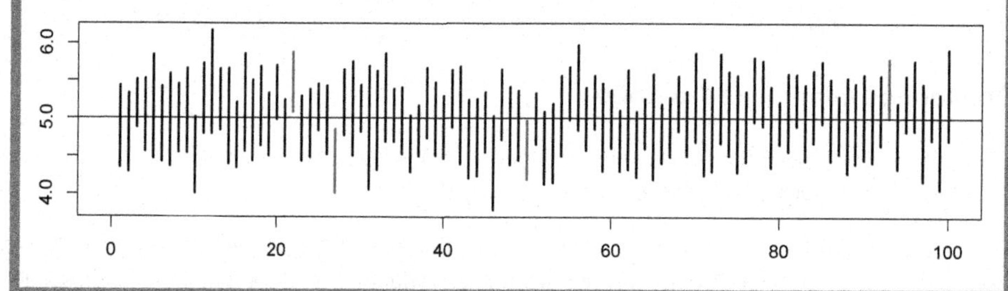

3.4 Statistical significance of a regression

In general, we consider the statistical significance of a *regression* separately from the statistical significance of its *predictors*. However, for simple linear regression (one predictor), these are one and the same. In the next chapter, where we build regression models using more than one predictor, the difference is critical. For now, let us focus the discussion on what it means for the *regression* itself to be significant.

Since the least squares criterion is used to estimate the regression coefficients, it makes sense to base significance on the sum of squared errors (SSE) of the model. The SSE of the naive model (where y is predicted to be the average value of y in the data, regardless of x) serves as the baseline. Review Figure 3.6 for a visual depiction of the errors made from the naive and regression models.

A regression using *any* predictor variable (even one that is completely unrelated to y) will *always* yield an SSE that is smaller than the SSE of the naive model (a line with a slope is flexible and will fit the data better than a rigid horizontal line). To be statistically significant, the reduction in SSE when using the regression needs to be substantially greater than the reduction in SSE that may happen "by chance" from a random, unrelated predictor. We can conduct a permutation test to determine what values of SSE could occur by chance. The permutation procedure was previously discussed in the study of associations in Sections 2.3.3, 2.4.2, and 2.6.3.

3.4.1 *p*-value approach

The significance of a regression model is gauged from its p-value. If the p-value is less than 5%, then the regression is statistically significant—x does a better job of predicting y than the naive model (i.e., using no additional information about the individuals).

> The p-value of your regression model is the probability that a model using a predictor unrelated to y would reduce the sum of squared errors (relative to the naive model) by at least as much as your model. If the p-value is small, then it is unlikely that the reduction in SSE has occurred "by chance"—x contributes *some* information about an individual's value of y. If the p-value is large, then the reduction in SSE is not impressive—x predicts y no better than a completely unrelated variable.

Refer back to Figure 3.6, where y is predicted by the naive model in the left panel and from the regression in the right panel. The SSE using the naive model is 1264 and 174 using the regression model. The reduction in SSE is $(1264 - 174) = 1090$. The reduction as a percentage of the original sum of squared errors is $1090/1264 = 86\%$ (which by definition is also R^2).

The decrease in SSE looks impressive, but is it more than what a random, unrelated predictor could do by chance? Let us use the **permutation procedure**.

1. Create an artificial dataset by shuffling up the observed values of y and randomly assigning them to individuals. Refer to the example in Table 2.4. Calculate the sum of squared errors made by the least squares regression line. By design, this procedure guarantees there is no underlying relationship between individuals' x and y values, so this value of the SSE is one that can occur "by chance."
2. Repeat this procedure many times to build up a distribution of values of the SSE that occur by chance.
3. Measure the SSE of the naive model (predict y from the overall average) and of your regression model. The (estimated) p-value of your regression is the fraction of these artificial datasets whose reduction in the SSE is at least as large as the reduction in SSE from your regression. See Figure 3.12.
4. If the p-value is less than 5%, your regression is statistically significant—it is unlikely that a predictor unrelated to y would predict y at least as well as x.

Figure 3.12 shows an example from the `BODYFAT` dataset (where we predict the body fat percentages of individuals based on various physical characteristics). An individual's age (`Age`) is a relatively poor predictor of body fat percentage (`BodyFat`) since $R^2 = 0.08$. Knowing someone's age only gets us about 8% of the way to knowing his or her body fat percentage. We may wonder if the regression is statistically significant, i.e., does age predict body fat percentages any better than an unrelated predictor?

Figure 3.12 — Evaluating significance of a regression model. To determine whether a regression model is statistically significant, we need to find the probability that a predictor unrelated to y would reduce the SSE by at least as much as our model. This can be estimated via the permutation procedure, where y values are shuffled up and randomly assigned to individuals.

The plot on the left shows the regression line when predicting someone's body fat percentage from his or her age in red. The grey and black lines are the regressions when predicting body fat percentage from an unrelated predictor (obtained by the permutation procedure). While the relationship between body fat percentage and age is definitely not strong ($R^2 = 0.08$), the regression is statistically significant. The regression using age as a predictor is noticeably more tilted than the regression using unrelated predictors.

The plot on the right shows the reduction in sum of squared errors (compared to the naive model) of the regression using age as a predictor (red line) and the regressions using unrelated predictors (histogram). The p-value of the regression is essentially 0 since none of the unrelated predictors manage (by chance alone) to reduce the SSE by anywhere near as much as age.

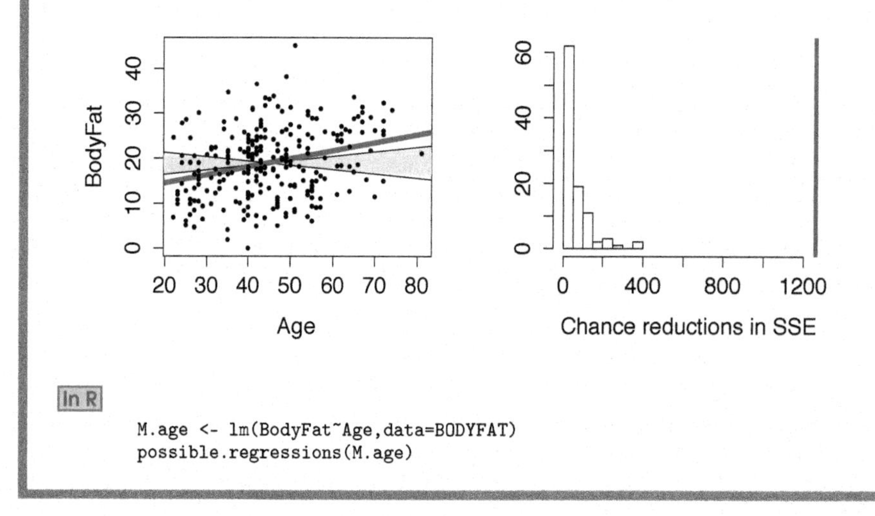

In R

```
M.age <- lm(BodyFat~Age,data=BODYFAT)
possible.regressions(M.age)
```

The permutation procedure reveals that age is a statistically significant predictor of body fat percentage. The observed regression line is noticeably more tilted (implying it has a stronger relationship) than the lines made with unrelated predictors. The reduction in the sum of squared errors when using age as a predictor is also noticeably larger than the reduction when using an unrelated predictor. Thus, it is very difficult for a predictor unrelated to body fat to produce a regression with an R^2 of 8% or more (none of the 100 random predictors come close).

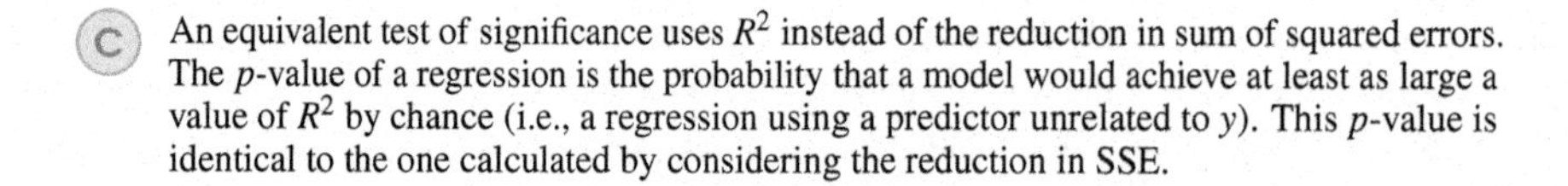

An equivalent test of significance uses R^2 instead of the reduction in sum of squared errors. The p-value of a regression is the probability that a model would achieve at least as large a value of R^2 by chance (i.e., a regression using a predictor unrelated to y). This p-value is identical to the one calculated by considering the reduction in SSE.

When the assumptions behind the regression model are true, it is possible to calculate the p-value with a formula (using the "**F test**"), so simulation is not necessary. However, the mechanics behind the procedure are sufficiently tedious that this discussion is omitted. In this work, this approximate p-value is used in lieu of performing the permutation procedure, so checking the assumptions of the regression is critical.

3.4.2 Confidence interval approach

It is also possible to gauge the statistical significance of a simple linear regression by using the confidence interval for the slope. If a regression is considered statistically significant when its p-value is less than α (usually 5%), then the regression is also statistically significant if a $100(1-\alpha)\%$ confidence interval (usually 95%) does *not* contain zero.

For the example in Figure 3.6, a 95% confidence interval for β_1 is $(2.45, 4.82)$. Since zero is outside the interval, we conclude the regression is statistically significant. When predicting an employee's salary from prior work experience (Figure 3.2), a 95% confidence interval for β_1 is $(-2.4, 23.3)$. Since zero is inside the interval, the regression is *not* significant (by itself, `Experience` does no better at predicting `Salary` than a typical variable unrelated to salary).

The reasoning is quite intuitive. The confidence interval gives a range of plausible values for β_1 based on the data. If zero is inside the interval, then zero is a plausible value for β_1. If $\beta_1 = 0$, then our regression model becomes $y_i = \beta_0 + 0 \times x + \varepsilon_i$ or $y_i = \beta_0 + \varepsilon_i$, i.e., the average value of y does not have a linear relationship with x.

3.4.3 Significance, sample size, and R^2

As discussed in Section 2.8, statistical significance and practical significance are two entirely different concepts. An association can be highly statistically significant but lack any sort of practical importance or value.

Review Figure 2.28, which shows a mosaic plot relating the interest in some product to the gender of the individual. The percentages of men and women who are interested in the product are essentially identical (70% vs. 68%) and has little to no practical importance. However, the p-value of the association was 0.0001, indicating the association was highly statistically significant.

Similarly, a simple linear regression may be highly statistically significant when the underlying relationship is so weak that it is of no practical value. For example, consider the `DONOR` dataset and the problem of predicting donation amounts to a charity. Let us predict a person's donation amount from the number of months since his or her last gift. Figure 3.13 shows the scatterplot.

The amount that someone donates in the `DONOR` dataset is not a good quantity to model with linear regression. The residuals have a strongly non-Normal distribution, so the assumptions behind regression are not quite met. However, with such a large dataset, the impact of the violation of Normality is fairly minimal.

The relationship is extremely weak and has $R^2 = 1.2\%$. The regression line is nearly horizontal, implying that the average donation amount hardly changes at all as the number of months since the last gift varies. However, the regression is highly statistically significant with a p-value of about 10^{-10}—the chance of winning Powerball is 100 times larger than the chance that a random predictor would reduce the SSE by as much as the model. While the regression model predicts y better than an unrelated, random predictor, the model is of little to no practical use.

Most discussions about regression spend *way* too much time on statistical significance and overemphasize its importance. Without context, a statistically significant regression means very little, only that it is unlikely that a random predictor would have reduced the sum of squared errors by as much as your model.

Figure 3.13 — Relationship between donation amount and length of time since last gift. The regression is significant since its p-value (3.2×10^{-10}) is much less than 5%. However, the relationship is of very little practical use for describing how the average donation amount is related to the number of months since someone last donated. $R^2 = 0.8\%$, so only about 1% of the variation in donation amounts can be attributed to the model. Thus, a statistically significant relationship may lack any sort of practical importance.

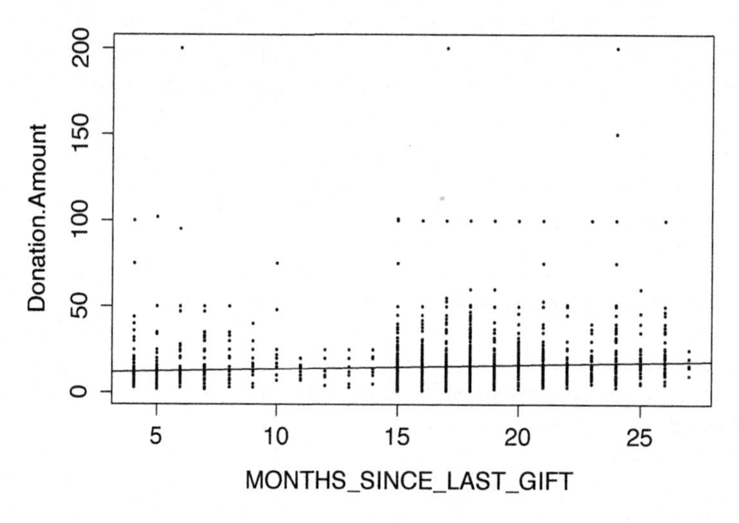

In R

```
M.amount <- lm(Donation.Amount~MONTHS_SINCE_LAST_GIFT,data=DONOR)
plot(Donation.Amount~MONTHS_SINCE_LAST_GIFT,data=DONOR,pch=20,cex=0.4)
abline(M.amount)
summary(M.amount)
Multiple R-squared:  0.008139,Adjusted R-squared:  0.007934
F-statistic: 39.72 on 1 and 4841 DF,  p-value: 3.187e-10
```

One drawback of statistical significance is its connection to sample size. The field of regression was developed when datasets were very small (a few dozen at most). Modern datasets, especially in business analytics, are extremely large. The value of n may be anywhere between a few thousand to a few million or beyond (some retailers like Walmart handle more than one million transactions per hour). Even the weakest (and uninteresting) linear relationship will be statistically significant for a large enough sample size, so it is always important to check R^2 and the $RMSE$ to gauge whether the relationship is strong or useful.

Statistical significance (and more specifically, the p-value) does *not* tell you whether the relationship is strong (you must gauge this with R^2 and $RMSE$) or even useful or important. Looking at R^2 and the $RMSE$ along with your personal judgment gives an idea of the practical significance of a regression model.

Further, statistical significance does not tell us whether the relationship is exploitable (e.g., do we need to increase or decrease x to get a larger value of y) since the regression equation is not a physical law. Similar to our discussion on associations, there may be a lurking variable that induces the relationship.

For example, consider the relationship between the number of wins and the number of fumbles in the `FUMBLES` dataset. The relationship looks like it could be well-modeled by a regression (Figure 2.18). The slope of the regression is -0.27, implying that teams that differ in the number of lost fumbles by four are expected to differ by about one win (more fumbles implies fewer wins). The regression is highly significant with a p-value of 7×10^{-11}. However, the relationship is rather weak ($R^2 = 11.5\%$), implying that knowing the number of lost fumbles gets you about 10% of the way to knowing the number of wins for the season.

Does this mean the coach should focus on techniques to avoid losing fumbles? While this would be a good idea regardless, the answer is an emphatic "no." The analysis does *not* mean that if a team fumbles four times in a game that it is going to lose. Remember that the slope is a comment on how individuals' y-values differ *from each other*, not what happens when an individual's value of x increases or decreases.

A sure-fire way to hardly ever fumble in a football game is to have the snap cover only a tiny distance to the quarterback, who then immediately kneels on the ground. This is also a sure-fire way to lose a game.

3.5 Checking assumptions

For the slope, R^2, p-value, etc., to have any legitimate meaning, the regression model needs to be an accurate reflection of reality. In other words, the critical assumption that the disturbances have a Normal distribution, $\varepsilon \sim N(0, \sigma)$, needs to hold.

- Linearity—the trajectory of the stream of points is well-described by a straight line.
- Equal spread—vertical deviations of points from the line are roughly the same everywhere.
- Normality—the distribution of residuals is approximately Normal.
- Independence—if the observations were taken in time sequence, the residuals must be independent from each other.

The main tool for checking assumptions is the **residuals plot**, which plots each individual's **fitted value** (predicted by the regression) on the horizontal axis with its residual (difference between observed and predicted value) on the vertical axis.

When the regression model is valid and assumptions are met, *there should be no interesting patterns* visible in the residuals plot. If there is a pattern, something about the relationship between x and y is *not* captured by the model.

Figure 3.14 — Good and bad residuals plots. A "good" residuals plot (indicative of the regression model being a reasonable reflection of reality) has no discernible pattern with the possible exception of unequal horizontal spread. It is acceptable if the points are concentrated unevenly from left to right since this only reflects the distribution of values of x (an artifact of the way data was collected or of the natural distribution of that variable) and not any aspect of the relationship between x and y. A "bad" residuals plot has unusual features or patterns: curvature, unequal vertical spread, or outliers.

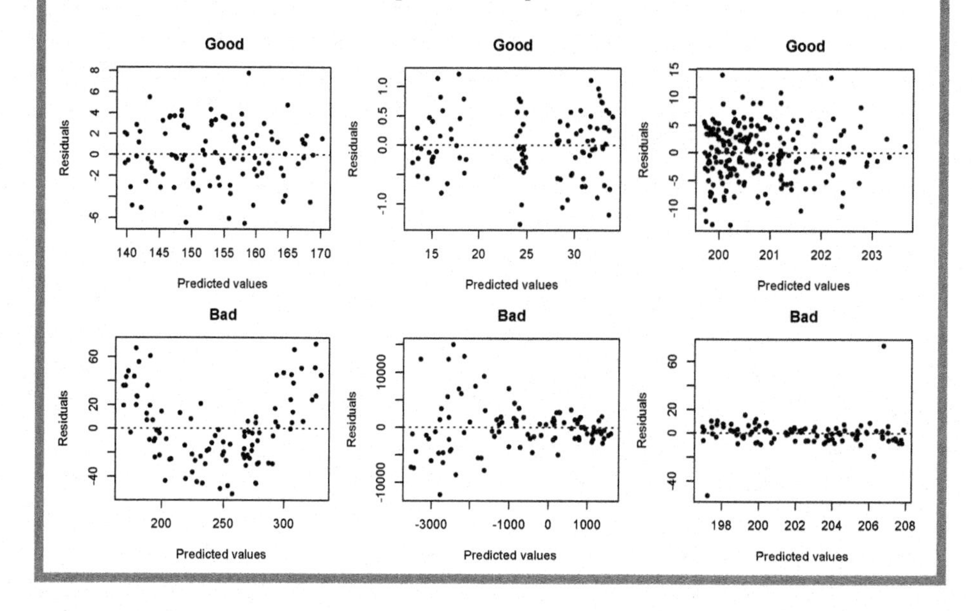

Figure 3.14 shows examples of "good" and "bad" residuals plots. With the exception of the middle panel, the "good" plots do not show any patterns. Residuals in the middle panel show "gaps" (a lack of residuals) in two areas. This (and only this) kind of pattern in the plot is acceptable—it does not matter whether the (horizontal) spread of the predicted values is the same everywhere.

Horizontal gaps and clumpiness in the residuals plot are artifacts of the distribution of x-values and either reflect the way the data was collected or the natural frequency of x-values. They do *not* indicate anything about the relationship between x and y, nor do they imply that the model has a problem.

Only the *vertical* spread of residuals matters when checking the validity of a model. The "bad" plots in Figure 3.14 show obvious patterns: curvature (indicative of nonlinearity), unequal vertical spread, and outliers.

For larger datasets (more than a few dozen observations), *small* violations of the assumptions of the regression model are typically inconsequential. The human eye is almost "too good" at finding small, inconsequential patterns. Often, you will look at a residuals plot and wonder whether something sticks out enough to be considered a pattern. Chances are, if you have to *ask* yourself this question, the answer is "no." Only *obvious* violations are deal breakers. One way to discern whether a potential pattern is important is to try visually removing a few points from it. If the pattern disappears without those points, it probably wasn't there to begin with.

From a purely statistical point of view, *any* violation or any pattern in the residuals, regardless of the sample size, means the model is invalid. However, remember that the *entire regression framework itself* is an approximation to reality. We know the real world is more complex than our model, and we should not expect the assumptions to hold up perfectly because our model isn't perfect—all models are wrong, some are useful. The good news is that statistical theory assures us that *small* violations do not affect the estimates of the coefficients, confidence intervals, or p-values (which are only approximate anyway) by much.

Statistical tests of the assumptions do exist but are generally only useful for small samples (less than a couple dozen). The tests become very sensitive to small, inconsequential violations for large datasets. Your eye really provides the best check for larger datasets!

The recommended procedure for checking assumptions is:

1. Check the results of the statistical tests. If they pass (p-values greater than 5%), then the model can be used.
2. If one or more of the tests are failed and there are fewer than $n \approx 25$ observations, stop. Regression is not appropriate for modeling the relationship. For larger datasets, check the residuals plot and see whether the violations are severe (in which case regression is not appropriate) or small enough to be ignored.

Linearity

The linear regression model assumes that the average value of y has a perfectly linear relationship with x. The interpretation of the slope hinges on this premise. This is the most important assumption to check since it makes no sense to model a curved relationship with a line! To check this assumption, look for bends in the residuals plot (e.g., lower-left panel in Figure 3.14).

Technically, this assumption checks the "mean zero" component of the requirement that $\varepsilon \sim N(0, \sigma)$. The location of the regression line is where the average value of y is supposed to be located at a given value of x. The residual is the distance from the line to a point. For the average value of y to have a linear relationship with x, the mean of the residuals must be zero to ensure that the average indeed falls on the line.

There are many formal statistical tests to check whether the relationship is exactly linear. We will use the "F test for linearity," which requires that at least two individuals share a common x-value. The test works by comparing two models: the regression model and a "saturated" model that predicts y to be the average value of y observed at each unique value of x. For example, imagine the data is

y	8	7	6	6	6	3	4
x	1	2	2	3	3	3	4
y_{pred}	8	6.5	6.5	5	5	5	4

The saturated model would predict y to be 8 when $x = 1$ (the "average" of the one observation at $x = 1$) and would predict y to be 6.5 when $x = 2$ (the average of the two observations at $x = 2$), etc.

The saturated model has more freedom compared to the regression model (which assumes a linear relationship between the average value of y and x), so it will fit the data better and will have a smaller sum of squared errors. When the linearity assumption is valid, the saturated model will not be *too much* better than the regression since the average really does vary linearly with x.

The "F test for linearity" checks where the decrease in sum of squared errors when going from the regression to the saturated model is statistically significant. If the p-value is less than 5%, then the reduction is significant—the saturated model is better than the regression, implying that the average value of y does not quite vary linearly with x. If the p-value is 5% or greater, then the saturated model is no better than the regression, implying that the assumption that the average value of y has a linear relationship with x is reasonable.

The "F test for linearity" is conducted in the same way as the test of significance for a linear regression model. A regression is statistically significant if the reduction in SSE when going from the naive model (predicting y from its overall average) to the regression model (predicting y from x) is "large," i.e., unlikely to be produced by chance. This significance test is also an F test, just with a different goal.

The top panels in Figure 3.15 show the relationships between responses to the question: "What percentage of your fellow students are you more attractive than?" and the same question regarding intelligence for 100 students in an introductory statistics class (SURVEY10 data). The regression is significant (p-value of 0.0005) but not very strong ($R^2 = 16\%$). The "F test for linearity" has a p-value of 21%, so the test is passed and, statistically, the relationship is linear. We are not required to check linearity using the residuals plot since the test is passed, but we see no hint of curvature.

The bottom panels in Figure 3.15 show the relationship between fuel efficiency and horsepower for a sample of 82 European cars (AUTO). The p-value of the "F test for linearity" is less than one in a million, so the test is failed—statistically, the relationship is not linear. Since this is a large sample, we look back to see if the violation is severe (remember, small violations are generally allowable). Indeed, we see a hint of curvature in the scatterplot and the residuals plot, so the simple linear regression model is not appropriate.

Equal vertical spread

The linear regression model assumes "equal vertical spread," i.e., that the typical distance of points from the line is the same everywhere. This assumption is secondary to linearity in importance. As long as the relationship is linear, the slope provides an accurate estimate of the average difference in y among two individuals who differ in x by one unit. However, if there is unequal vertical spread, the formula for the standard error of the slope (and confidence interval) is wrong.

Figure 3.15 — Assessing the linearity assumption. The p-value of the F test for linearity in the top panels is 21%, implying that the relationship is statistically linear. Although a check of the residuals plot is unnecessary in this case, we see no curvature. The p-value of the F test for linearity in the bottom panels is 2×10^{-11}, so statistically the relationship is not linear. Since the number of observations is large, we look at the residuals plot to see if the violation is severe enough for us to abandon the model. Obvious curvature is apparent, so indeed the linear regression model is not appropriate here.

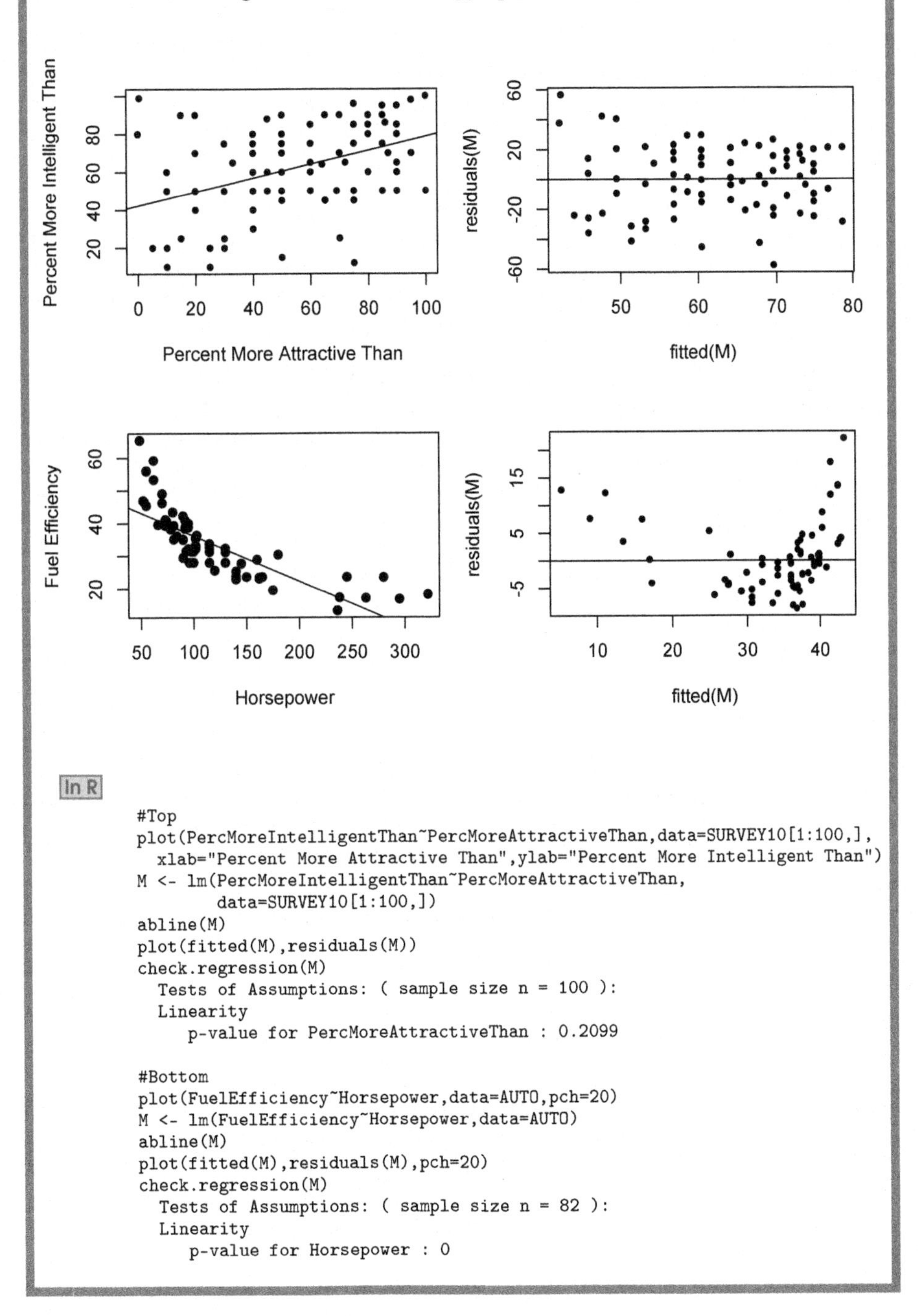

In R

```
#Top
plot(PercMoreIntelligentThan~PercMoreAttractiveThan,data=SURVEY10[1:100,],
  xlab="Percent More Attractive Than",ylab="Percent More Intelligent Than")
M <- lm(PercMoreIntelligentThan~PercMoreAttractiveThan,
        data=SURVEY10[1:100,])
abline(M)
plot(fitted(M),residuals(M))
check.regression(M)
  Tests of Assumptions: ( sample size n = 100 ):
  Linearity
     p-value for PercMoreAttractiveThan : 0.2099

#Bottom
plot(FuelEfficiency~Horsepower,data=AUTO,pch=20)
M <- lm(FuelEfficiency~Horsepower,data=AUTO)
abline(M)
plot(fitted(M),residuals(M),pch=20)
check.regression(M)
  Tests of Assumptions: ( sample size n = 82 ):
  Linearity
     p-value for Horsepower : 0
```

Technically, this assumption checks the σ component of the requirement that $\varepsilon \sim N(0,\sigma)$. The standard deviation σ of the Normal curve describes how far individuals are away from the average. The model assumes this value does not vary with x or y. If it did vary, then the precision with which predictions are made depends on x.

For example, examine the bottom middle panel of Figure 3.14. The y-values are much closer to the line when $x \approx 500$ than they are when $x \approx -500$, implying that the predictions made by the model are much more precise for larger values of x than for smaller values of x.

To visually check this assumption, scan the residuals plot from left to right and see if the scatter up and down is about the same everywhere (it is in the top panels of Figure 3.14). If the scatter is smaller in some places than in others (like in the bottom middle panel of Figure 3.14), then the relationship is **heteroscedastic** (unequal vertical spread), and any confidence intervals for the slope or for predictions will be incorrect.

The Breusch-Pagan test is a standard test for unequal vertical spread. This test fits a regression model predicting the *squared* residuals of the original regression with x as the predictor variable. If the spread is equal, then this regression should not be statistically significant (the size of the residual has no relationship with x). If the p-value of this test is at least 5%, the test is passed and, statistically, the residuals can be considered to have equal vertical spread.

Consider Figure 3.16. The top panels show the scatterplot and residuals plot for a model predicting 272 eruption times of Old Faithful (`faithful`) from the waiting times between eruptions. The *horizontal* spread is not constant (there are hardly any observations near eruption times of 3.0 or fitted waiting times of 65), but this is never of any concern. The *vertical* spread looks about the same everywhere. Indeed, the p-value of the equal spread (Breusch-Pagan) test is about 95%, implying that, statistically, the vertical spread is the same everywhere.

Contrast this with the bottom panels in Figure 3.16. Here, a scatterplot and residuals plot are presented for a model predicting 309 total domestic movie grosses from their opening-weekend grosses (`MOVIE`). While the relationship looks linear, the vertical spread is clearly not a constant. The variation in residuals is very small for small predicted values and large for big predicted values. The p-value of the Breusch-Pagan test is much less than one in a billion, confirming that, statistically, the relationship does not have equal spread.

The violation is so severe that, even with 309 observations, the regression model does not reflect reality. While the slope still gives an accurate estimate of the difference in total domestic grosses for two movies that differ in opening-weekend gross by one million, confidence intervals for the slope or for predictions will be inaccurate. If we ignore this violation and proceeded normally, we would *overestimate* how far points are from the line at small values of opening-weekend gross and *underestimate* how far points are from the line for larger values of opening-weekend gross.

Normality

The linear regression model assumes that distances of points to the line (i.e., the difference between an individual's value of y and the average value of y) are Normally distributed. This assumption (like equal spread) is secondary to linearity in importance and only comes into play when we want reliable confidence intervals for the slope or for predictions. Even when residuals are not Normal, the point estimate of the slope still provides an accurate estimate of the difference in y values between two individuals who differ in x by one unit.

Figure 3.16 — Assessing the equal spread assumption. To assess the equal spread assumption, look at the *vertical* scatter around the regression line and in the residuals plot. In the top panels, the vertical spread looks to be about the same everywhere, so this assumption holds. The horizontal spread is certainly not the same, and data is concentrated in two clumps. This is just an artifact of the natural distribution of eruption times and *not* of the relationship between x and y.

In the bottom panels, the vertical spread is not constant: small for low values of opening weekend and large for high values of opening weekend. While the value of the slope is still meaningful, confidence intervals for the slope or for predictions are wrong.

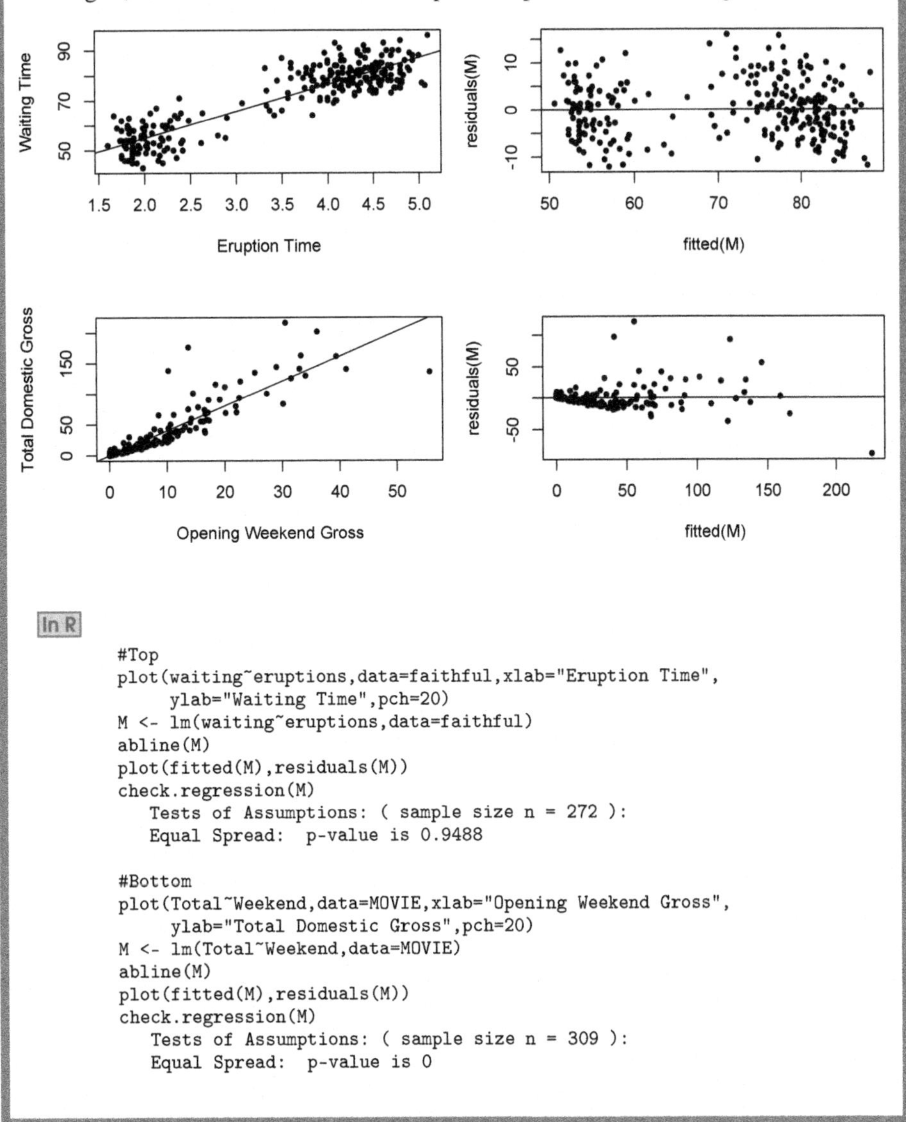


```
#Top
plot(waiting~eruptions,data=faithful,xlab="Eruption Time",
     ylab="Waiting Time",pch=20)
M <- lm(waiting~eruptions,data=faithful)
abline(M)
plot(fitted(M),residuals(M))
check.regression(M)
   Tests of Assumptions: ( sample size n = 272 ):
   Equal Spread:  p-value is 0.9488

#Bottom
plot(Total~Weekend,data=MOVIE,xlab="Opening Weekend Gross",
     ylab="Total Domestic Gross",pch=20)
M <- lm(Total~Weekend,data=MOVIE)
abline(M)
plot(fitted(M),residuals(M))
check.regression(M)
   Tests of Assumptions: ( sample size n = 309 ):
   Equal Spread:  p-value is 0
```

Technically, we should check whether the residuals are Normal at *every* observed value of x in the data. However, this is usually impractical since only a few (if any) observations share a common value for x. Rather, we check this assumption by looking at the distribution of the residuals *as a whole*. Assessing Normality is done by looking at a histogram of residuals in tandem with a **QQ-plot**.

A QQ-plot essentially plots the *observed* values of the residuals vs. the values they *should* have had if they were Normally distributed. When the residuals have a Normal distribution, these two values should match up, and the points should fall on the diagonal line of "perfect agreement." Review Section 2.1.2.

However, just like we don't expect the slope we measure from a regression to exactly equal β_1, we don't expect points to fall *exactly* on the line. Curved vertical bands are drawn on the QQ-plot to give the points some leeway. When points are inside the bands and there is no systematic curvature away from the line, we can consider the distribution to be approximately Normal. See Figure 3.17 for some examples.

If a statistical test is necessary (fewer than a few dozen observations), the Shapiro-Wilk and Kolmogorov-Smirov tests are commonly used. Again, if the test is failed (p-value less than 5%) and you have more than a few dozen data points, check the histogram and QQ-plot to see if the violation is severe enough to invalidate the model.

3.6 Transformations

When the assumptions behind regression are invalid, the model must be abandoned since it does not do a good job reflecting reality. However, there may be a simple "fix" that can be applied that allows us to approach the relationship between x and y in a different manner.

> A key insight is that y and x in a regression model are completely arbitrary values. While they are typically the measured quantities in the data (amounts, weights, etc.), they can be derived quantities, e.g., the logarithm of amount, the square root of weight, or even the product of amount times weight.

For example, it may be the case that the relationship between y and x is nonlinear while the relationship between the quantity y^2 and the quantity $1/x$ is linear. In this case, a "linear" regression would look like

$$y_i^2 = \beta_0 + \beta_1(1/x_i) + \varepsilon_i$$

The technique of using quantities derived from those that were originally measured is called **transformation of variables**. What is used as inputs to the regression model is very flexible.

In fact, we have already employed this trick when studying the relationship between the tip percentage and bill amount at a restaurant (`TIPS` data). The waiter at the restaurant did not record the percentage of the bill left as a tip and instead only wrote down the bill and tip amounts. The tip percentage is $100 \times Tip/Bill$, and it has been used as the y variable previously in this chapter.

Figure 3.17 — Histogram of residuals and QQ-plot. The top panels display a histogram and QQ-plot of residuals to a model predicting self-assessed intelligence from self-assessed attractiveness (see Figure 3.15, which uses the SURVEY10 data). While the histogram may not look all that Normal, the points in the QQ-plot fall close to the diagonal line and stay within the bands with no obvious curvature. Indeed, the p-value of the test of Normality is 61%, so the assumption is met.

The bottom panels display a histogram and QQ-plot of residuals to a model predicting the amount someone donates to a charity from the length of time since his or her last donation (see Figure 3.13, which uses the DONOR data). The histogram looks quite non-Normal, and there is obvious curvature away from the line in the QQ-plot. The violation of Normality is severe, and the regression model is not appropriate.

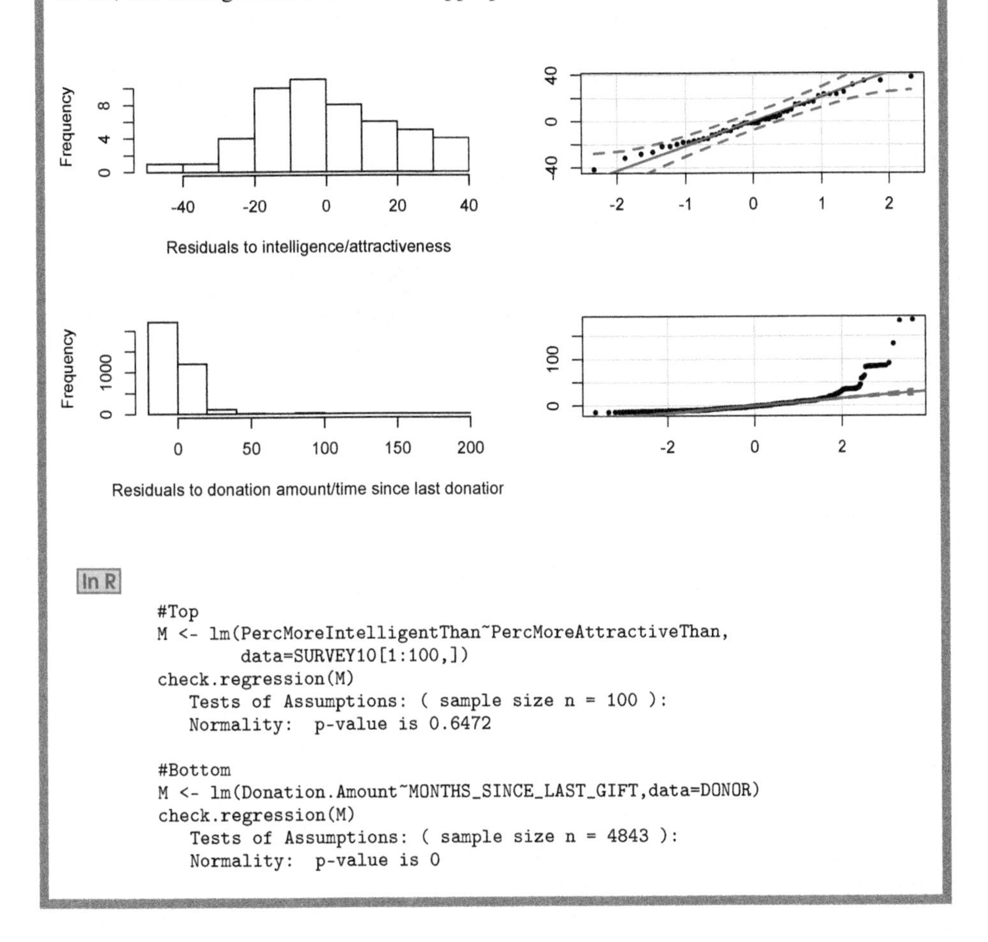

In R

```
#Top
M <- lm(PercMoreIntelligentThan~PercMoreAttractiveThan,
        data=SURVEY10[1:100,])
check.regression(M)
   Tests of Assumptions: ( sample size n = 100 ):
   Normality:  p-value is 0.6472

#Bottom
M <- lm(Donation.Amount~MONTHS_SINCE_LAST_GIFT,data=DONOR)
check.regression(M)
   Tests of Assumptions: ( sample size n = 4843 ):
   Normality:  p-value is 0
```

Consider Figure 3.18. The scatterplot clearly shows that a linear regression is not appropriate for modeling the relationship between x and y—the stream of points is curved and there is unequal vertical spread. However, the relationship between the quantities $1/x$ and y^2 looks quite linear. Indeed, the residuals plot of a regression predicting the quantity y^2 from the quantity $1/x$ looks great—no curvature and the vertical spread is about the same everywhere.

Figure 3.18 — Fixing a regression using transformations of variables. The relationship between x and y is nonlinear and has unequal vertical spread. However, the regression framework does not care *what* we consider to be x and y, and it turns out that the relationship between the quantities y' and x' is linear if we take $y' = y^2$ and $x' = 1/x$. The residuals plot for the regression using the transformed variables looks great. There are more values on the left than on the right (unequal horizontal spread). However, recall that this is not a violation of the assumptions and is just an artifact of the natural distribution of the predictor variable.

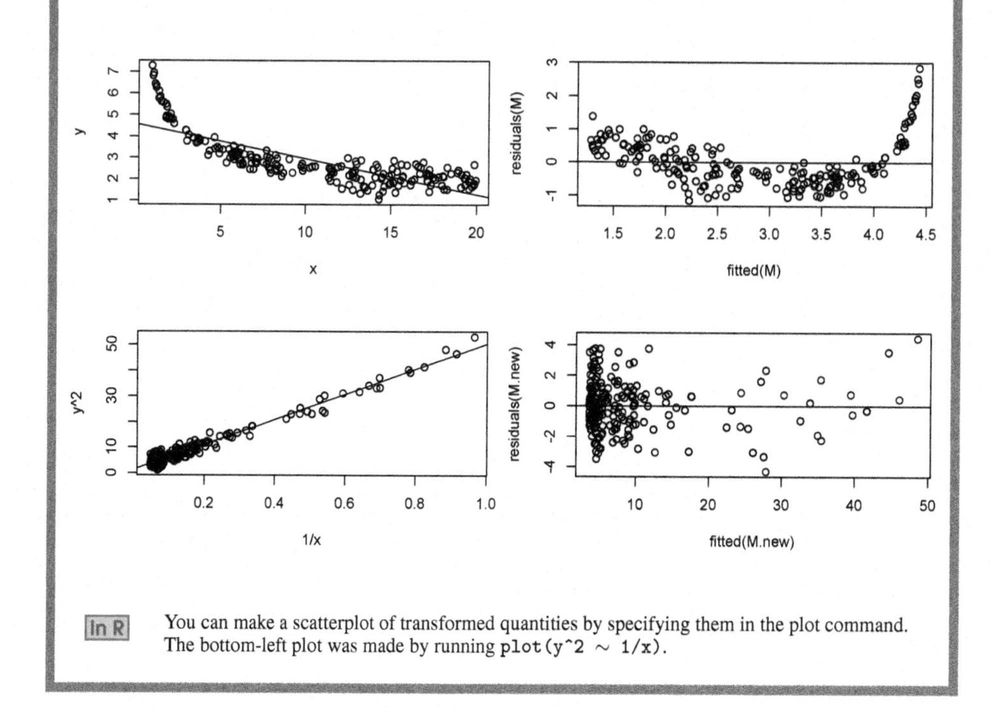

In R: You can make a scatterplot of transformed quantities by specifying them in the plot command. The bottom-left plot was made by running `plot(y^2 ~ 1/x)`.

Strategy

If the relationship between x and y cannot be modeled with a linear regression, what (if any) transformations can?

> Our strategy will be to consider *all* simple transformations of x and y (basically raising them to some power) and picking the one whose resulting R^2 is largest. If this transformation looks appropriate, we select it. If not, we can consider the second best, etc.

Specifically, let us consider taking $y^{-3}, y^{-2.75}, y^{-2.5}, \ldots, y^{2.75}, y^{3.0}$ and the same transformations for x. However, we will use $\ln y$ (the natural logarithm) instead of y^0 (which would equal 1 regardless of the value of y).

For example, let us try to fix the regression predicting fuel efficiency from horsepower (originally seen in Figure 3.15) in the `AUTO` dataset. What follows is a table of attempted transformations and the R^2 of the resulting models.

In R

```
M <- lm(FuelEfficiency~Horsepower,data=AUTO)
find.transformations(M)

  y is FuelEfficiency
  x is Horsepower
  No transformation yields rsquared of 0.624

   x.power y.power rsquared
   -0.75     0.5    0.847
    -0.5    0.25    0.847
   -0.75    0.75    0.846
    -0.5     0.5    0.846
      -1    0.75    0.844
      -1       1    0.843
   -0.25   log10    0.843
```

In this case, it looks like the best way to model the data is by raising `FuelEfficiency` to the 0.5 power and `Horsepower` to the -0.75 power (or `FuelEfficiency` to the 0.25 power and `Horsepower` to the -0.5 power) since this gives us the largest value of R^2. The model becomes:

$$(FuelEfficiency)^{\frac{1}{2}} = \beta_0 + \beta_1 \cdot \frac{1}{Horsepower^{3/4}}$$

Figure 3.19 shows that these transformations seem to work. The stream of points now looks linear, and the residuals plot has no obvious patterns. With a little algebra, we can rewrite the equation as:

$$FuelEfficiency = \left(\beta_0 + \beta_1 \cdot \frac{1}{Horsepower^{3/4}}\right)^2$$

Although this equation is that of a (quite sophisticated) curve, we can still estimate the coefficients β_0 and β_1 using a linear regression by taking y to be $FuelEfficiency^{0.5}$ and x to be $Horsepower^{-0.75}$. Linear regression is indeed a very powerful framework that actually allows us to fit *curves* to relationships!

Figure 3.20 shows transformations for the `MOVIE` dataset (which was plagued by unequal vertical spread). By the numbers, the transformations look promising—the highest R^2 is 99.6%! However, this transformation is unacceptable because of extreme outliers induced by the transformations. In this case, some of the original values are close to zero (e.g., 0.001). The transformations that yield the highest R^2 take the values and raise them to the -3 power. This converts a 0.001 into a 10^9.

log-log transformation

One very common and useful "fix" for nonlinearity and/or unequal vertical spread is the log-log transformation. Here, the natural (or base 10) logarithms of the original values are used as x and y. Figure 3.21 shows the log-log transformation on the `AUTO` and `MOVIE` datasets. This transformation seems to work well when predicting fuel efficiency from horsepower, but there are still issues with unequal vertical spread when predicting the total gross of a movie based on its opening-weekend performance.

Figure 3.19 — The "fixed" regressions after transformation for `AUTO` **data.** Instead of considering x and y themselves, we pick the transformation of x and of y whose resulting R^2 is biggest. This fixes the nonlinearity present in the original relationship between horsepower and fuel efficiency.

The relationship between cars' horsepowers and fuel efficiencies is nonlinear (top-left plot). We see that many transformations of these variables yield relationships that are linear with roughly equal vertical spread.

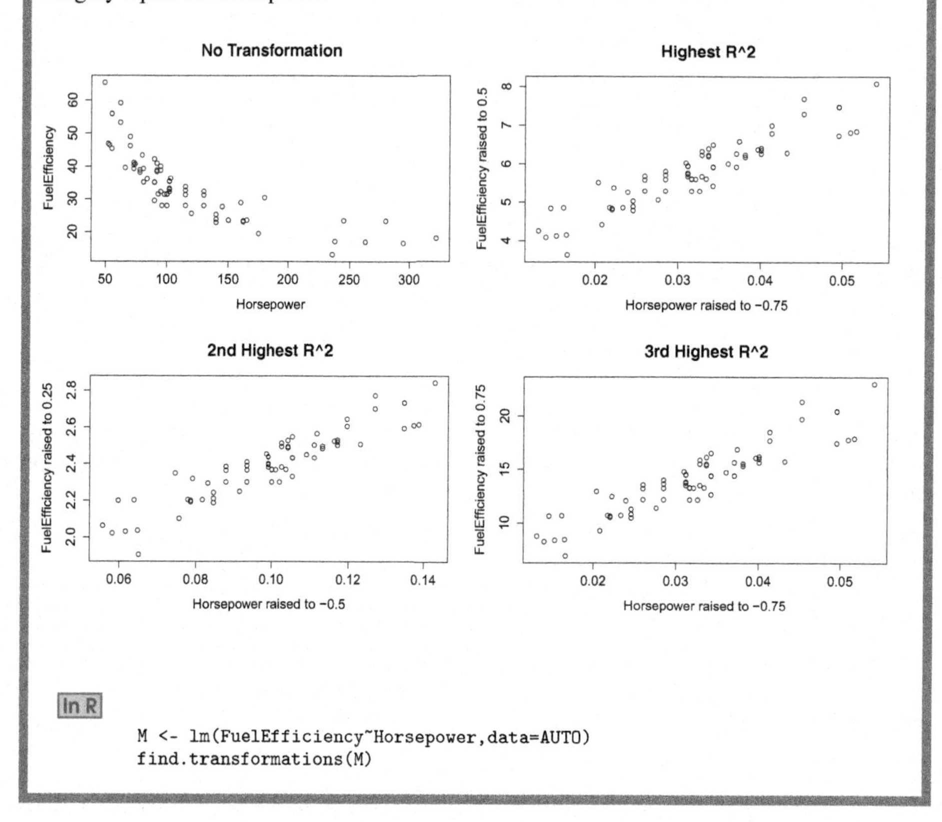


```
M <- lm(FuelEfficiency~Horsepower,data=AUTO)
find.transformations(M)
```

One appealing property of the log-log transformation is that it essentially fits a **power-law** curve to the stream of points.

$$\log_{10} y = \beta_0 + \beta_1 \log_{10} x \rightarrow y = c \times x^{\beta_1} \tag{3.9}$$

In the equation, c is just a number that depends on b_0. Thus, the log-log transformation has y vary with the β_1 power of x. In the fuel efficiency dataset, we find that $\ln(FuelEfficiency) = 2.9 - 0.67\ln(Horsepower)$, implying that the fuel efficiency of a car is proportional to its horsepower raised to the $-2/3$ power.

Figure 3.20 — The "fixed" regressions after transformation for `MOVIE` data. The three transformations with the highest R^2 do not yield relationships that are well-modeled by a linear regression. In this case, some values of opening and total gross are very small, near 0.001. Taking 0.001 and raising it to the -3 power yields 10^9, thereby creating outliers. Better (though not ideal) transformations here are to take logarithms or square roots of both quantities (a common thing to do for business-related datasets), which can be seen in the bottom panels.

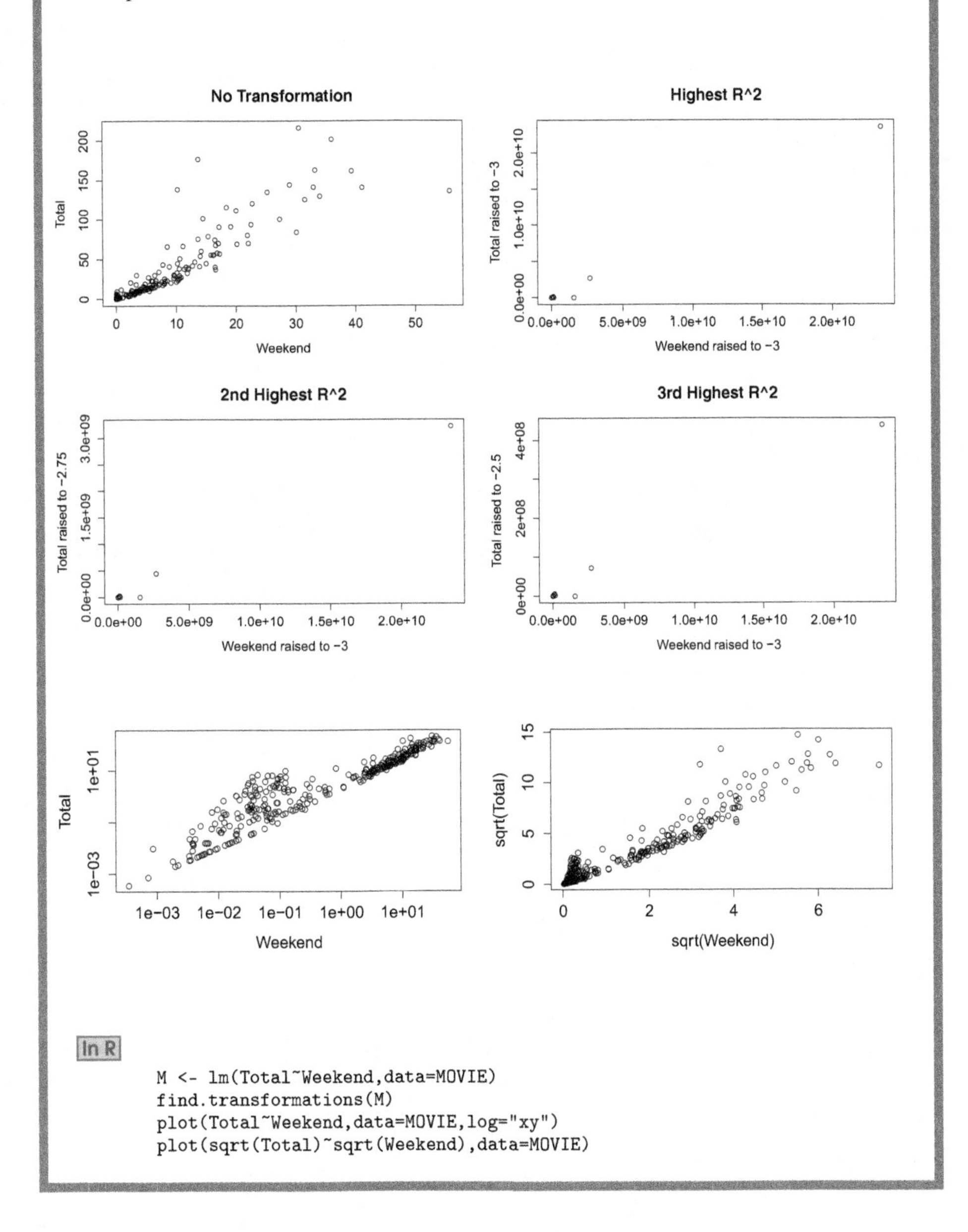


```
M <- lm(Total~Weekend,data=MOVIE)
find.transformations(M)
plot(Total~Weekend,data=MOVIE,log="xy")
plot(sqrt(Total)~sqrt(Weekend),data=MOVIE)
```

Figure 3.21 — The log-log transformation. The relationship between the logarithm of `Horsepower` and the logarithm of `Fuel Efficiency` is quite linear, and the scatterplot shows no issues (no curvature and equal vertical spread). The relationship between the logarithm of opening-weekend gross and the logarithm of total domestic gross is linear but still has issues with unequal vertical spread. It may be wise to model movies with high and low grosses separately.

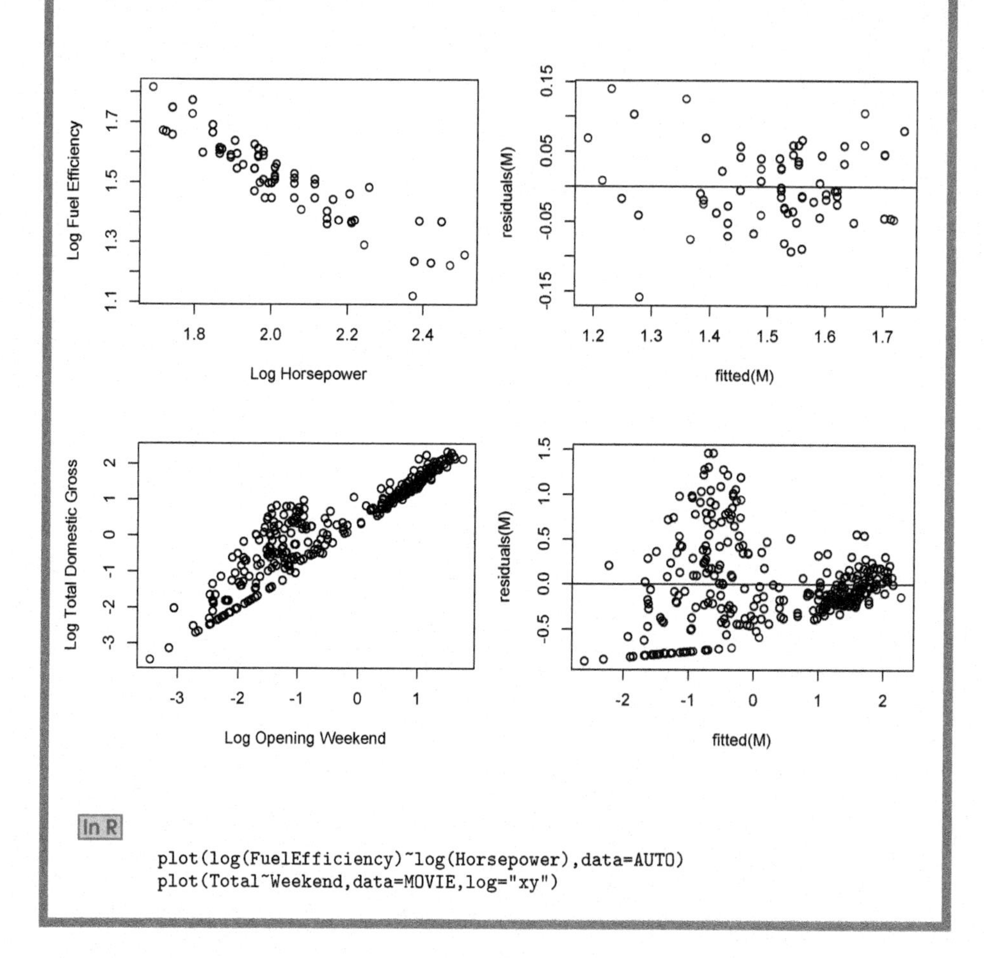


```
plot(log(FuelEfficiency)~log(Horsepower),data=AUTO)
plot(Total~Weekend,data=MOVIE,log="xy")
```

Comments and advice

The coefficients of a regression using transformed variables are typically of little importance (is the expected difference in $y^{0.25}$ between individuals who differ in $1/x^2$ by one unit interesting?). Instead, we look at the *powers* of the optimal transformation. Often, we "untransform" the regression equation so that we can write $y = \ldots$ (some function of x).

For example

$$y^{0.5} = \beta_0 + \beta_1 x^2 \longrightarrow y = (\beta_0 + \beta_1 x^2)^2$$

We *could* expand this out further, but since it looks simple in this form we will leave it as is and just say that the relationship is a fourth-order polynomial. For another example:

$$y^{-1} = \beta_0 + \beta_1 x^{-1} \longrightarrow y = \frac{1}{\beta_0 + \beta_1 x^{-1}} = \frac{x}{\beta_1 + \beta_0 x}$$

Finally, when hunting for a good transformation, there will often be *many* models that have R^2 very close to each other. Any transformations with R^2 within a few fractions of a percent are essentially equivalent, and any of them would be a valid selection (as long as outliers have not been induced by the transformation). One rule of thumb is to treat all models whose values of R^2 (between 0 and 1) are within 0.005 as valid and to pick your favorite (perhaps the one that is easiest to work with mathematically).

3.7 Predictions

The main goal of a descriptive model is to estimate the coefficients of the predictors with as much precision as possible and to mathematically describe the relationship between x and y. However, the model can also be used to predict values of y at new values of x.

Making a prediction is as easy as plugging a value for x into the regression equation and evaluating the result.

$$\hat{y} = b_0 + b_1 x \tag{3.10}$$

To make it clear that a prediction is being made, the symbol $\hat{y}$ (pronounced y-hat) is used. The predicted value $\hat{y}$ is a **point estimate**, i.e., the best guess of what y will be.

For example, imagine predicting a product's sales from its amount of advertising. It is found that $b_0 = 12.3$ and $b_1 = 0.5$. If we want to predict sales when advertising is 10, then our point estimate is $\hat{y} = b_0 + b_1 x = 12.3 + 0.5(10) = 17.3$.

Since the estimated coefficients of the regression are likely off from "the truth," there is some amount of uncertainty regarding the predictions. Once the standard errors of the coefficients of the model are known, the standard errors of predictions can also be calculated. However, to quantify the amount of uncertainty in a prediction, it is necessary to specify exactly *what* is trying to be predicted.

- Do we want to predict the *average* value of y at some value of x ($\mu_{y|x}$)? For example, what will be the average college GPA among all graduating high school students who have a GPA of 3.2? What is the average salary among all new employees with seven years of experience?
- Do we want to predict an *individual's* value of y given he or she has a particular value of x? For example, what will Jane's college GPA be given she has a high school GPA of 3.2? What will Kelly's salary be given that he has one year of experience?

While the point estimate of y is the *same* regardless of whether we are predicting the average or an individual's value of y, the amount of uncertainty is not. The precision of a individual's predicted value is smaller than the precision of the predicted average because, even if the average was known exactly, an individual deviates from the average by a random amount.

To find confidence and prediction intervals, the assumptions behind the linear regression must hold, i.e., $\varepsilon \sim N(0, \sigma)$. In other words, the relationship between the average value of y and x must be linear, the distribution of residuals (i.e., how far individuals deviate from the line) must be Normal, and the vertical spread of the residuals must be the same regardless of where the prediction is being made.

3.7.1 Predicting average values

First, let us focus on the $\mu_{y|x}$, the *average* value of y among all individuals who share some common value of x. For example, what is the average donation amount among all individuals whose household incomes are \$100,000?

The value of $\hat{y}$ obtained from plugging x into Equation 3.10 is our point estimate for $\mu_{y|x}$, the "true" average value of y at that value of x. When all assumptions of the regression model hold, $\hat{y}$ is a predictable distance from $\mu_{y|x}$. Let us run a simulation to illustrate this point.

Imagine "the truth" is that $y_i = 3 + 5x_i + \varepsilon_i$, $\varepsilon_i \sim N(0, 2)$. When $x = 1$, we have that $\mu_{y|x} = 8$, and at $x = 4$, we have that $\mu_{y|x} = 23$. Imagine we create a dataset where five observations are collected at each $x = 1, 2, \ldots, 10$ (so the sample size is $n = 50$). Using the estimated regression equations from each sample, let us predict $\hat{y}$ at $x = 1$ and again at $x = 4$. Figure 3.22 shows the distribution of the values of $\hat{y}$ over 10,000 rounds of this procedure.

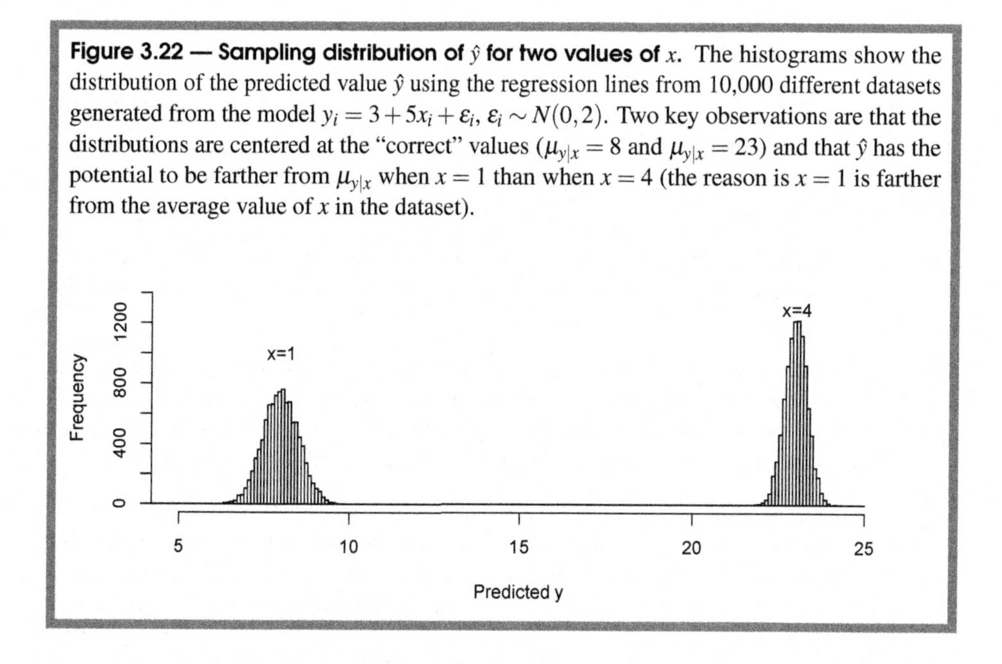

Figure 3.22 — Sampling distribution of $\hat{y}$ for two values of x. The histograms show the distribution of the predicted value $\hat{y}$ using the regression lines from 10,000 different datasets generated from the model $y_i = 3 + 5x_i + \varepsilon_i$, $\varepsilon_i \sim N(0, 2)$. Two key observations are that the distributions are centered at the "correct" values ($\mu_{y|x} = 8$ and $\mu_{y|x} = 23$) and that $\hat{y}$ has the potential to be farther from $\mu_{y|x}$ when $x = 1$ than when $x = 4$ (the reason is $x = 1$ is farther from the average value of x in the dataset).

The distributions are centered at the true values of $\mu_{y|x}$, which is good news. Interestingly, the amount by which the predicted values differ from the truth depends on the value of x where predictions are being made. In this example, the predicted values at $x = 4$ are more tightly packed around $\mu_{y|x} = 27$ than the predicted values at $x = 1$ are around $\mu_{y|x} = 8$.

In general, predictions made at values of x that are close to $\bar{x}$ (the average value of x in the data used to build the model) have less uncertainty than predictions made at values of x that are far from $\bar{x}$. In other words, the standard error of the predicted value increases as the difference $x - \bar{x}$ grows in magnitude.

This peculiar fact is reflected in the formula for the standard error of $\hat{y}$ (the predicted average value of y among all individuals who share some common value of x):

$$SE_{\hat{y}} = RMSE\sqrt{\frac{1}{n} + \frac{(x-\bar{x})^2}{(n-1)SD_x^2}} \tag{3.11}$$

C Remember the **standard error** of a quantity is the typical difference between what is measured from a dataset and "the truth."

The quantity $(x-\bar{x})^2$ gets larger as x is increasingly further away from its average. This is the reason that the standard error and amount of uncertainty grows when making predictions at values of x progressively farther from its average. The formula also shows that as the sample size n gets larger, the amount of uncertainty gets smaller.

Finally, the formula has an implication for experimental design, i.e., how to collect data. The standard error gets *smaller* as the standard deviation of the x-values *increases*. Thus, to minimize the amount of uncertainty when making predictions, try collecting data at values of x that are as spread out as possible. A similar observation was found regarding the precision of the slope in Equation 3.8.

So why should the uncertainty about the predicted average value depend on the difference between x and $\bar{x}$? To illustrate, let us run another simulation. Take "the truth" to be that $y_i = 3 + 5x_i + \varepsilon_i$, $\varepsilon_i \sim N(0,2)$. Let us create a dataset by generating a single y-value at each $x = 3, 4, \ldots, 7$ using the model. Figure 3.23 shows the estimated regression lines from 100 different samples using this scheme.

Since the regression line itself *is* the predicted average value for y, the spread in the possible lines reflects the amount of uncertainty regarding the predicted average value. Near $\bar{x} = 5$, the lines are fairly close together. At values of x farther from 5, the lines diverge more and more. Consequently, the standard error and amount of uncertainty regarding the predicted average value is larger when making a prediction at an x farther from $\bar{x}$.

The standard error can be used to make a 95% confidence interval for $\mu_{y|x}$ in a similar manner to making a 95% confidence interval for β_1 (see Section 3.3.2).

An approximate 95% confidence interval for $\mu_{y|x}$, the average value of y among all individuals with a common value x, is:

$$\hat{y} \pm 2 \times SE_{\hat{y}} \tag{3.12}$$

The number in front of $SE_{\hat{y}}$ (which is always calculated by software) may be a little smaller or larger than 2 depending on the sample size.

Figure 3.23 — Uncertainties when predicting averages. Each sample has $x = 3, 4, \ldots, 7$ so that $\bar{x} = 5$. Looking at the regression lines from 100 different random samples, we see that most of the lines are fairly close to each other around $x = 5$. The farther away we look from $\bar{x}$, the more the lines diverge from each other. The uncertainty in where the "true line" falls (and thus in the average value of y) increases the further we look from $\bar{x}$.

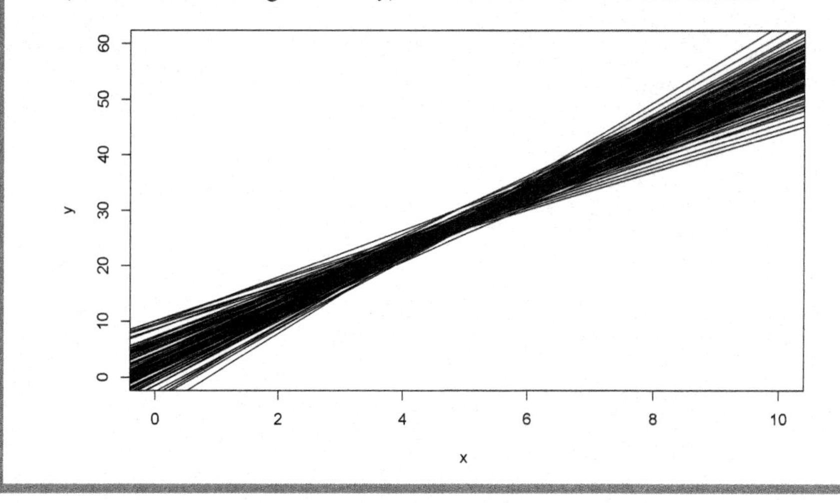

The interpretation of the confidence interval is: "We are about 95% confident that the average value of y among all individuals with the common value of x is between ________ and ________," where the blanks represent the lower and upper limits of the confidence interval.

Aside 3.1 — Example confidence interval for $\mu_{y|x}$. Imagine we want to predict the average tip percentage on a \$20 and \$40 ticket based on the TIPS dataset. The regression equation is

$$TipPercentage = 20.68 - 0.23Bill$$

- The point estimate at $x = 20$ is $20.68 - 0.23 \times 20 = 16.0$
- The point estimate at $x = 40$ is $20.68 - 0.23 \times 40 = 11.4$

By plugging numbers into the formula for the standard error (the RMSE is 5.8, $n = 244$, $\bar{x} = 19.79$, and $SD = 8.9$) or by using software, it is found that $SE_{\hat{y}} = 0.369$ when $x = 20$ and $SE_{\hat{y}} = 0.916$ when $x = 40$. Not surprisingly, the latter is bigger since $x = 40$ is much farther from $\bar{x}$ than $x = 20$ (the average tip percentage in the data is 16%).

An approximate 95% confidence interval for $\mu_{y|x}$ for \$20 tickets is

$$16.0 \pm (2 \times 0.369) = 16.0 \pm 0.7$$
$$(15.3, 16.7)$$

We are thus about 95% confident that the average tip percentage when the bill is \$20 is between 15.3% and 16.7%. Following similar calculations, we find the approximate 95% confidence interval at $x = 40$ is 11.4 ± 1.8.

3.7.2 Predicting individual values

Quite often, predicting an individual's value of y is more interesting than predicting the average. What will *your* neighbor donate to a charity if her income is $100,000? What will *your* salary be if you have six years of education?

Once again, when all assumptions of the regression model hold, the predicted value for an individual (let us call this y_p) is obtained from plugging x into the regression equation (Equation 3.10). This value will be a predictable amount away from that individual's actual value. The standard error gives the typical difference between the predicted and actual values.

$$SE_{y_p} = RMSE\sqrt{1+\frac{1}{n}+\frac{(x-\bar{x})^2}{(n-1)SD_x^2}} \tag{3.13}$$

The equation for the standard error looks very much like Equation 3.11, except there is an additional "1 +" under the square root sign, implying that the standard error is *always larger* when predicting an *individual's value* when compared to predicting the *average value.*

A larger value for the standard error is logical since there are *two* sources of uncertainty regarding an individual's value of y—the uncertainty about $\mu_{y|x}$, the average value of y, plus the *additional* uncertainty of how far away the individual will be from the average. Even if we *knew* $\mu_{y|x}$, the individual will differ from the average by an unknown, random amount.

> An approximate 95% prediction interval for an individual's value of y is
>
> $$y_p \pm 2 \times SE_{y_p} \tag{3.14}$$
>
> Again, the number in front of SE_{y_p} will be either a little smaller or larger than 2 depending on the sample size.

The prediction interval is interpreted by saying: "There is about a 95% chance that the individual's y-value will be between _______ and _______," where the blanks represent the lower and upper limits of the prediction interval.

> **Aside 3.2 — Example prediction interval.** Let us revisit the `TIPS` data. Imagine you are a server and your table has a bill of $20. What do you predict *your* tip percentage to be, and what is the approximate 95% prediction interval?
>
> - The point estimate is $y_p = 20.68 - 0.23Bill = 20.68 - 0.23 \times 20 = 16.0$ (same as the point estimate for the average).
> - The standard error is 5.77 (found either through software or plugging the relevant quantities into Equation 3.14.
>
> $$16.0 \pm (2 \times 5.77)$$
>
> $$(4.7, 27.4)$$
>
> There is about a 95% chance the tip percentage will be between about 5 and 27%. This interval is *much* wider than the 95% confidence interval for the average (15.3 to 16.7). Because tip percentages are highly variable at a given bill amount, there is a lot of uncertainty about just how far your tip percentage will be from average.

Figure 3.24 displays the confidence interval for the average value of y and the prediction interval for an individual's value of y for the `TIPS` dataset and illustrates the larger uncertainty for individual vs. average values. The confidence bands are fairly narrow. By design, the prediction intervals need to encompass 95% of the data points, so the prediction bands are understandably quite wide.

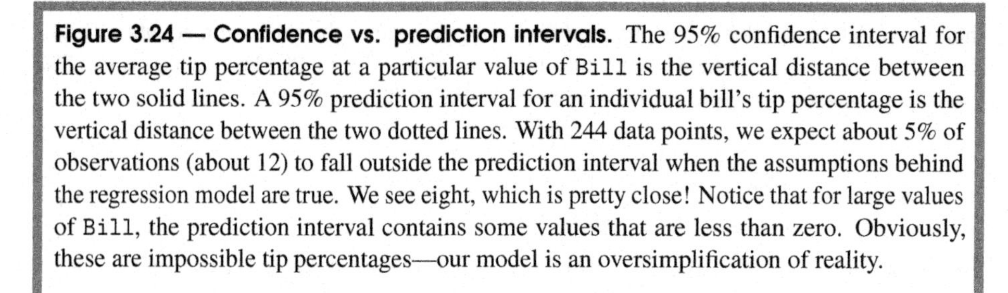

Figure 3.24 — Confidence vs. prediction intervals. The 95% confidence interval for the average tip percentage at a particular value of `Bill` is the vertical distance between the two solid lines. A 95% prediction interval for an individual bill's tip percentage is the vertical distance between the two dotted lines. With 244 data points, we expect about 5% of observations (about 12) to fall outside the prediction interval when the assumptions behind the regression model are true. We see eight, which is pretty close! Notice that for large values of `Bill`, the prediction interval contains some values that are less than zero. Obviously, these are impossible tip percentages—our model is an oversimplification of reality.

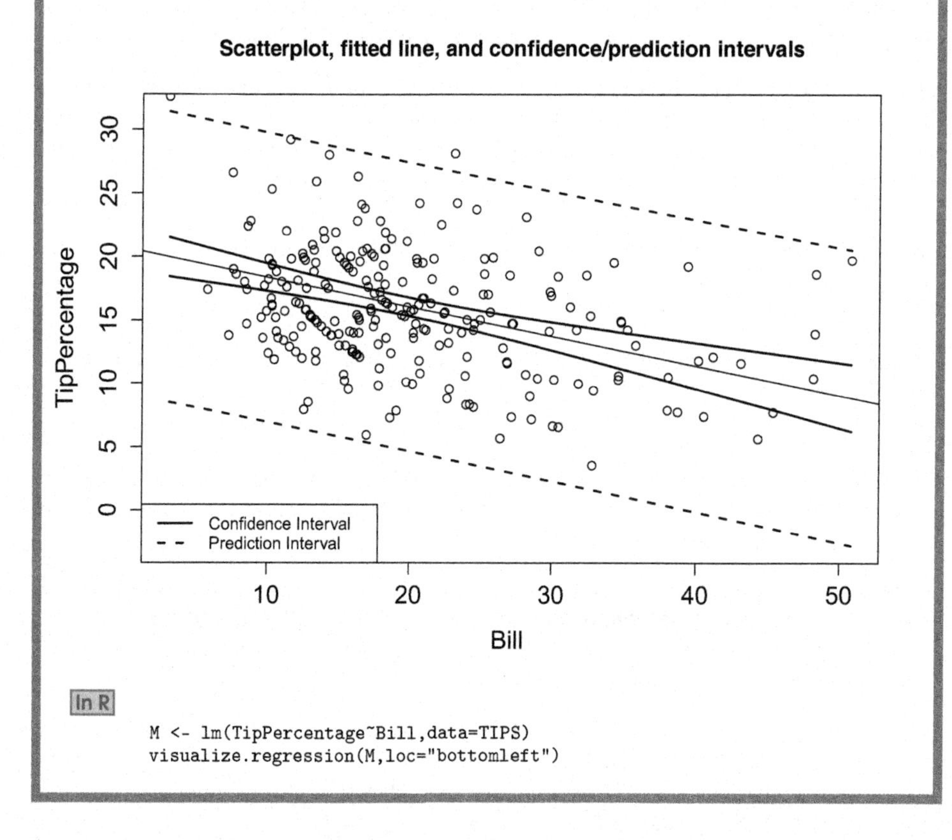

In R

```
M <- lm(TipPercentage~Bill,data=TIPS)
visualize.regression(M,loc="bottomleft")
```

As expected, the amount of uncertainty increases for predictions that are farther away from the average bill size of about $20. In fact, for bill sizes of about $40, the uncertainty is so large that negative values are included in the prediction interval. These values are impossible and imply that the model "breaks down" for large bill sizes—it doesn't take into consideration that the minimum possible tip percentage is 0. As the mantra goes: all models are wrong, some are useful!

3.7.3 Confidence vs. prediction intervals

You may have noticed that the term "confidence interval" is used regarding inferences about an average. The term "prediction interval" is used when inferring an individual's y-value. The interpretations of these two intervals are fundamentally different.

The average value of y among all individuals who share a common value of x is $\mu_{y|x}$. This quantity is unknown to us, but it does represent a *fixed* number. If we "knew" the value, every time we collected data and checked its value, it would be the same number.

The confidence interval for $\mu_{y|x}$ itself is a *random* quantity because it depends on the specific values in the data that was collected. If a new set of data was obtained, the confidence interval would most surely be different. Thus, the uncertainty in a 95% confidence interval refers to the interval itself, not to $\mu_{y|x}$. The "confidence" in "confidence interval" refers to the probability that the *procedure* building the interval gets it right. In the long-run, 95% of 95% confidence intervals are correct and contain $\mu_{y|x}$, we just don't know which ones.

An individual's value of y at some value of x, by definition, *is* a random quantity: $y_i = \beta_0 + \beta_1 x_i + \varepsilon_i$. Since y_i is random, it is acceptable to talk about the *probability* that it will be inside an interval (if we check another individual, the actual y-value may or may not be in the interval). Revisiting Section 3.3.1 and Figure 3.11 (which discuss confidence intervals for the slope, the *average* difference in y for individuals who differ in x by one unit) may be quite useful in illustrating these concepts.

3.7.4 Extrapolation

Regression models have limits, and extrapolation occurs when we try to make predictions outside these limits.

> Extrapolation occurs when we predict y at a value of x that is outside the range of x-values used to build the model. This is dangerous because there is no guarantee the model will still be valid at values of x that have not been seen.

For example, consider a person's weight over the course of a multi-week, rigorous diet and exercise regimen. Figure 3.25 shows the weight recorded each day for the first 35 days on the left (along with the regression line and 95% prediction intervals) and a comparison of extrapolated and actual values after 90 days.

The recorded weights in the first 35 days are very well-modeled by a linear regression. However, the model should not be used to predict what the weight will be too far beyond day 35 because there is no guarantee that the linear trend will continue. Indeed, the right panel in Figure 3.25 compares the predictions of the model on days 90-120 with the actual weights. The prediction intervals get it wrong because the fundamental nature of the relationship between weight and time changed at some point beyond day 35. Intuitively, we know that weight loss can't continue indefinitely. At some point, the individual's weight is going to level out (hopefully at the goal weight). Our model is not psychic and won't be able to predict where this happens!

Figure 3.25 — Extrapolation. In the first 35 days of an exercise and diet regimen (left), the weight steadily decreased by about 0.37 pounds per day (DIET data). The behavior looks to be well-modeled by a linear regression, but the weight loss cannot be assumed to continue indefinitely into the future. Imagine trying to extrapolate what the weight will be 90-120 days after the diet has started. On the right, the regression line is extended to these values along with the prediction intervals, but there is a mismatch between what is predicted and what actually happened (at some point, the weight levels out at around 135). Extrapolation is dangerous because it assumes the model and trend will continue at values of x that have not been seen before. This may not be the case!

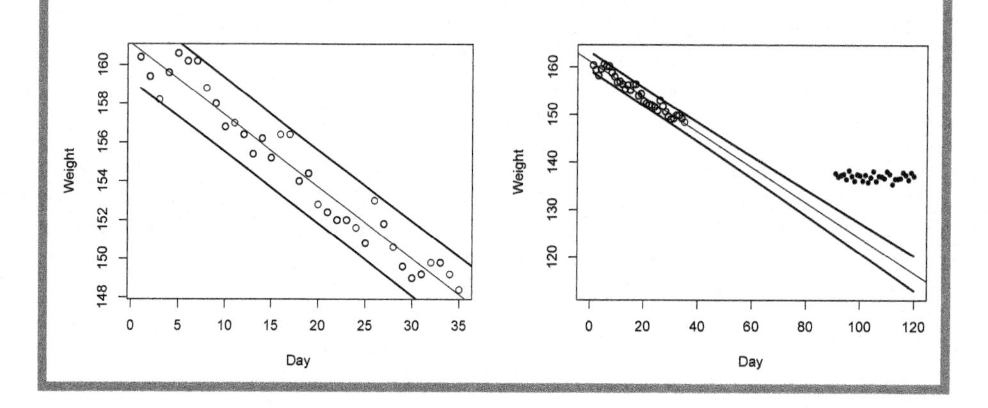

3.8 Simple linear regression using R

For the sake of discussion, imagine the data frame that contains the data is DATA and that the y and x variables are named y and x, respectively.

Plotting

Always begin by making a scatterplot

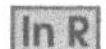

```
plot(y~x,data=DATA,xlim=c(lower,upper),ylim=c(lower,upper),pch=20,cex=1)
```

- `xlim` and `ylim` are optional arguments used to change the range of values displayed on the x and y axes. If the default values are unsatisfactory, you can add the `xlim` and/or `ylim` arguments and replace `lower` and `upper` with the desired values.
- `pch` is an optional argument that controls the type of point. By default, points are open circles. Adding the argument `pch=20` makes the points filled circles. The numbers 1-20 all give different-looking points.
- `cex` is an optional argument that controls the size of the points. Numbers smaller than 1 shrink the point size, and numbers larger than 1 make the points larger.

Note: it is possible to plot transformations of the original variables. For powers of x, surround the transformation with `I()`.

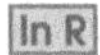

```
plot(sqrt(y)~log10(x),data=DATA)
plot(y^0.3~I(x0.2),data=DATA)
```

Fitting the model

There are many ways to fit a simple linear regression in R, but the standard is to use the `lm()` command (which stands for linear model). It is customary to name the model before using it. By convention, M (perhaps followed by a period and short description) is used in this work.

In R

```
M <- lm(y~x,data=DATA)
```

Note: as with plotting, it is possible to use transformations of variables. If x is being raised to a power, it must be surrounded by `I()`.

In R

```
M.logs <- lm(log(y)~log(x),data=DATA)
M.powers <- lm(y^0.3~sqrt(x),data=DATA)
M <- lm(1/y~I(x^(.2)),data=DATA)
M <- lm(y~I(1/x),data=DATA)
```

Numerical output and summary of the model

To obtain b_0, b_1, R^2, the RMSE, and the p-value of the regression, run `summary()` on the model.

In R

```
M <- lm(TipPercentage~Bill,data=TIPS)
summary(M)
Call:
lm(formula = TipPercentage ~ Bill, data = TIPS)

Residuals:
    Min      1Q  Median      3Q     Max
-10.791  -3.316  -0.314   2.449  52.005

Coefficients:
            Estimate Std. Error t value Pr(>|t|)
(Intercept)  20.6807     0.9000  22.979  < 2e-16 ***
Bill         -0.2325     0.0415  -5.602 5.74e-08 ***
---
Signif. codes:  0 '***' 0.001 '**' 0.01 '*' 0.05 '.' 0.1 ' ' 1

Residual standard error: 5.758 on 242 degrees of freedom
Multiple R-squared:  0.1148,Adjusted R-squared:  0.1111
F-statistic: 31.38 on 1 and 242 DF,  p-value: 5.743e-08
```

- The intercept of the line b_0 is the value located in the row (Intercept) under the column heading Estimate. In this example, the intercept is 20.68.
- The slope b_1 is the value located in the row named after the predictor variable x (in this case Bill) under the column heading Estimate. In this example, the slope is -0.2325.
- The standard error of the slope SE_{b_1} is the value located in the row named after the predictor variable x (in this case Bill) under the column heading Std. Error.
- R^2 is referred to as the Multiple R-squared, and in this example it is 11.48%.
- The root mean squared error (RMSE) is referred to as the Residual standard error, and in this example it is 5.758 (the number in front of the "degrees of freedom" reveals the effective number of observations used to estimate the typical size of the residual).
- The p-value of the regression is the last number of the output located after p-value. In this case it is 5.743×10^{-8}.

Visualizing and checking assumptions of the model

None of the numerical outputs of a regression model are meaningful unless the model provides a reasonable reflection of reality.

In package regclass, the command visualize.model(M) provides a scatterplot with fitted line, confidence, and prediction intervals, while the command check.regression(M) provides the residuals plot, histogram and QQ-plot of residuals, and statistical tests of assumptions.

In R

```
#See regression line, confidence, and prediction intervals
visualize.model(M)

#See diagnostics plots and statistical tests of assumptions
check.regression(M)
Tests of Assumptions: ( sample size n = 352 ):
Linearity
   p-value for FumblesLost : 0.8575
   p-value for overall model : 0.8575
Equal Spread:  p-value is 0.0231
Normality:  p-value is 0.0425
```

In the above example, the model M is for predicting Wins from FumblesLost in the FUMBLES dataset. We see that the model passes the test for linearity but fails tests for equal spread and Normality. However, since the sample size is large, $n = 352$, a visual examination of the diagnostics plots will let us know if violations are small and inconsequential.

In the standard installation of R, it is possible to make a few of these plots by using the commands residuals(M) and fitted(M) to get the residuals and fitted (predicted) values for the model.

In R

```
#See regression line
plot(y~x,data=DATA)
M <- lm(y~x,data=DATA)
abline(M)

#See some diagnostic plots
plot(fitted(M),residuals(M))
hist(residuals(M))
```

Confidence intervals for the slope

A 95% confidence interval for the slope is roughly $b_1 \pm 2SE_{b_1}$. For this and other levels of confidence, it is possible to use the `confint(M,level=)` command. For example, here is a 98% confidence interval for the coefficient of `Bill` when predicting `TipPercentage`.

In R

```
M <- lm(TipPercentage~Bill,data=TIPS)
confint(M,level=0.98)
                   1 %        99 %
(Intercept) 18.5730413 22.7883141
Bill        -0.3296338 -0.1352829
```

The confidence interval for the slope is the range between the two numbers in the row labeled after the x variable. In this case, we are 98% confident that β_1 is between $(-0.330, -0.135)$. Note: the *difference* in the percentages given in the column names reveals the level of confidence associated with the interval. In this example, 99% - 1% = 98%.

Predictions

Making predictions for a regression model can take a bit of work. First, a data frame containing the values of x for which predictions are to be made must be constructed (or read in from a file). For illustration, let us call the new data frame `TO.PREDICT`.

In R

```
TO.PREDICT <- data.frame(x=6)
TO.PREDICT <- data.frame(Bill=c(23.3,12.5,36.87))
```

It is imperative that the name of the column in `TO.PREDICT` matches up exactly with the name of the predictor variable in the regression.

In the first example, the data frame is set up where x is the name of the predictor variable, and we are interested only in predicting when x equals 6. In the second example, the data frame has `Bill` as the name of the predictor. We are interested in predicting at bill amounts of 23.3, 12.5, and 36.87.

Once the `TO.PREDICT` data frame has been defined, the `predict()` command can be used. The following examples use the regression predicting tip percentage from bill amount.

In R

```
#Predicting average tip percentages left on bills
predict(M,newdata=TO.PREDICT,interval="confidence",level=0.95)
       fit      lwr      upr
1 15.26440 14.48349 16.04531
2 17.77495 16.83581 18.71409
3 12.10994 10.53600 13.68388


#Predicting individual tip percentages left on bills
predict(M,newdata=TO.PREDICT,interval="prediction",level=0.90)
       fit      lwr      upr
1 15.26440 5.733647 24.79515
2 17.77495 8.234170 27.31573
3 12.10994 2.510596 21.70928
```

- The interval= argument must be either "confidence" (confidence interval for the average) or "prediction" (prediction interval for an individual's value).
- The level= argument is optional and specifies the level of confidence (if omitted, the default is 0.95).
- The values under the column fit give the point estimates (i.e., the values had you plugged those values of x into the regression equation) of each value in the TO.PREDICT data frame (in row order).
- The values under the lwr and upr give the lower and upper limits of the desired confidence or prediction interval.

In this example, we are 95% confident that the average tip percentage left on bills of size $23.30 (the first row of TO.PREDICT) is between 14.48% and 16.05%. There is a 90% chance that the tip percentage left on a bill of size $23.30 is between 5.73% and 24.80%.

Transformations

When the scatterplot or residuals plot shows that linear regression is not appropriate for modeling the relationship, it may be possible to model transformations of the original variables. If M is the name of the original (inappropriate) model, then run:

In R

```
find.transformations(M,powers=seq(from=-3,to=3,by=.25))
y is TipPercentage
x is Bill
No transformation yields rsquared of 0.115

 x.power y.power rsquared
    -0.5     0.5    0.167
   -0.25    0.25    0.167
```

- powers is an optional argument that specifies to what powers x and y will be raised. By default, it is a sequence from -3 to 3 in steps of 0.25. Note: instead of raising something to the 0 power, logarithms are used.
- The output gives the R^2 of the original model with no transformation and a list of transformations with large R^2. One heuristic is to choose any model that has an R^2 within 0.005 of the absolute highest since there is typically no strong statistical justification to prefer one versus another.
- The graphical output shows the original scatterplot and the scatterplots of the three best transformations. Always check the scatterplots to make sure the high R^2 is not induced by outliers.

Typical analysis

A typical analysis involves plotting the data to make sure regression is appropriate, then viewing and visualizing the results and checking assumptions.

In R

```
plot(y~x,data=DATA) #initial plot
M <- lm(y~x,data=DATA) #fit model
visualize.model(M) #see the model and prediction/confidence intervals
check.regression(M) #see if assumptions behind model hold
summary(M) #view the numerical output of the regression
```

3.9 Summary

The linear regression framework is extremely flexible and gives the ability to model linear relationships and, through the use of transformations, curved (monotonic) relationships.

Equation and model

- The regression equation is $\mu_{y|x} = \beta_0 + \beta_1 x$. In other words, the average value of y has a linear relationship with x.
- The regression model is $y_i = \beta_0 + \beta_1 x_i + \varepsilon_i$ where $\varepsilon_i \sim N(0, \sigma)$. In other words, an individual's value of y is equal to $\mu_{y|x}$ (the average value of y of all individuals with the common value of x) plus a "disturbance" ε_i.
- Disturbances represent how much individuals differ from the average and are taken to be Normally distributed with a constant standard deviation everywhere (i.e., individuals vary from the average by about the same amount regardless of their particular x- and y-values).
- Regression tells us *nothing* about what happens to an individual's y-value when his or her x increases by one unit. The regression equation is not a physical law and does not establish cause and effect.

Coefficients

- The quantity β_1 is the slope of the regression line and is interpreted by saying: "Two individuals who differ (for whatever reason) in x by one unit are expected to differ in y by β_1 units. If β_1 is positive, the individual with the larger x is expected to have the larger y, etc."
- The quantities β_0 and β_1 are properties of the real world and are inherently unknown unless one can obtain a census. They are approximated by b_0 and b_1, the intercept and slope of the regression line built on the sample.
- b_0 and b_1 are found using the least squares criterion. Of all possible straight lines, these give the one with the smallest possible sum of the squared errors (the residuals, or difference between actual and predicted values).

Standard errors, confidence intervals, and prediction intervals

- When the assumptions of the regression hold, the measured slope is a predictable amount from the "true" slope β_1. The typical difference is called the standard error of the slope SE_{b_1}, and it can be estimated from the data itself (without even knowing β_1). This fact is exploited to make a confidence interval for β_1. We can be about 95% confident that β_1 is somewhere in the interval $b_1 \pm 2SE_{b_1}$.
- When the assumptions of the regression hold, the predicted value for an individual and for the average value among all individuals are predictable amounts away from the "true" values. The standard errors of these predictions depend on the sample size (smaller errors for larger samples), RMSE (larger errors when the stream of points has more scatter), and the distance from the average value of x at which the predictions are made (larger errors farther from the average). The uncertainty regarding an individual's value is always larger than the uncertainty regarding the average because an individual differs from the average by a random amount.

Goodness of fit of a regression

- R^2 gives the percentage of the variability in y that can be attributed to or "explained" by the model (for whatever reason). For simple linear regressions, this value is equivalent to the square of Pearson's correlation, r^2.

- The root mean squared error *RMSE* gives the typical error made by the regression, i.e., the typical size of the residual.
- The values of R^2 and *RMSE* indicate how well the model fits the data, but not whether the model is appropriate.

Statistical significance and p-values

- The p-value of the regression is the probability that a predictor unrelated to y would reduce the sum of squared errors (compared to the SSE of the naive model) by at least as much as your model.
- Alternatively, the p-value is the probability that a regression using a predictor unrelated to y would yield a value of R^2 at least as high as your regression.
- If this p-value is less than 5%, the regression is statistically significant. x predicts y "better" than a random, unrelated predictor or no predictor at all.
- The p-value does *not* reveal the strength of the relationship (refer to R^2 or the *RMSE*).

Checking assumptions

- Always first check the statistical tests of the assumptions. If the p-values are all greater than 5%, the regression model can be used since (statistically) it appears to be a reasonable reflection of reality. If any are failed and the sample size is small (fewer than 25 or so), the model is invalid and must be abandoned. If any are failed and the sample size is large, visually check the assumptions.
- To visually gauge whether the assumptions of the regression hold, check the residuals plot (predicted values vs. residuals).
  - The residuals plot should have no *obvious* pattern (careful, your eyes are "too good" at recognizing small, inconsequential patterns).
  - There should be no curvature in the residuals plot.
  - The vertical spread should be about the same everywhere (the concentration of values horizontally does not matter).
  - The histogram of residuals should look symmetric and roughly Normal.
  - Points on the QQ-plot should fall within the bands and have no systematic curvature away from the diagonal line.
- Small violations of assumptions can be tolerated when there are more than a few dozen data points. For smaller datasets, formal tests of the assumptions must be made (F-test of linearity, equal spread, Normality tests).
- When the regression model is not appropriate, it may be possible to instead fit transformations of the original values with a regression. Since x and y are arbitrary, it may be the case that something like $\ln Weight$ and $\sqrt{Height}$ have a linear relationship.

3.10 Exercises

1: Use `EX3.NFL` for the following problems. The number of wins for each NFL team over the course of 11 years is tabulated (column `Wins`) along with well over 137 potentially useful statistics about offense, defense, team changes, etc. Imagine you are in charge of "sports analytics" and are tasked with investigating which variables help to predict the number of wins. Your results can shape how players are recruited and how pre-season training proceeds. This type of analysis is everywhere in business analytics—a quantity we're interested in (sales, percent of people who respond to an ad, etc.) clearly should be predictable by *something*, but by what we don't know until we analyze data!

a) Technically, predicting the number of Wins (which can range from 0 to 16) is *not* a task for which we can use regression because the number of wins is an *integer* amount. Why does y being integer-valued violate the assumption that $\varepsilon \sim N(0, \sigma)$? Hint: read up about the Normal distribution and what kind of numbers it describes. Although a more sophisticated model is more appropriate, we can still learn a good deal about relationships between these variables, so let's proceed.

b) Using `all.correlations()`, find the six variables that have the strongest correlations with `Wins`. Note: this command may take a while to finish. Note: XP in this dataset is an abbreviation for "extra point."

c) Many of the variables that have the strongest correlations with Wins are not interesting to analyze (obviously, teams that make more touchdowns are going to win more), so let us examine the relationship between `Wins` and `X1.Off.Tot.Yds`. Make a scatterplot and fit a simple linear regression. The units of x are "one hundred yards." If you saw a value of 30, this means the team had $30 \times 100 = 3000$ yards for the season.

   1) Include the scatterplot with the regression line on it (make this manually or with `visualize.model`). Is the trajectory of the stream of points linear enough so that a regression model is appropriate for describing the relationship?
   2) Examine the results of running `summary()` on the model. Write out the regression equation, but round the coefficients to two decimal places. Remember, use actual variable names, not x and y.
   3) Interpret the intercept as if you were speaking to your boss. Is the intercept a meaningful quantity in this case? Why or why not?
   4) Interpret the slope as if you were speaking to your boss. Begin your sentence with the phrase, "Two teams that differ by 100 in ..."
   5) Quote the value of the root mean squared error of the regression. Interpret its value as if you were speaking to your boss.
   6) Quote the value of R^2. Interpret its value as if you were speaking to your boss.
   7) Quote the value of the standard error of the slope. Interpret its value as if you were speaking to your boss.

d) What is the reduction in the sum of squared errors when a regression model is used to predict `Wins` from `X73.Off.2pt.Conv.Made` rather than the naive model (predicting `Wins` from the overall average in the data)? Is this reduction statistically significant? Explain why or why not. Hint: look at `anova(M)`. Note: the reduction is the number in the `Sum Sq` column in the row named after the x-variable.

e) Obtain a 95% confidence interval for the slope of the regression predicting `Wins` from `X82.Def.Fumbles.Recovered`. Does the interval suggest the regression is statistically significant? Explain.

f) Is there a statistically significant relationship between `Next.Years.Wins` and `Wins` (i.e., this year's wins)? Quote the relevant evidence. If there is a statistically significant relationship, is the relationship *useful* and exploitable (e.g., for the purposes of being within one win when placing bets on the number of wins a team gets next year)?

2: The following questions review important statistical terms that are used quite often.

a) The fundamental model in regression (what we are assuming to be true about the world) is that

$$y_i = \beta_0 + \beta_1 x_i + \varepsilon_i$$

The quantity "$\beta_0 + \beta_1 x_i$" represents the average value of y in the population among all individuals with the same common value of x. What do the ε_i's represent, and what do we assume about their possible values?

b) What does it mean when we say that the coefficients of a regression have been estimated using "least squares" criteria?
c) What is the difference between the RMSE (root mean squared error) and the standard error of the slope (SE_{b_1}) when discussing simple linear regression?
d) From the ANOVA table, we find the p-value of the regression is 0.03. Explain precisely what this p-value means.
e) Explain why the p-value of the regression does not give any information about how *strong* or how *useful* the relationship between x and y is (and comment on what number we look at to quantify these two properties).
f) If we had data on every entity in the population (a census) and fit a least squares regression, should we call the coefficients b_0 and b_1 or should we call them β_0 and β_1? What about if we had a random sample of size $n = 100$?
g) Imagine a 95% confidence interval for the slope is $(-0.1, 1.2)$.
   1) What do we mean when we say: "We are 95% confident that the 'true' slope is between -0.1 and 1.2"? Hint: we do *not* mean that there's a 95% *chance* that the true slope is between these values, since the true slope is a numerical fact about the population, not a random quantity.
   2) Since the interval contains 0, the relationship is not statistically significant. Would it be correct to say that there is a 95% chance that there is no relationship between x and y? Why or why not?
   3) If the goal of analysis is to estimate the coefficient as precisely as possible (small standard error for the slope), which is better?
      - A sample of size 50 or a sample of size 100?
      - Collecting 10 observations at $x = 5, 6, 7$ or collecting 3 observations at $x = 1, 2, \ldots, 10$?

3: Use `EX3.ABALONE` for the following questions. An abalone is a fancy kind of clam with a very pretty shell. (`http://en.wikipedia.org/wiki/Abalone`) Let us predict `Meat.Weight` (the meat is a delicacy) from `Diameter`.

a) Make the relevent scatterplot, using the additional arguments `pch=20` and `cex=0.3` to see the points better. Explain why we cannot model this relationship with a linear regression.
b) Fit the linear regression anyway and look at it using `visualize.model`, then produce a list of possible transformations that may "fix" the issues by running `find.transformations`. Is the log-log model one of the choices (how do you know)?
c) Choose the transformation with the highest R^2. Fit this transformed model and run `summary()`. Write out the regression equation of this transformed model, then "untransform" it to get an equation of the form Meat Weight = ...
d) Check whether the transformed model reasonably reflects reality by running `check.regression`. Statistically, which assumptions (if any) are satisfied?
e) The residuals plot is hard to digest since most points are clustered on the left. Assuming you have saved your transformed regression as `M.trans`, we can manually made a residuals plot with arbitrary axes by changing the limits displayed with `xlim` and `ylim`. Run the following command, and based on your visual assessment, address whether we have "fixed" the regression or whether there are still violations.

```
plot(fitted(M.trans),residuals(M.trans),
   xlim=c(1.5,6),ylim=c(-4,4),pch=20,cex=0.3)
```

4: Use `EX3.HOUSING` for the following questions. This dataset tabulates the selling prices and square areas of over 500 houses in Massachusetts. Companies like Zillow and Trulia employ statistical modelers to incorporate basic information about the house and neighborhood to come up with a reasonable estimate of what a house will sell for. Unfortunately, the relationship is not well-described by a linear regression.

a) A very common transformation pair is the log-log pair. Although it is not the transformation pair that gives the highest R^2, let us use it. Fit this transformed model and examine the results of `visualize.model` and `check.regression`. Are the statistical tests of the assumptions passed? If not, does it look like linear regression is appropriate for modeling this transformation (why or why not)?
b) Verify that the regression equation is $\log_{10} PRICE = 1.21 + 1.26 \log_{10} AREA$ by using `summary()` on the transformed model. Untransform the equation to be in the form PRICE $= \ldots$

5: Use `EX3.BODYFAT`. We want to predict someone's body fat percentage (`Fat`) based on their triceps skinfold thickness (`Triceps`).

a) Predict (and examine 95% confidence and prediction intervals) the body fat percentage when Triceps equals 18 and when it equals 31.
b) Which of the intervals is appropriate if you want to predict your friend's body fat percentage given he has a triceps measurement of 18? Which interval is appropriate if you wanted to predict the average body fat percentage of all males whose triceps measurements are 31?
c) Can we use this model to predict the body fat of a body builder whose triceps measurement is 45? Why or why not?

6: Rewrite each equation below so that it is in the form $y =$. Note: you do not need to simplify any further except for (c).

a) $\sqrt{y} = 3 + 4/x$
b) $\log_{10} y = 1 - 2x^2$
c) $\log_{10} y = 2 + 3\log_{10} x$
d) $1/y^2 = 1 - 2x^2$
e) $y^2 = -4 + 8\sqrt{x}$

Scatterplot and correlation matrices
The multiple regression model
Checking assumptions
Goodness of fit: $\mathbf{R}^2$ and $\mathbf{R}^2_{adj}$
Interpretation of coefficients
Coefficients are model-dependent
Inference
The standard error of a coefficient
Confidence interval for β_i
Variance inflation factor and collinearity
Examples: salary and body fat data
Statistical Significance
of model
of subset of predictors
of individual predictors
Quirks of coefficients and *p*-values
Increasing the flexibility of a model
Polynomial models
Variable creation
Interaction variables
Influential points and outliers
Predictions with multiple regression
Summary
Multiple Regression in R
Exercises

4. Multiple Regression for Descriptive Modeling

Two people have just been hired to fill one of five openings on the analytics team at a major company. The older employee has five years of work experience and three years of education while the younger employee has four years of both. Who would we expect to garner a higher salary? If we had data on other employees, one strategy for answering this question could be to fit two simple linear regressions to predict salary—one using educational level and one using prior work experience. If the slope of the model with educational level is greater, then we would expect the younger employee to have the higher salary. Unfortunately, such a strategy may not work. The slopes of the two linear regressions may be misleading if there is a correlation between educational level and prior work experience.

To see why, imagine that this company only has executives and interns. People either have large amounts of both education and experience or hardly any of either. Imagine that the coefficient of educational level in a simple linear regression is 100. This implies that two employees who differ in education by one year are expected to differ in salaries by $100 (with the person with more education having the higher salary). Imagine the coefficient of the number of years of prior work experience is 50. On the surface, the younger employee (more education) should have the higher salary.

However, educational level and prior work experience are (positively) correlated at this company. When two employees differ in educational level by one year, they likely also differ in prior experience by some amount. The expected difference of $100 in these two individuals' salaries *could* be due to differences in their educational background, but it *could* be due to differences in their prior work experience as well. A simple linear regression alone cannot separate the association between salary and educational level from the association between salary and prior work experience.

Thus, we cannot directly compare the expected difference of $100 to the expected difference of $50 to guess which of the two employees has the higher salary. To truly isolate the relationship between salary and educational level, we first need to *account* for differences in employees' prior experiences.

Multiple regression, where we predict y from numerous x's, is a tool that allows us to study the association between y and a particular predictor of interest while accounting for the existence of other variables and associations. Multiple regression is a standard technique in research when many "common causes" or lurking variables may influence the relationship between y and x. When you read an article and see that researchers "accounted for" various factors, this typically means they fit a multiple regression model to isolate their relationship of interest. Some recent examples include:

- A 2013 study showed that liver transplant success varied by race. Researchers accounted for "social and economic" status since it *could* have been the case that one race in the study was typically poorer, had worse diets, were in generally poorer health, etc., than the other (which obviously would affect transplant success).[1]
- A 2014 study showed that aggressiveness toward your spouse is associated with blood-glucose levels through an interesting experiment involving participants stabbing voodoo dolls of their spouses in secret. Researchers accounted for differences in marital satisfaction, which could have also explained the variation in aggression levels.[2]
- A 2014 study linked childhood abuse and neglect to increased risk of obesity, diabetes, and other health problems (via hormone imbalances). Researchers took into account differences in diet, exercise, and other lifestyle factors since these could alternatively explain the increased health risks.[3]
- A 2015 study showed that being bullied during adolescence was associated with depression during early adulthood. Researchers accounted for potential alternative factors for depression such as behavioral problems, social class, child abuse, and family history of depression.[4]
- Many studies look at the impact of music education on academic achievement and find that playing an instrument in high school is associated with a higher GPA[5]. Such studies are complicated because they *should* account for gender (girls tend to have higher GPAs and are more likely to play an instrument), race (some minorities tend to have lower GPAs and are less likely to play an instrument), and other factors such as socioeconomic status, but most do not.

Multiple regression provides a technique to compare the average value of y between two individuals who differ in x but who are "otherwise identical" in terms of other (potentially lurking) variables. In this chapter, we discuss how multiple predictors can be incorporated into a regression model along with what specific questions such a model can and cannot answer. Emphasis is placed on fitting and interpreting a regression model with *pre-determined* predictor variables. Choosing *which* variables to include in the model is addressed in Chapter 7. Specific goals for the chapter include:

- Learn how to precisely interpret a coefficient in a multiple regression model.
- Learn how to gauge statistical significance of the model and of an individual predictor along with understanding what significance truly means.
- Learn how to check whether a multiple regression model provides an adequate description of reality.
- Learn how to improve a model by creating new variables, including "interaction" terms.
- Learn how to check for outliers and influential points.

---

[1] Google "liver transplant success varies by race".

[2] `http://www.pnas.org/content/early/2014/04/09/1400619111.abstract`

[3] Google "webmd childhood abuse lead adulthood illness".

[4] `http://www.bmj.com/content/350/bmj.h2469`

[5] `http://www.issaquah.wednet.edu/documents/highschool/schedule/arts/achievement.pdf`

Unfortunately, many researchers act as if accounting for these potential "common cause" or lurking variables allows them to draw cause and effect inferences. To do so, the study must be carefully designed so that the *only* differences between the individuals are in the variables measured. Any differences left unaccounted for may be the "real" reason for the association between y and x. Review Section 2.7 (the relationship between height vs. number of piercings is induced by gender). This begs the question of how we can *ever* be sure that we are measuring all ways in which individuals could differ. Most likely, we can't, which once again reiterates that a regression equation is not a physical law and can almost never be used to establish cause and effect.

4.1 Scatterplot and correlation matrices

In multiple regression, it is important to understand *both* the relationships between y and the predictor variables as well as the relationships between the predictor variables themselves. The **scatterplot matrix** allows us to simultaneously visualize how each pair of variables in the data is related.

Figure 4.1 shows the scatterplot matrix for the monthly salary data (`SALARY`). There are three predictors of `Salary`: `Education` (years of education post-high school), `Experience` (years in the workforce), and `Months` (number of months at the company).

To study the relationship between y and the x's, we focus on the *row* where y is labeled (so y is on the vertical axis). Since we wish to predict someone's monthly `Salary`, we scan the top row to see how it is related with each predictor. The vertical axes for each of these plots are `Salary`, and the horizontal axes are the relevant predictor variables. Here, we see the relationships between `Salary` and each predictor look roughly linear (no obvious curvature) and are good candidates for simple linear regressions (and as we will see, multiple regression as well). Note: the *column* where y is labeled presents these same graphs (a mirror image flipped across the diagonal) and can be ignored.

The other plots show how the x's are related. Here, the three predictor variables do not appear to be strongly related to each other since the scatterplots do not have any obvious patterns. This is actually good news, since strong relationships between predictor variables make precise estimates of coefficients difficult. Further, when relationships exist between the predictor variables, it will be imperative to account for them when trying to isolate the association between y and a particular x.

The motivating example in this chapter imagined a company where the educational level and years of prior work experience are strongly and positively correlated. In this company, their correlation of -0.10 has a p-value of 0.33 and is thus not significant.

A secondary tool to gauge the strength of the relationship between the variables is the **correlation matrix**. This matrix is a table that gives the Pearson (or Spearman rank) correlations of each pair of variables. The matrix is symmetric because the correlation between y and x and between x and y are the same.

Figure 4.1 — Scatterplot matrix of SALARY data. A scatterplot matrix shows the relationships between every pair of variables in the data. To find a scatterplot for a particular relationship, e.g., `Months` and `Experience`, first identify the variable that plays the role of y (let it be `Months` in this case) and find the row with the relevant name (fourth row here). This row shows the scatterplots of y vs. x in the usual orientation. Then, find the column labeled with the x variable (third column here). The scatterplot where the row and column intersect is the desired scatterplot. Here, the plot in the fourth row/third column shows the relationship between $y =$ `Months` and $x =$ `Experience`.

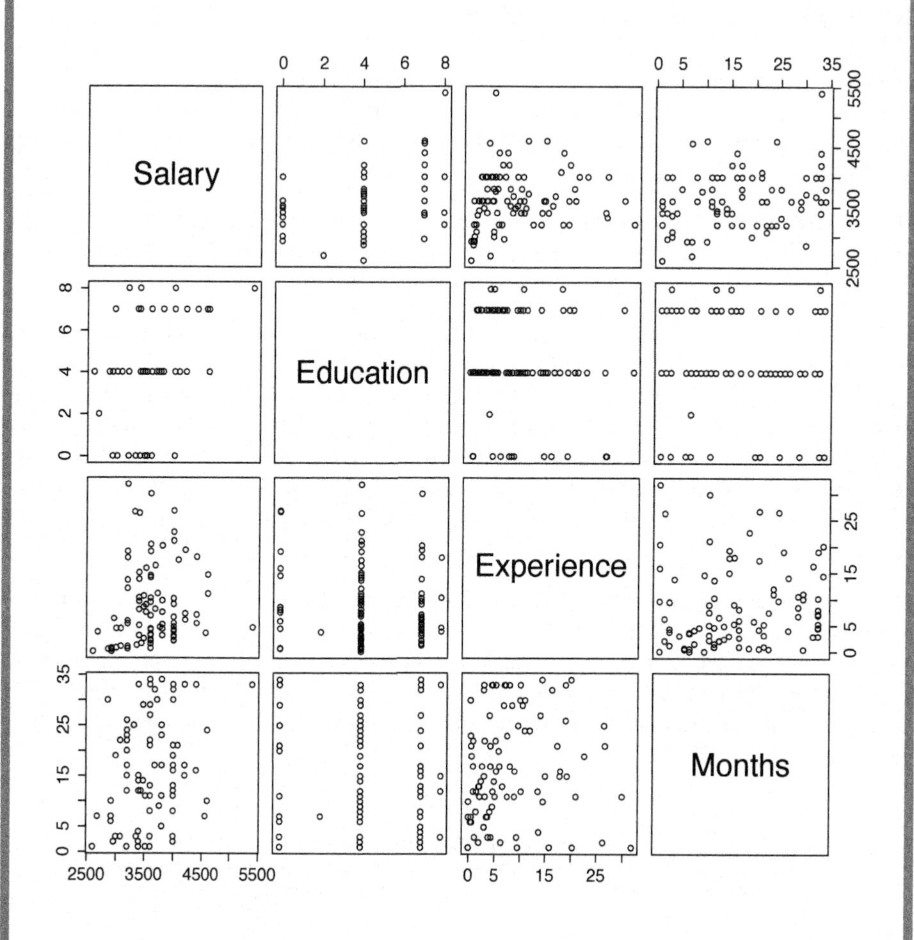

In R

```
pairs(Salary~Education+Experience+Months,data=SALARY)
#Put the y variable before the ~
#This way, the top row of plots show the relationships between y
#and the x's
```

For example, in the SALARY data, we see that the correlation between Salary and Education is fairly strong ($r = 0.41$), while the correlation between Salary and Experience is relatively weak ($r = 0.17$). The correlation between Education and Experience is -0.10. A negative value here implies that, for this company, employees with above-average education have lower than average experience (though the association lacks statistical significance).

```
cor.matrix(SALARY)

           Salary Education Experience Months
Salary      1.000     0.412      0.167  0.286
Education   0.412     1.000     -0.102 -0.060
Experience  0.167    -0.102      1.000  0.077
Months      0.286    -0.060      0.077  1.000
```

Sometimes, the number of variables in the data is extremely large, and a matrix of all correlations is difficult to process. Instead, we can look at the correlations in the form of a list, potentially sorted from most negative to most positive or by a particular variable of interest.

```
all.correlations(SALARY)
```

4.2 The multiple regression model

The multiple regression model is a straightforward extension of the simple linear regression model and allows us to incorporate relationships between multiple quantities simultaneously. Let there be a total of k predictor variables $x_1, x_2, \ldots, x_k$. Each predictor variable has a coefficient β_1, β_2, etc. The model assumes that for each individual in the population:

$$y_i = \beta_0 + \beta_1 x_1 + \beta_2 x_2 + \ldots + \beta_k x_k + \varepsilon_i \qquad \varepsilon_i \sim N(0, \sigma) \tag{4.1}$$

In essence, the multiple regression model says:

- The average value of y among all individuals with a common set of characteristics (i.e., a particular combination of x-values) is essentially a weighted sum of predictor variables (with weights given by the coefficients).
- An individual's value of y differs from the average by a random amount ε_i, the **disturbance**.

Unless a census is available, the coefficients of the model are estimated from the data using the least squares criterion and are denoted b_0, b_1, ..., b_k. Among all possible choices for the coefficients, these minimize the sum of squared residuals and in a sense give the model that "best" fits the data.

(C) Amazingly, a concise set of equations can be written down that produces the estimates b_0, b_1, etc. However, the formulas are difficult to work with by hand and are usually evaluated using a computer. If you are familiar with matrices (an advanced mathematical construct that is beyond the scope of this book), you can write $\mathbf{Y}$ as an $n \times 1$ matrix containing the values of y, $\mathbf{X}$ as an $n \times (k+1)$ matrix where the first column is all ones and the remaining columns are values of the x's, and β as a $(k+1) \times 1$ matrix that contains the values b_0, b_1, ..., b_k that we want to estimate. The least squares estimates are $\hat{\beta} = (\mathbf{X}^T\mathbf{X})^{-1}\mathbf{X}^T\mathbf{Y}$, where $\mathbf{X}^T$ and $\mathbf{X}^{-1}$ are the transpose and inverse of $\mathbf{X}$.

Finally, what we call y and x is completely arbitrary. They can be the original measurements in the data, e.g., *Salary*, or they can be any function of them, e.g., $\ln(Salary)$, $1/Salary$, $Salary^2$. In fact, predictor variables can be functions of two or more measurements, e.g., $x = Education \times Experience$. The latter variable is said to be the *interaction* between *Education* and *Experience*. Transformations are useful to "fix" nonlinearities or other issues in the regression, and interactions are useful when the strength of the relationship between y and a predictor depends on the value of another variable.

4.2.1 Checking assumptions

As with simple linear regression, the model assumes that the distribution of possible values for the disturbances is Normal, i.e., $\varepsilon_i \sim N(0, \sigma)$. The consequences of this assumption, and the requirements for the model to be valid, are:

1. The relationship between y and *each* x needs to be linear (this addresses the requirement that the average value of ε be zero for all combinations of x's).
2. The typical difference between an individual's value and the average is the same regardless of the individual's particular combination of x's (this addresses the requirement of equal vertical spread, i.e., σ is the same for all combinations of x's).
3. The distribution of residuals as a whole is Normal.
4. If data was collected over time, residuals are independent.

Checking the assumptions is critical to using the model. As with simple linear regression, we first check the assumptions with statistical tests. If any are failed (and there are more than a couple dozen observations), we look at the residuals plot (checking for curvature and unequal spread) and histogram/QQ-plot of the residuals (checking for Normality) to see if violations are minor and can be ignored. Nothing about the model can be trusted until we are sure the model provides a reasonable reflection of reality. Section 3.5 reviews how to visually and statistically check the major assumptions.

For multiple regression models, an additional set of plots involving residuals must be checked—**residual vs. predictor plots**. These plots show the relationship between the residuals of the models and the x-values for each predictor. There should be no interesting patterns in these plots. If there is a pattern, some important component of the relationship between y and that predictor is not being captured by the model.

> If there is curvature in the residual vs. predictor plots, you must either try a transformation of the predictor, e.g., x^2, $\ln x$, $\sqrt{x}$, etc., or fit it with a polynomial model in x (see Section 4.5.1). If there is unequal vertical spread, you must try a transformation of y. Unequal horizontal spread is not an issue since this is only an artifact of how the data was collected or the natural distribution of x-values.

For example, consider a multiple regression model predicting monthly salary from the three available predictors in the `SALARY` data. To determine whether the model provides an accurate reflection of reality, we first check the statistical tests. The only test that is failed is linearity with `Experience`. Small violations are allowed when datasets are large ($n = 93$ here), so we check its residual vs. predictor plot. See Figure 4.2. There is no hint of curvature or any other pattern, so whatever violation is present must be small and can be ignored. As expected, the other diagnostic plots look great. The model looks like a valid reflection of reality.

Figure 4.2 — Checking the Salary model. The statistical tests of assumptions are passed except for linearity with `Experience` (the linearity of the model itself cannot be checked since no two individuals share the same combination of predictor variables). Since the sample size is large, we check the plots to see if the violation is small and can be ignored.

The diagnostics plots of the model look great. The residuals plot (top left) shows equal vertical spread and no apparent curvature. The histogram (top middle) shows a roughly Normal distribution for residuals. The QQ-plot (top right) has points within the upper and lower bands, further indicating that the distribution of residuals is Normal. The bottom three panels are the residual vs. predictor plots. We focus on the residuals vs. `Experience` plot since it failed the linearity test. There is no hint of any leftover curvature, so whatever violation is small and can be ignored. The model looks like it provides a reasonable reflection of reality.

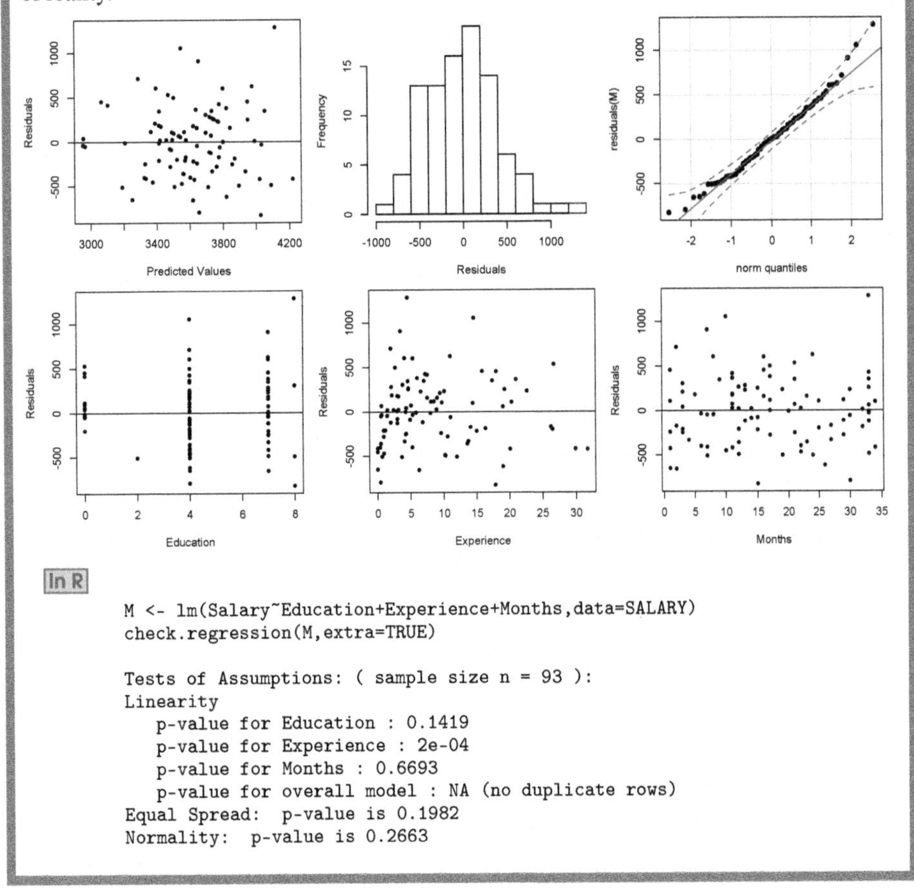

In R

```
M <- lm(Salary~Education+Experience+Months,data=SALARY)
check.regression(M,extra=TRUE)

Tests of Assumptions: ( sample size n = 93 ):
Linearity
   p-value for Education : 0.1419
   p-value for Experience : 2e-04
   p-value for Months : 0.6693
   p-value for overall model : NA (no duplicate rows)
Equal Spread:  p-value is 0.1982
Normality:  p-value is 0.2663
```

Now consider the `BULLDOZER` data, where we try to predict `SalePrice` (the selling price at auction) based on five different predictors. See Figure 4.3. All statistical tests of the assumptions are failed. The nonlinearity in the residuals plot is likely due to the nonlinear relationship of selling price with the model year of the vehicle. Had we been diligent and made a scatterplot matrix of the variables before attempting to build a model (see Figure 4.8), we would have seen that a multiple regression model using `YearMade` as a predictor would not be appropriate.

Figure 4.3 — Checking the Bulldozer model. All statistical tests of assumptions are failed when a model predicting the sales price of a bulldozer is created using the provided variables. Since the sample size is large, we check the diagnostic plots to see if the violation is small and can be ignored.

The diagnostics plots of the model have serious issues. There is obvious curvature in the residuals plot (violation of linearity is severe), and the histogram and QQ-plot of the residuals show distinct non-Normality (the "dip" in the lower left of the QQ-plot corresponds to an unusual clump of residuals with a size of about $-25,000$).

An examination of the residual vs. predictor plots shows that there are approximately linear relationships between the selling price and the predictors with the exception of `YearMade`. We cannot use this regression model until these violations are "fixed" (we will see how to do this soon by using a polynomial model in `YearMade`).

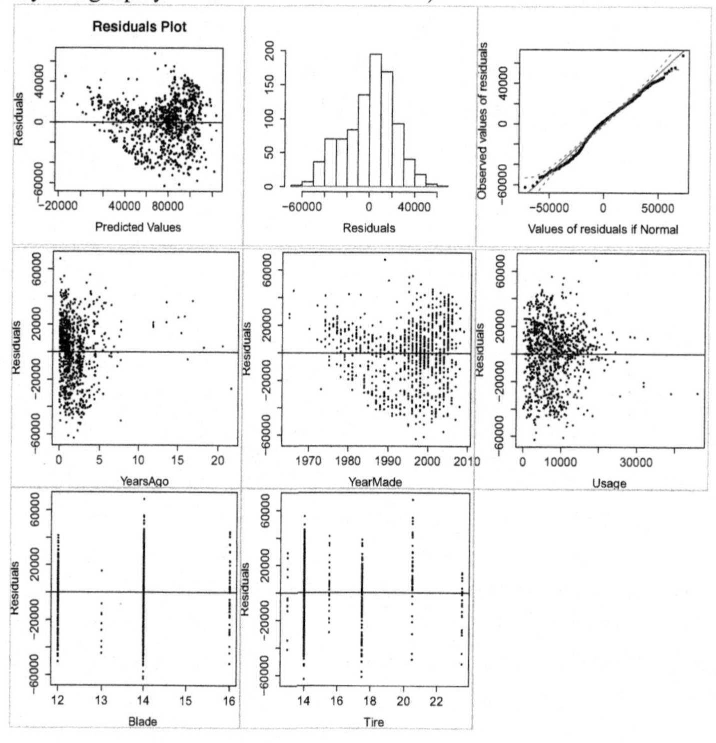

In R

```
M <- lm(SalePrice~.,data=BULLDOZER)
check.regression(M,extra=TRUE)

Tests of Assumptions: ( sample size n = 924 ):
Linearity
   p-value for YearsAgo : 0
   p-value for YearMade : 0
   p-value for Usage : 0.0061
   p-value for Blade : 0
   p-value for Tire : 0
   p-value for overall model : 0
Equal Spread:  p-value is 0
Normality:  p-value is 0
```

4.2.2 Goodness of fit: R^2 and R^2_{adj}

Assuming the multiple regression model provides a decent reflection of reality, often the first thing that is checked is how well the model fits the data. In the context of simple linear regression, we measured R^2 (Section 3.2.4) and interpreted the value as the percentage of the variation in y that can be attributed to the model. While the interpretation is the same in the context of multiple regression, the value of R^2 may be quite misleading. A related measure, R^2_{adj}, is preferred.

R^2

R^2 is calculated by comparing the sum of squared errors when predicting y from the regression model to the sum of squared errors when predicting y from the naive model (i.e., from its overall average $\bar{y}$). Let SSE_{naive} (also referred to as the total sum of squares) be the sum of squared errors made by the naive model:

$$SSE_{naive} = \text{sum of squared errors using } \bar{y} \text{ to predict } y = \sum_{i=1}^{n} (\bar{y} - y_i)^2 \quad (4.2)$$

If $\hat{y}_i$ is the predicted value of y for individual i using the regression equation, then the sum of squared errors using the regression SSE_{reg} is:

$$SSE_{reg} = \text{sum of squared errors using regression to predict } y = \sum_{i=1}^{n} (\hat{y}_i - y_i)^2 \quad (4.3)$$

R^2 gives the fractional decrease of the total variation in y when going from the naive to the regression model:

$$R^2 = \frac{SSE_{naive} - SSE_{reg}}{SSE_{naive}} \quad (4.4)$$

The value of R^2 can range from 0 (equivalent to the naive model) up to 1 (a perfect fit). In most contexts, an R^2 of 80% or higher is very impressive, though an R^2 of 40-60% is more common in business analytics and an R^2 of 20-40% is often seen for models of human behavior (e.g., spending). A large value of R^2 implies the model fits the data quite well, but it does *not* imply that the regression is suitable for modeling the data since nonlinear relationships can sometimes have $R^2 \approx 1$ (review Figure 3.7).

In multiple regression models, R^2 may give a misleading impression of how well the model fits the data. Adding an additional predictor to a model *always* decreases the model's sum of squared errors (the model has more wiggle room to fit the data) and makes the value of R^2 increase. This is true even when that additional predictor has no real relationship with y.

In fact, when the data contains n cases, it is possible to get a perfect fit ($R^2 = 100\%$) using *any* $n-1$ predictor variables, even if they are completely unrelated to y! For example, consider the following experiment. Ten random values of y are generated between 0 and 1 along with nine random "junk" predictor variables. Figure 4.4 shows how the value of R^2 increases as more junk predictors are added to the model. With nine variables, the model achieves $R^2 = 100\%$ (no error), even though *none* of the predictors have any relationship with y.

Figure 4.4 — Artificially increasing R^2 by adding junk predictors. The addition of any predictor to a model, even one with no relationship to y, will always increase R^2. Here, all nine predictor variables are independent of y, but the value of R^2 (open dots and solid line) creeps up to 100% when enough are added to the model. R^2_{adj} penalizes the value of R^2 by its complexity (the number of terms in the model) and does not share this deficiency (solid dots and dashed line). When using a multiple regression, focus on R^2_{adj}.

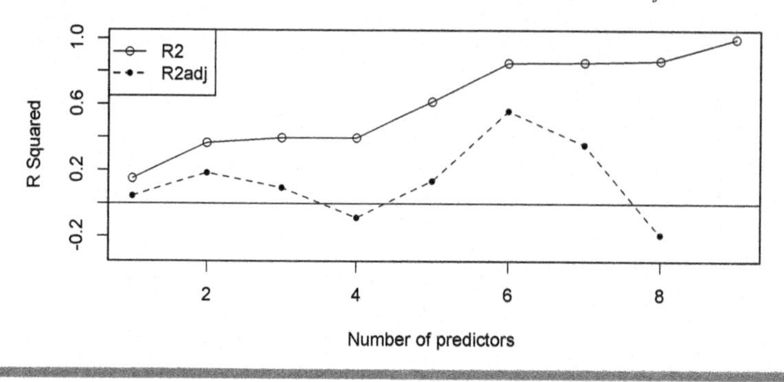

R^2_{adj}

A fairer measure of how well the model fits the data is the **adjusted R^2**, or R^2_{adj}, defined as:

$$R^2_{adj} = R^2 - (1 - R^2)\frac{k}{n-k-1} = \text{original } R^2 - \text{penalty term} \tag{4.5}$$

In effect, R^2_{adj} is the value of R^2 after applying a penalty based on the number of predictors. As more predictors are added to the model, the value of R^2 naturally increases. However, the penalty term increases as well. The increase in R^2 will be canceled out by the increase in penalty term unless the new predictor adds additional information about y that the model did not already contain. Thus, R^2_{adj} only increases when the added predictor is "good."

Unlike R^2, R^2_{adj} does not have a nice interpretation. In fact, it is possible to have a *negative* R^2_{adj} if it is a *really* bad model (the maximum value of R^2_{adj} is still 100%). Thus, R^2_{adj} gives an informal, but far more honest assessment of the fit of a multiple regression model than R^2.

4.2.3 Interpretation of coefficients

The coefficients in a multiple regression have a *very* precise meaning and are often misunderstood and misinterpreted. Imagine that a particular predictor x_i has an estimated coefficient of b_i. One key property of the interpretation of b_i is that it is *model-dependent* and always must be put in the context of what other variables are present in the model.

We interpret b_i by saying: "Two individuals who differ in x_i by one unit but who are otherwise identical (in terms of the other predictors in the model) are expected to differ in y by b_i units." If the coefficient is positive, the individual with the larger value of x_i is expected to have the larger value of y, etc.

Thus, multiple regression allows us to account for other factors before studying the association between y and x. All that is required is to put these other factors in the multiple regression model and to examine the coefficient of the predictor of interest.

- To study the expected difference in salary between two individuals who differ in educational levels by one year, we need to compare individuals with identical values of previous work experience, months at the company, etc., since these other factors can influence salary.
- To study the expected difference in GPA between students who play instruments and students who do not, we need to compare students with otherwise identical backgrounds. Thus, we can put gender, race, family income, socioeconomic status, etc., into the model to account for their potential to influence GPA.

As always, regression discusses the *differences* in the y-values between individuals. The coefficients *never* tell us what will happen to an individual when his or her x_i increases by one unit since that is a statement about cause and effect and regression is not a physical law.

Example—`TIPS`

In the `TIPS` dataset, the tip percentage (`TipPercentage`, 0-100) left on bills for a particular waiter have been recorded along with the bill amount (`Bill`) and the number of people in the party (`PartySize`). Figure 4.5 shows that the relationships between tip percentage and these variables are roughly linear. Multiple regression is an appropriate model for this problem.

Figure 4.5 — Scatterplot matrix for TIPS dataset. The relationships between the y variable (`TipPercentage`) and both x_1 = `Bill` and x_2 =`PartySize` look roughly linear, so a multiple regression model should be appropriate. There is a positive correlation between `Bill` and `PartySize` (a bill will be larger when more people are ordering food and drinks).

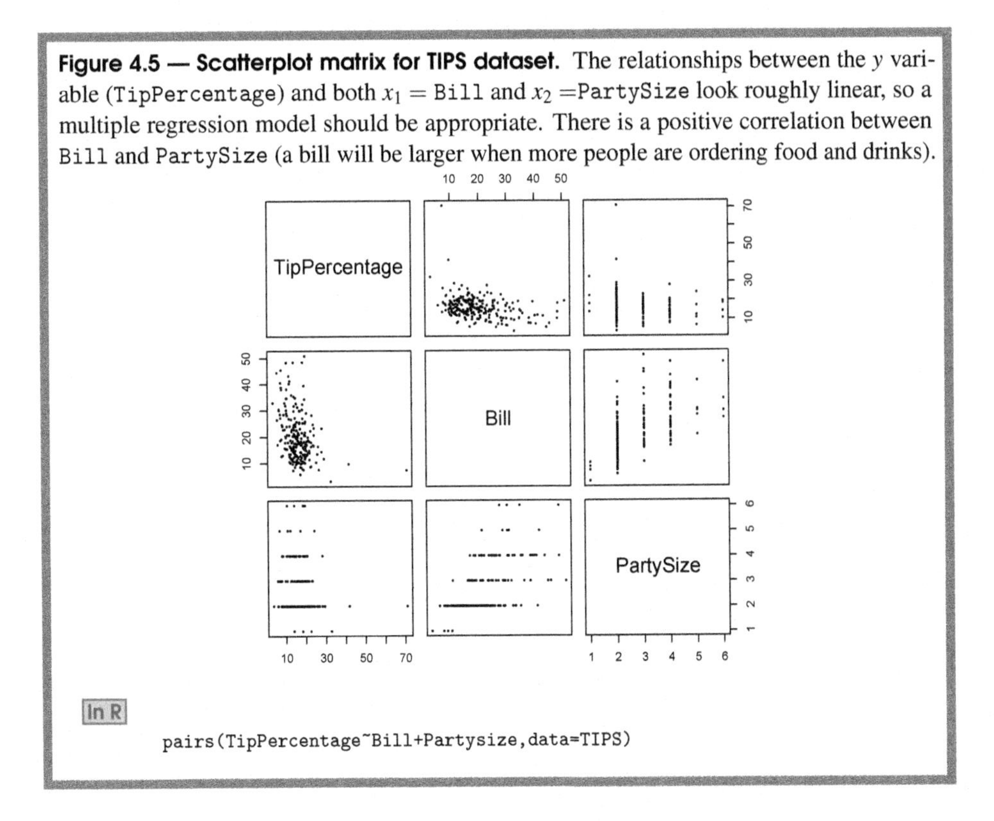

In R

```
pairs(TipPercentage~Bill+Partysize,data=TIPS)
```

Let us fit a multiple regression model predicting the tip percentage from these two variables and interpret the output.

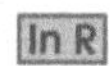

```
M <- lm(TipPercentage~Bill+PartySize,data=TIPS)
summary(M)

             Estimate Std. Error t value Pr(>|t|)
(Intercept) 19.90159    1.09886  18.111  < 2e-16 ***
Bill        -0.27062    0.05173  -5.231 3.66e-07 ***
PartySize    0.59704    0.48421   1.233    0.219

Multiple R-squared:  0.1203,Adjusted R-squared:  0.113
```

Writing the regression equation, we find:

$$TipPercent = 19.90 - 0.27Bill + 0.60Partysize$$

We interpret the coefficients as follows:

- The coefficient of Bill is -0.27. Two tables whose bill amounts differ by \$1 (but which are identical in terms of `PartySize`) are expected to differ in tip percentage by 0.27% (the units of `TipPercent` are percentage points, from 0-100). Since the coefficient is negative, the larger bill is expected to have a smaller tip percentage.
- The coefficient of `PartySize` is 0.60. Two tables whose party sizes differ by one (but which are identical in terms of total bill amount) are expected to differ in tip percentage by 0.6%. Since the coefficient is positive, the bigger party is expected to leave a higher tip percentage.

The model is not a great fit to the data—R^2 is 0.12 and R^2_{adj} is only 0.113. Thus, bill amount and party size are relatively poor predictors of the tip percentages. Convention is to leave between 15-20% of the bill as a tip, regardless of the size of the bill and regardless of the number of people in the party, so we should not be surprised that these variables are poor predictors of tip percentages.

Perhaps other predictors would do a better job, or it could be the case that tip percentages are so variable and subjective that for all intents and purposes they appear nearly random. It would be interesting to use people's income levels, savings/checking account balances, amount they donate to charity, etc., but collecting this sort of information for the study is not feasible.

Example—Education analytics

In the education analytics dataset (`EDUCATION`), the college GPA of a student is recorded along with information about that student from high school, e.g., GPA (`HSGPA`), ACT score (`ACT`), and the number of clubs to which the student belonged (`ClubsInHS`). Let us fit a multiple regression model predicting college GPA from these three variables.

Figure 4.6 — Scatterplot matrix for EDUCATION dataset. The relationship between College GPA and other variables looks roughly linear, so a multiple regression model may be appropriate. There may be some positive correlations between the predictor variables.

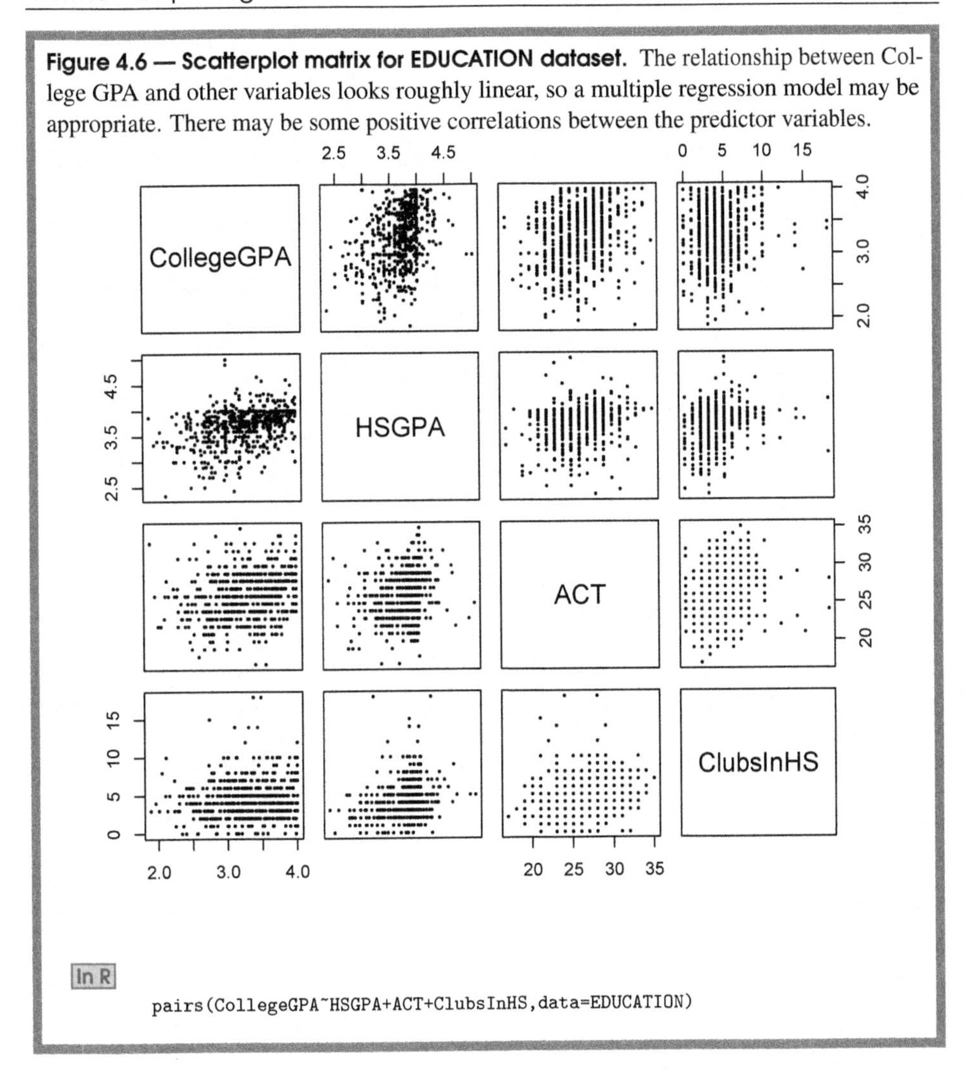

In R

```
pairs(CollegeGPA~HSGPA+ACT+ClubsInHS,data=EDUCATION)
```

In R

```
M <- lm(CollegeGPA~HSGPA+ACT+ClubsInHS,data=EDUCATION)
summary(M)

                Estimate Std. Error t value Pr(>|t|)
(Intercept)  1.106064   0.200499   5.517 5.14e-08 ***
HSGPA        0.418864   0.049595   8.446 2.26e-16 ***
ACT          0.023710   0.005559   4.265 2.32e-05 ***
ClubsInHS   -0.001885   0.007030  -0.268    0.789

Multiple R-squared:  0.1665,Adjusted R-squared:  0.1624
```

Writing out the regression equation:

$$CollegeGPA = 1.106 + 0.419HSGPA + 0.024ACT - 0.002ClubsInHS$$

Figure 4.6 shows that the relationship between college GPA and each predictor is roughly linear. Thus, multiple regression should be an appropriate model. We interpret the coefficients (quite verbosely) as follows:

- The coefficient of HSGPA is 0.42. This means that two students whose high school GPAs differ by one point (but who are identical in terms of ACT score and number of clubs) are expected to differ in college GPA by 0.42 points. Since the coefficient is positive, the student with the higher high school GPA is also expected to have a higher college GPA.
- The coefficient of ACT is 0.02. This means that two students whose ACT scores differ by one point (but who are identical in terms of high school GPA and number of clubs) are expected to differ in college GPA by 0.02 points. Since the coefficient is positive, the student with the higher ACT score is expected to have a higher college GPA.
- The coefficient of ClubsinHS is −0.002. This means that two students who differed in the number of high school clubs by one (but who are identical in terms of high school GPA and ACT score) are expected to differ in college GPA by 0.002 points. Since the coefficient is negative, the student who participated in more clubs is expected to have a lower college GPA.

4.2.4 Coefficients are model-dependent

The *value* and *meaning* of b_i will change depending on what other predictors are in the model. These changes occur because there is correlation, i.e., redundancy, between predictors. Only when predictors are independent (which will only occur for carefully designed experiments) will coefficients remain the same regardless of what other variables are in the model.

Logically, we should *expect* this behavior. By definition, we interpret b_i as the expected difference in y among two "otherwise identical individuals" who happen to differ in x_i by one unit. The "otherwise identical" means the same values for the other x's in the model. If we compare the coefficient of x_i in one model to its coefficient in another, then the two sets of individuals under comparison are potentially quite different.

For example, the coefficient of `HSGPA` in a model with `ACT` and `ClubsInHS` was found to be 0.42. In a model without `ACT`, the coefficient becomes 0.47. You may wonder which is the "right" coefficient, but the answer is "both."

- In the first model, we are comparing two students who have the same ACT scores and who belong to the same number of clubs.
- In the second model, we are only comparing two students who belong to the same number of clubs (they may or may not have the same ACT scores).
- The types of students in the first comparison may be quite different than the types of students in the second, so we should not be surprised when the difference in GPAs is different.

Example—`SALARY` data

Imagine we are interested in figuring out how much an additional year of education "buys" an employee in terms of extra salary. Since salary is connected to educational level and to previous job experience, and because these two quantities may be correlated, it is necessary to first account for the effect of prior experience on salary if we truly wish to isolate the association between salary and education (or vice versa).

Consider first a simple linear regression predicting `Salary` from `Education` in the `SALARY` dataset.

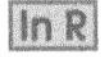

```
M <- lm(Salary~Education,data=SALARY)
summary(M)

             Estimate Std. Error t value Pr(>|t|)
(Intercept)  3228.83      99.88  32.327  < 2e-16 ***
Education      85.39      19.80   4.313 4.08e-05 ***
```

The regression equation is:

$$Salary = 3229 + 85Education$$

The slope of the line is 85, implying that two individuals who differ in their education by one year are expected to differ in their monthly salary by $85 (with the more educated person receiving the higher salary).

Now consider a multiple regression model predicting salary from education and experience.

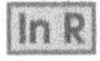

```
M <- lm(Salary~Education+Experience,data=SALARY)
summary(M)

             Estimate Std. Error t value Pr(>|t|)
(Intercept)  3097.93     113.82  27.218  < 2e-16 ***
Education      89.83      19.47   4.613 1.31e-05 ***
Experience     13.17       5.87   2.244   0.0273 *
```

The regression equation is:

$$Salary = 3100 + 90Education + 13Experience$$

The coefficient of `Education` is now 90. Thus, two employees with the same prior work experience but who differ in their education by one year are expected to differ in monthly salary by $90.

Notice that the coefficient of `Education` has changed from 85 in the simple linear regression to 90 in the multiple regression. Why the discrepancy? According to the simple linear regression, a difference of one year of education is associated with a difference of $85 in salary, but *some* of this expected difference can be attributed to varying levels of prior work experience. Recall that these two variables have a negative correlation in the data, so the person with the higher amount of education is expected to have a lower amount of experience. Since `Experience` is not in the model, there is no guarantee that the two individuals we are comparing have the same prior work experience.

The multiple regression makes the more *specific* (and interesting) comparison between two employees who differ in `Education` by one year *and* who have the same amount of prior experience. See Aside 4.1 for further exposition.

To compare the impact of `Education` and `Experience` on `Salary`, we can compare their coefficients in the multiple regression.

- The coefficient of experience is 13. Two employees who differ in experience by one year (but who are identical in terms of education) are expected to differ in salary by $13.
- The coefficient of education is 90. Two employees who differ in education by one year (but who are identical in terms of experience) are expected to differ in salary by $90.

Since the coefficient of education is larger (more accurately, farther from zero), it appears that an additional year of education is "worth" more to this company than an additional year of experience.

We would overstep the scope of the model if we were to say that an additional year of education *makes* someone's salary go up by $90. A coefficient in a multiple regression model describes the average difference in y among two otherwise identical individuals who happen to differ in x by one unit, *not* what happens when an individual's value of x increases by one unit. A regression equation is not a physical law, so we cannot make any statements about cause and effect.

Aside 4.1 — Understanding why coefficients are model-dependent. To further grasp why coefficients are model-dependent, consider the following deterministic example. Imagine the company uses the following equation exactly when determining salary:

$$Salary = 5000 + 20Education + 10Experience$$

Thus, two employees who differ in Education by one year (but who have the same amount of prior experience) will differ in Salary by exactly $20.

Now imagine that, for whatever reason, the company employs only two types of individuals:

- Education = 0 and Experience = 4 (no education but highly experienced)
- Education = 4 and Experience = 0 (no experience but highly educated)
- Education and Experience are perfectly correlated (if you know the value of Education, then you know the value of Experience, and vice versa)

If the company operates this way, then there are only two possible values for Salary: 5040 (no education but highly experienced) or 5080 (no experience but highly educated). Thus, a dataset of company salaries would look very simple:

Salary	Education	Experience
5040	0	4
5080	4	0

A simple linear regression predicting Salary from Education has the equation (plug in numbers to verify):

$$Salary = 5040 + 10Education$$

The coefficient of Education has gone from 20 to 10 because the effect of Education is getting "canceled out" due to its correlation with Experience. People with higher education at this company have less experience, so the effect of Education on Salary gets diminished.

Thus, the simple linear regression misses how Salary and Education are truly connected. The multiple regression model, where we can account for Experience, is necessary to understand what is really going on.

Example—Body Fat data

An individual's body fat percentage is best measured by "hydrostatic testing"—a process that requires submersion of the individual in a tank of water. The procedure is time consuming and expensive. The goal of the BODYFAT dataset is to develop a model that can predict someone's body fat percentage from more easily obtainable physical measurements such as the circumferences of the neck and abdomen. Figure 4.7 shows the scatterplot matrix of some of the variables in the dataset. Imagine we are interested in describing the relationship between someone's body fat percentage (BodyFat) and his or her neck circumference (Neck).

Figure 4.7 — Scatterplot matrix of BODYFAT data. We want to predict someone's body fat percentage from the circumferences of various body parts. The relationships between body fat and the predictors (top row) look to be linear, so a multiple regression is appropriate. However, the coefficients will be challenging to interpret and will have large standard errors because of the extreme amount of correlation between the predictors.

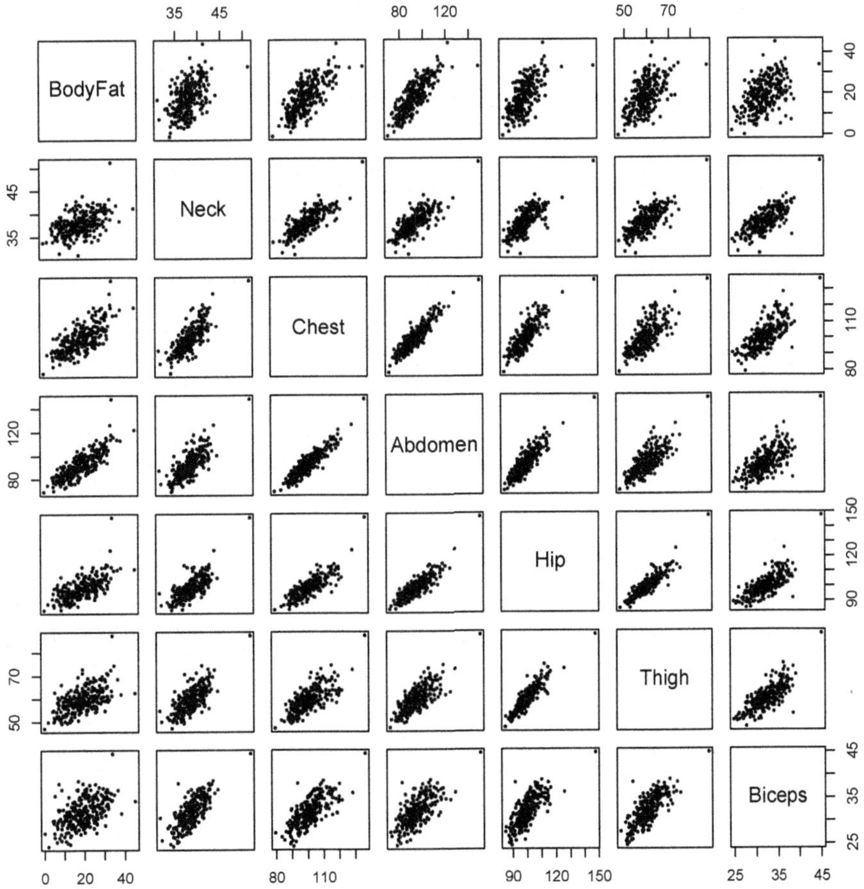

In R

```
pairs(BodyFat~Neck+Chest+Abdomen+Hip+Thigh+Biceps,data=BODYFAT)
```

Let us begin by fitting a simple linear regression. The units of BodyFat are in percentage points (0-100) and the units of Neck are centimeters. The coefficient of Neck turns out to be 1.57.

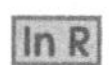

```
M <- lm(BodyFat~Neck,data=BODYFAT)
summary(M)

             Estimate Std. Error t value Pr(>|t|)
(Intercept) -40.5985     6.6857  -6.072 4.66e-09 ***
Neck          1.5671     0.1756   8.923  < 2e-16 ***
```

Thus, two people who differ in their neck circumferences by 1cm are expected to differ in their body fat percentages by 1.57% (wider neck implies a higher body fat percentage). However, people who differ in neck circumference may also differ in other physical measurements. Let us account for differences in abdomen circumferences (Abdomen) by fitting a multiple regression model.

```
M <- lm(BodyFat~Neck+Abdomen,data=BODYFAT)
summary(M)

(Intercept) -15.1075     4.4370  -3.405 0.000771 ***
Abdomen       0.7383     0.0382  19.329  < 2e-16 ***
Neck         -0.9026     0.1694  -5.327 2.23e-07 ***
```

The coefficient of Neck is now -0.90. Thus, two people who differ in neck circumference by 1cm (but who have identical abdomen sizes) are expected to differ in their body fat percentages by 0.90% (wider neck implies a *lower* body fat percentage).

The results of the multiple regression appear confusing at first. The coefficient of Neck is negative, while in the simple linear regression it was positive (an apparent contradiction). Further, a negative coefficient for Neck seems to fly in the face of intuition—we envision people with thicker necks as having a higher body fat percentage (as the simple linear regression suggests).

To resolve these "contradictions," we must remember that coefficients in a regression model are commenting on how *individuals differ from each other*, not what happens when *an individual's value* of x increases by one unit. The negative coefficient of Neck means that among people (in this dataset) with identical abdomen sizes, wider necks are associated with lower body fat percentages.

(C) The negative sign of Neck in the multiple regression *may* have a logical justification. Imagine that this data consists of 35-year-old white males, and let's focus specifically on men who have abdomen sizes of 32 inches. Among these specific men, neck size variation is probably due to the amount of *muscle* the man has on his body. If a guy has a thick neck but a small, 32-inch abdomen, he probably has a more muscular frame overall and thus a lower body fat percentage.

Lesson and implications

Coefficients being model-specific is a fundamental reason why many studies that you may read about in the news contradict each other. For example, if you Google "diet soda" and "weight gain," many hits will be to studies linking diet soda to *gaining* weight. Most pages refer to the San Antonio Heart Study, which followed more than 5000 adults over seven or eight years. This study compared people who drank diet soda to people who drank sugar-sweetened soda and found it was more likely that diet soda drinkers became obese.

Of course, it could have been the case that people who were on the path to becoming obese tried to slow the process down by drinking diet soda. If so, it was obesity that "caused" diet soda drinking instead of the other way around. Another alternative explanation could be (though it seems far-fetched) that people with poor diets (and thus who are likely to be obese) prefer diet soda for whatever reason.

However, a 2014 (industry-funded) study claims that diet soda helps weight *loss*. This study compared water drinkers to diet soda drinkers and found that diet soda drinkers tended to lose more weight. In essence, the first study found the sign of the coefficient of diet soda drinking to be positive, while the second found the coefficient to be negative. Thus, the results of the studies appear to contradict each other. Is one study "wrong" while the other is "right"? It may be the case that *both* studies can be correct.

Read the study at `http://www.cnn.com/2014/05/27/health/dietsoda-weight-loss/`

The contradiction between studies (assuming they were conducted correctly) can be resolved by examining what other variables were accounted for by the researchers' models. If they controlled for a different set of variables (e.g., one controlled for overall level of health, age, race, and profession while the other controlled for age, gender, and income level), then it's very possible to naturally obtain different signs for the same coefficient. This is what happened in the `BODYFAT` dataset—the coefficient of `Neck` is positive when predicting `BodyFat` by itself (accounting for nothing else), while it was negative when predicting `BodyFat` after accounting for `Abdomen`.

In order to meaningfully compare the typical value of y between two groups, the only significant difference between groups must be the one factor being studied. Any other differences are lurking variables and provide an alternative explanation for why the groups may differ.

Most of the time, it is impossible to ensure otherwise identical groups. However, multiple regression allows us to do this (at least artificially) by putting these lurking variables into the model and accounting for them. The key to a good study is accounting for the "right" set of variables so that the coefficient of your predictor of interest actually answers the question being posed.

In the case of the water vs. diet drink study, the researchers took about 300 adults who regularly had diet soda to drink and told half to continue their diet soda drinking and half to only drink water. Could there be differences in the groups besides what they were drinking?

- Overall diet? The random assignment into groups likely ensures there is no systematic difference in overall diets between water drinkers and soda drinkers.
- Exercise? The random assignment into groups likely ensures there is no systematic difference in the exercise between water drinkers and soda drinkers.
- Willpower? Although all people were coached regarding their choice of meals and exercise, it could be the case that the water-only drinkers had a tougher time making healthier choices since they were the only group that had to *change* their habits.
- Something unanticipated?

It is unclear whether *either* diet drink study accounted for *every* important difference between diet soda drinkers and non-diet soda drinkers. Who really knows the "right" set of variables to include in the multiple regression to solve this problem? Thus, neither study represents the final word about a connection between diet soda drinking and weight loss. Further, the results are not actually contradictory because they use different sets of "lurking" variables in the model (the water study did not account for any other variables, while the San Antonio study accounted for "baseline BMI" and "demographic/behavioral characteristics").

4.3 Inference

The estimated coefficient b_i found with least squares is the **point estimate**, i.e., "best guess," for β_i. As with simple linear regression, we don't expect our estimate to *exactly* equal "the truth," but it should be close.

The standard error of the estimated coefficient, abbreviated SE_{b_i}, measures how far off we think b_i may be from β_i, i.e., how far our estimate is from "the truth." The amount of uncertainty in an estimated coefficient depends not only on how well the model fits the data as a whole (via R^2), but also on the amount of correlation and redundant information in the predictors. Review Section 3.3.1 for a discussion on standard errors in the context of a simple linear regression.

4.3.1 The standard error of a coefficient

It is possible to write the equation for the standard error of the slope b_1 in a simple linear regression (Equation 3.8) in terms of the standard deviations of x and y and the R^2 of the regression:

$$\text{Simple Linear Regression:} \quad SE_{b_1} = \frac{SD_y}{SD_x}\sqrt{\frac{1-R^2}{n-2}} \tag{4.6}$$

An analogous formula for the standard error of the coefficient b_i in a multiple regression model exists. First, let us consider a model that predicts x_i from *all other* predictors.

$$x_i = a_0 + a_1x_1 + a_2x_2 + \ldots a_{i-1}x_{i-1} + a_{i+1}x_{i+1} + \ldots + a_kx_k$$

Let us define R_i^2 as the value of R^2 for this multiple regression. Then,

$$\text{Multiple Regression:} \quad SE_{b_i} = \frac{SD_y}{SD_{x_i}}\sqrt{\frac{1-R^2}{(1-R_i^2)(n-k-1)}} \tag{4.7}$$

The same insights regarding the standard error for simple linear regression still apply.

- SE_{b_i} is smaller when the values of x_i are more spread out (i.e., SD_{x_i} is larger)
- SE_{b_i} is smaller when the fit is better (higher R^2)
- SE_{b_i} is smaller when there is more data (larger n)

However, the formula for SE_{b_i} in multiple regression has an additional component that measures the "redundancy" of the predictor x_i. If x_i can be predicted accurately from the other x's (i.e., R_i^2 is large), then much of the information that x_i provides about y may already be given by the other predictors. If this is the case, it is difficult to disentangle the "effect" of x_i on y from the effects of the other x's on y, making the standard error of b_i larger than it would have been had the predictors been independent.

When x_i is well-predicted by the other x's, the quantity $1 - R_i^2$ will be close to zero, so the denominator in the formula for the standard error will be very small. Dividing by a number close to zero makes the result very large, so the standard error will be large.

This effect can also be understood by remembering how to interpret b_i. The coefficient tells us the expected difference in y between two otherwise identical individuals who differ in x_i by one unit. When x_i is highly correlated with some of the other predictors, it becomes difficult to find or envision individuals who differ in x_i but not in any other variables since they all change together.

For example, imagine predicting the price of tomatoes based on the price of oil and the price of gas (each factor into the transportation costs of bringing the food from a farm to the store). The prices of oil and gas are highly correlated. The coefficient of gas price in the model is interpreted as the expected difference in the price of tomatoes on days where gas prices differ by one unit but oil prices are the same. Although such days surely exist, they are relatively rare since gas and oil prices go hand in hand. Thus, the amount of uncertainty regarding the coefficient should be large.

Aside 4.2 provides additional non-obvious insights gained from analyzing the formula for the standard error. In addition, it provides justification for performing multiple (instead of simple) linear regression and for tweaking what variables exist in the model once it has been fit.

4.3.2 Confidence interval for β_i

As with simple linear regression (Section 3.3.1), when the assumptions regarding the disturbances are true, i.e., $\varepsilon \sim N(0, \sigma)$, b_i will probably only be up to about two standard errors away from "the truth," β_i. Thus, an approximate 95% confidence interval for β_i is:

$$b_i \pm 2SE_{b_i} \tag{4.8}$$

The number in front of SE_{b_i} may be a little larger or smaller than 2 depending on the number of predictors in the model as well as the sample size. Software should be used to calculate the exact number.

Although we have previously discussed the meaning of "confidence" and what a confidence interval does and does not tell us, a reminder never hurts. By design, the *procedure* (taking b_i and calculating $\pm 2SE$) for making a 95% confidence interval has a 95% chance of being correct (β_i is inside the interval) and a 5% chance of being wrong. While you will never know if a particular confidence interval contains β_i, in the long-run 95% of the time your intervals will. This statement is what we mean when we say we have "confidence" in an interval.

Aside 4.2 — Some insights about the standard error of coefficients. The formula for SE_{b_i} yields some interesting and useful insights that are not immediately obvious.

- If the other x's are "good" predictors of y and are not too strongly correlated with x_i, then SE_{b_i} in the multiple regression model will be *smaller* than SE_{b_1} in the simple linear regression. Informally, this is because the multiple regression model removes the extraneous variation of y from the other x's (i.e., the variation not associated with x_i), making our estimate of how y and x_i vary together more precise. This is a key reason why people do multiple regression!

  (C) Mathematically, this occurs when the value $(1-R^2)/(n-k-1)$ term is smaller than the $(1-R^2)/(n-2)$ term in the simple regression formula. For the standard error to be smaller in the multiple regression, the increase in R^2 when adding the other predictors in the model must be enough so that the decrease in the denominator $n-k-1$ results in a smaller number.

- If x_i is strongly correlated with the other x's, then SE_{b_i} in the multiple regression model *may be higher* than it is in the simple linear regression model. Informally, this is because the model attempts to compare individuals who differ in x_i but who are identical in the other x's, i.e., it tries to disentangle the effect of x_i from the other variables. If all the x's change together, this is difficult, and the coefficients cannot be nailed down with much precision.

  (C) The quantity $1-R^2$ always gets smaller when going from simple to multiple regression. If x_i is highly correlated with the other x's, it may be the case that $(1-R_i^2)(n-k-1)$ is small enough that the fraction of the two make the standard error larger.

- If the other x's are not good predictors of y, then SE_{b_i} in the multiple regression model can be *larger* than SE_{b_1} from the simple linear regression. This is an argument for "kicking out" unimportant variables, and we will return to this when we discuss model selection.

  (C) Mathematically, this is because the increase in R^2 when adding in the other x's is not enough to offset the increase in the number of variables, i.e., the quantity $(1-R^2)/(n-k-1)$ actually gets bigger.

Confidence intervals in a multiple regression model require some special consideration. When there are many predictors, there is a pretty good chance that *at least one* of the confidence intervals is wrong. For example, with five predictors there is about a 23% chance that at least one is wrong. With 10 predictors, this increases to 40%. With 20 predictors, the chance that at least one is wrong is 64%, and with 50 predictors, this increases to about 92%. In fact, we *expect* 5% of 95% confidence intervals to be incorrect. The unfortunate part is that we will never know *which* 5%.

(C) The calculations presented assume that each predictor is independent of one another. The probability that at least one is wrong is $1 - P(\textit{all correct}) = 1 - (0.95)^k$.

Multiple regression works best when there is a single question being asked: what is the expected difference in y between two (otherwise identical) individuals who differ in x_i by one unit, and how uncertain are we about the expected difference? The answer to this question is b_i along with its standard error or confidence interval.

4.3.3 Variance inflation factor and collinearity

The standard error of an estimated coefficient b_i depends on how well x_i can be predicted from the other x's. Large values of R_i^2 (the value of R^2 in a regression predicting x_i from the other x's) indicate that the information about y contained in x_i may be redundant with the information provided by the other variables. Consequently, the model has a hard time disentangling the association between y and x_i from the associations between y and the other predictors. The net result is that SE_{b_i} can be much larger than it would have been had x_i been independent of the other x's.

This "inflation" in the standard error can be explained from another angle. Imagine that we are predicting y from x_1 and x_2. The correlation between x_1 and x_2 is high, so some of the information about x_1 is contained in x_2 and vice versa. When both x_1 and x_2 are in the model, there is *less* overall information about y than if both predictors were independent. Thus, the amount of uncertainty (and thus standard error) regarding the coefficients is larger when x_1 and x_2 are correlated than when x_1 and x_2 are independent (and two independent sets of information are available).

The **variance inflation factor**, or VIF, quantifies the increase in standard error (relative to the case where the predictors are independent) due to the correlation among the predictors. If R_i^2 is the value of R^2 for the regression predicting x_i from the other x's, then:

$$VIF_i = \frac{1}{1-R_i^2} \tag{4.9}$$

A VIF of 1.0 means that x_i is uncorrelated with the other x's. The value $\sqrt{VIF}$ tells us how many times larger the correlation among predictors has made the standard error compared to the case where x_i is independent of them. For example, if x_i has a VIF of 9, this means that SE_{b_i} is $\sqrt{9} = 3$ times larger than it would have been had x_i been independent of the other predictors.

A VIF of about 5-10 or larger is universally accepted as indicative of a large amount of redundancy between predictors. An alternative threshold is given by $1/(1-R^2)$, where R^2 is from the multiple regression predicting y.

C If $VIF_i > 1/(1-R^2)$, then the x's do a better job at predicting x_i than they do at predicting y.

If a variable has a *very* large VIF (greater than 10), then it is said to be nearly *collinear* with the other predictors, i.e., essentially a weighted sum of the other x's. If many variables have large VIFs, then we say the regression suffers from **multicollinearity**.

The scatterplot matrix provides a quick check for seeing how strongly predictors are related. However, it may be the case that complex three-way or higher dependencies exist, so looking at the VIFs is necessary.

> Large VIFs and the presence of multicollinearity do *not* invalidate a model. Rather, they indicate that the model is having difficulty pinning down the coefficients of the predictor variables.

Consequences of large VIFs are as follows:

- Standard errors of the coefficients are much larger than they would have been had the predictors been independent. They may even be larger than the corresponding standard errors found in simple linear regressions.
- Coefficients may be very sensitive to the particular set of *data* on which the model was built. Addition or deletion of a data point may drastically change the coefficients.
- Coefficients are very sensitive to the set of *predictors* used in the model. Adding or removing a predictor in the model can drastically change the coefficients.
- Predicted values and their standard errors are not affected by multicollinearity.

Dealing with multicollinearity is difficult. Multiple regression is best when the goal is to estimate one particular coefficient while accounting for other sources of extraneous variation. If that variable has a large VIF and is nearly collinear with the other predictors, either the experiment was designed poorly (next time, choose x-values that minimize the correlation between the predictors) or the correlations between predictors is built-in from nature. Ridge regression and the lasso method minimize a penalized sum of squared errors (with penalty proportional to the size of the coefficients) and provide somewhat of a recourse for this situation, but those are topics for a more advanced course.

4.3.4 Examples: salary and body fat data

Let us revisit the `SALARY` and `BODYFAT` datasets and study the effects of correlation among the predictors.

Salary

The regression model is $Salary = \beta_0 + \beta_1 Education + \beta_2 Experience + \varepsilon$. The coefficient of `Education` in this model is estimated to be about 90, implying that people who differ in one year of education (but whose years of prior work experience are the same) are expected to differ in salary by $90. Thus, 90 is our point estimate and "best guess" for β_1.

The standard error of the estimate is about 19.50, implying that the measured coefficient is likely off from "the truth" by about 19.5 or so. An approximate 95% confidence interval for the coefficient is $90 \pm (2 \times 19.5)$, or $(51, 129)$. Thus, we are about 95% confident that, when comparing two individuals with equal work experience but who differ in education by one year, the expected difference in salaries is between $51 and $129.

A more careful calculation done by software reveals that the "2" in the formula for the confidence interval should be 1.987. After rounding the final results to the nearest integer, the more precise confidence interval is no different than the one we calculated.

How much has the (weak) correlation between `Education` and `Experience` inflated the standard error relative to the case where they are independent?

- If we make a simple linear regression predicting `Education` from `Experience` (or vice versa), we find that $R^2 = 0.01031$ (very low).
- The VIF for `Education` is $1/(1-R^2) = 1.01$.
- The standard error is $\sqrt{VIF} = \sqrt{1.01} \approx 1.005$ times larger than it would have been had `Education` and `Experience` been independent.

Thus, the coefficient of `Education` is well-estimated, and its standard error is essentially the smallest it could have been. Further, since the VIFs are very low, the coefficients of these variables in the multiple regression should be about the same as they are in simple linear regressions (they are—the coefficient of `Education` in a simple linear regression is 85.4, and the coefficient of `Experience` in a simple linear regression is 10.4).

Body fat

Figure 4.7 shows that all predictor variables (circumferences of body parts) are highly correlated with each other. We anticipate the VIFs to be large. Further, we would not be surprised if the coefficients in the multiple regression are quite different than the coefficients in simple linear regressions. Table 4.1 shows the relevant information for the simple and multiple regressions for each predictor.

Table 4.1 — Coefficients for single and multiple regression models using Body Fat data. The predictors are highly correlated, and their VIFs in the multiple regression model are large. Thus, we are not surprised when a coefficient is quite different than its value in a simple linear regression.

	Coefficient in		Standard Error in		
Term	Simple LR	Multiple LR	Simple LR	Multiple LR	VIF
Neck	1.57	-0.79	0.18	0.19	3.1
Chest	0.65	-0.09	0.04	0.09	7.6
Abdomen	0.58	0.95	0.03	0.07	8.6
Hip	0.68	-0.46	0.05	0.11	9.0
Thigh	0.83	0.19	0.08	0.12	5.9
Biceps	1.26	0.14	0.14	0.15	3.1

Indeed, the VIFs of the predictors are fairly large. The R^2 for the multiple regression is about 72%, so if x_i has a VIF larger than $1/(1-R^2) = 3.6$, then the x's are doing a better job predicting x_i than predicting y. Indeed, multicollinearity is an issue in this dataset since all but two VIFs exceed this threshold.

As expected, many coefficients change dramatically from the simple to multiple regression. For example, the coefficient of `Biceps` increases by nearly a factor of 10, while the coefficients of `Neck`, `Chest`, and `Hip` flip from positive to negative.

Unlike the `SALARY` data, the standard errors in the multiple regression are *larger* than they were in the simple linear regressions because of the multicollinearity. For example, it is difficult for the model to discern what variation in body fat percentage should be attributed to differences in `Abdomen` vs. `Hip`. `Abdomen` has a VIF of 8.6, implying its standard error is $\sqrt{VIF} = 2.9$ times higher than it would have been had `Hip` been independent of the other predictors.

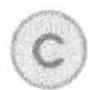

Because of the large VIFs and inflated standard errors, confidence intervals for the coefficients are wider than they would be had the variables been independent.

At this point, you may be asking yourself what we are actually gaining by using a multiple regression to model body fat percentage since the standard errors are larger than in the simple linear regression case. The answer is that if you *really* want to study the association between y and x, you do need to account for other "common cause" and lurking variables that are associated with both y and x. Otherwise, the coefficient of your predictor of interest can be horribly biased.

Recall that when we predicted the top speed of a car from its weight (`AUTO` dataset), the coefficient of its weight was positive (contrary to what is expected from real-world experience); see Figure 2.27. Without accounting for horsepower (which is related to both the weight and top speed of a car), the estimated coefficient was biased!

If the goal of our study is to pin down how `Hip` and `BodyFat` are associated, it would be naive to use a simple linear regression. Variation in body fat percentage is due to *many* different factors. By accounting for these other factors in a multiple regression, we are more accurately answering the question being posed. The question of how body fat percentage varies with physical measurements is particularly tricky.

Finally, let us address the fact that there are negative coefficients (e.g., `Hip`) in the model, which at first glance seem counterintuitive. The model *does not* imply that people with wider hips have lower body fat percentages. Rather, the model implies that *among people with the same* neck, chest, abdomen, thigh, and biceps circumferences, people with wider hips tend to have lower body fat percentages (for whatever reason). Remember that coefficients are *never* a comment on how y and x_i are causally connected—regression equations are not physical laws. Rather, they are comments on how individuals in *your* data happen to differ.

4.4 Statistical Significance

In a simple linear regression, the regression (and thus the predictor) is statistically significant if it reduces the sum of squared errors (relative to the naive model) by more than what is expected "by chance," i.e., by a predictor unrelated to y (Section 3.4). In multiple regression, the significance of the model and the significance of the predictors are treated separately. There are three scenarios:

- The model is not significant (none of the predictors in the model help to predict y).
- The model is significant, and at least one of the predictors is statistically significant.
- The model is significant, but none of the predictors are statistically significant.

The last possibility appears confusing at first glance. Before we can understand how that can be the case, we need to learn exactly what it means for the model and for a predictor to be significant.

4.4.1 Significance of the model

Recall that R^2 of a model tells us the fractional reduction in the sum of squared errors (SSE) compared to the naive model (Equation 4.3):

$$R^2 = \frac{SSE_{naive} - SSE_{regression}}{SSE_{naive}}$$

We have seen that *any* predictor (even one unrelated to y) will reduce the sum of squared errors (and thus increase R^2) when added to a model. To be considered statistically significant, a multiple regression model must reduce the SSE by "significantly" more than the reduction expected from a model predicting y from an equal number of unrelated predictors.

Since R^2 and the sum of squared errors are connected, we can also consider a multiple regression model to be significant if its value of R^2 is significantly larger than the values of R^2 that are produced by models containing predictors unrelated to y. Let us take the p-value of the model to be the probability of observing a value of R^2 at least as large as our model's "by chance." If this probability is less than 5%, the model is statistically significant—*something* in the model helps to predict y. We can estimate this probability by using the permutation procedure (see Aside 4.3).

- Make an artificial dataset by shuffling up the values of y and randomly assigning them to each individual in the dataset. Note: the x-values of the individuals stay the same during this procedure. The random assignment ensures that there is no underlying relationship between y and any of the predictors while respecting the existing correlations between the predictors.

Original			Permutation 1			Permutation 2		
y	x_1	x_2	y	x_1	x_2	y	x_1	x_2
3.2	1.1	7	12.8	1.1	7	3.2	1.1	7
12.8	3.3	6	4.4	3.3	6	9.2	0.5	1
9.2	0.5	1	3.2	0.5	1	4.4	2.0	2
4.4	2.0	2	9.2	2.0	2	12.8	3.3	6

- Calculate the reduction in SSE (or the R^2) for the regression on the artificial dataset and repeat the procedure many times.
- The p-value of the regression is the fraction of models on these artificial datasets that reduce the SSE by at least as much (or have an R^2 at least as high) as that of the original model.
- If the p-value is less than 5%, the model is statistically significant. It is unlikely that a model containing predictors unrelated to y would fit the data at least as well as your model.

Alternatively, when all assumptions of the regression model are true (linearity, equal spread, Normality), we can approximate the p-value with a formula rather than from the permutation procedure. Letting n be the number of observations in the data and k be the number of predictors, the F statistic is defined as:

$$F = \frac{(SSE_{naive} - SSE_{reg})/k}{SSE_{reg}/(n-k-1)} = \frac{n-k-1}{k}\frac{R^2}{1-R^2} \tag{4.10}$$

The numerator of the F statistic is the average reduction in the sum of squared error per predictor in the model. The denominator is essentially the average squared error of the regression. Thus, F is related to the average percentage reduction in sum of squared errors per predictor in the model. A model containing predictors unrelated to y is expected to have an F near 1.0. Large values of F are evidence that *something* in the regression helps to predict y.

Aside 4.3 — Simulating the *p*-value of a regression model. Consider predicting the number of wins of an NFL team based on its "longest" statistics: longest pass, rushing, punt return, kickoff return, and punt. The naive model's sum of squared errors of $SSE_{naive} = 3327$. The sum of squared errors using the regression is $SSE_{reg} = 3278$, a reduction of only 49 (yielding $R^2 = 1.484\%$).

Is the model statistically significant? Does *anything* in the model contain information about the number of wins for the season? Let us estimate the p-value of the model using the permutation procedure. What is the probability that a model with five predictors unrelated to the number of wins would produce a value of R^2 of at least 1.484%?

To run the simulation, we shuffle up the observed values of wins and randomly assign them to teams. This process ensures there is no systematic relationship between the number of wins and the predictors, so the resulting value of R^2 is one that has occurred "by chance." Let us perform 10,000 rounds of the procedure and plot the distribution of R^2 values that occur.

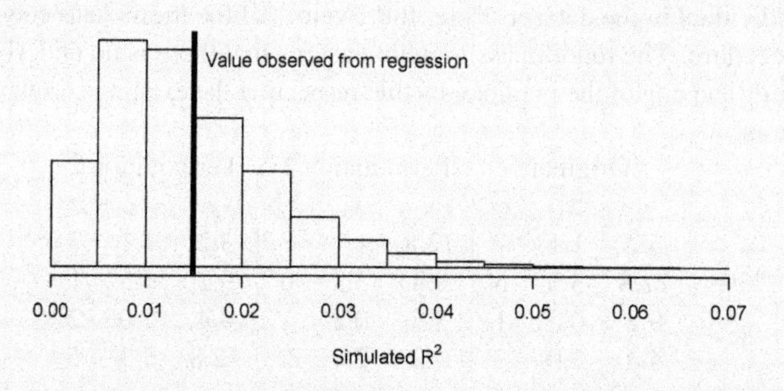

After 10,000 permutations, 3937 "random" models have $R^2 \geq 1.484$. Thus, the p-value of our regression is about 40%. It is fairly likely that a random model that contains no information about the number of wins will have R^2 at least as large as our model, so the regression is not statistically significant.

For the NFL analytics example in Aside 4.3, the value of F is 1.042. The p-value using the formula approximation is 0.3926 (compared to the simulated p-value of 0.3937). Indeed, the approximation gives quite an accurate p-value.

(C) Since the number of wins of an NFL team is an integer between 0 and 16, the Normality assumption is automatically violated. Numbers that come from a Normal distribution can be positive or negative integers, fractions, and decimals. It is somewhat remarkable that the F statistic still yields the correct p-value even though one of the assumptions of the model is violated.

When the regression model is significant, you may then gauge the statistical significance of a subset of predictors or even an individual predictor.

4.4.2 Significance of a subset of predictors (Partial F test)

All else being equal, a simpler model is preferred over a complex model. If possible, it is a good idea to eliminate variables from your model when doing so does not cause its performance to suffer. How can we gauge whether adding a set of variables (thus making the model more complex) is justified from a statistical point of view? We can test whether the *additional* reduction in sum of squared errors when they are added to the model is statistically significant, i.e., more than what would be expected "by chance."

To formalize the procedure, let us define:

- SSE_{simple} as the sum of squared errors when the simpler (fewer variables) regression is used to predict y
- $SSE_{complex}$ as the sum of squared errors when the complex (more variables) regression is used to predict y
- S and C as the number of variables in the simpler and complex regressions, respectively
- n as the number of observations in the data (i.e., the sample size)

Let us consider the quantity:

$$F_{complex} = \frac{(SSE_{simple} - SSE_{complex})(C-S)}{SSE_{complex}/(n-C-1)} = \frac{(R^2_{complex} - R^2_{simple})/(C-S)}{(1-R^2_{complex})/(n-C-1)} \quad (4.11)$$

The numerator in this equation is the reduction in the sum of squared errors when the set of variables is added to the simple model divided by the number of additional predictors and can be thought of as the *additional reduction in SSE per added variable*. The denominator is essentially the average squared error of the complex model. Thus, $F_{complex}$ is related to the percentage reduction in the sum of squared errors per additional variable added to the model. If this quantity is "large," then the model improves significantly when the set of new variables is added. If this quantity is "small," the model doesn't improve when the set of predictors is added by any more than what would be expected by chance.

Alternatively, it is possible to write $F_{complex}$ in terms of the R^2's of both models. $F_{complex}$ is a measure of how much R^2 increases when going from the simple to complex model. This increase needs to be "big enough" per predictor added for the set of variables to be considered significant.

To obtain the p-value of $F_{complex}$, we can once again perform a permutation procedure to find what values of $F_{complex}$ occur by chance. However, when the assumptions of the regression model are true, the p-value can be found via a formula instead.

> A test of significance of a *set* of predictors (in the "complex" model) is called the **partial F test**. If the p-value of the test is $< 5\%$, then the set of predictors is statistically significant. The predictors are "worth" including in the model since they reduce the sum of squared errors by more than what would be expected "by chance." If the p-value is $\geq 5\%$, then the set of predictors is not significant and all of them can be omitted from the model.

For example, in the `OFFENSE` dataset, we wish to predict the number of wins per season of an NFL team from basic offense statistics (first downs, passing yards, interceptions, rushing yards, fumbles, and field goal attempts). The output of the model is in Aside 4.4.

Aside 4.4 — Model for Wins in NFL. Output for regression model predicting the number of wins in a season based on some offensive statistics.

In R

```
M.complex <- lm(Win~.,data=OFFENSE)
summary(M.complex)
                       Estimate Std. Error t value Pr(>|t|)
(Intercept)          -2.0985150  1.5966798  -1.314 0.189626
FirstDowns            0.0175679  0.0081365   2.159 0.031534 *
PassingYards          0.0008370  0.0004881   1.715 0.087327 .
Interceptions        -0.1882616  0.0276628  -6.806 4.52e-11 ***
RushingYards          0.0018488  0.0005589   3.308 0.001039 **
Fumbles              -0.0518398  0.0210173  -2.467 0.014133 *
X1to19FGAttempts      0.3445560  0.1829584   1.883 0.060515 .
X20to29FGAttempts     0.1540869  0.0403779   3.816 0.000161 ***
X30to39FGAttempts     0.1154927  0.0395026   2.924 0.003690 **
X40to50FGAttempts     0.0315441  0.0385457   0.818 0.413725
---
Residual standard error: 2.184 on 342 degrees of freedom
Multiple R-squared:  0.5097,Adjusted R-squared:  0.4968
F-statistic:  39.5 on 9 and 342 DF,  p-value: < 2.2e-16
```

A simpler model without field goal information has:

In R

```
M.simple <- lm(Win~FirstDowns+PassingYards+Interceptions+
            RushingYards+Fumbles,data=OFFENSE)
summary(M.simple)

                 Estimate Std. Error t value Pr(>|t|)
(Intercept)    -0.0301010  1.5597110  -0.019 0.984614
FirstDowns      0.0191109  0.0083629   2.285 0.022906 *
PassingYards    0.0009137  0.0005017   1.821 0.069410 .
Interceptions  -0.2043880  0.0282056  -7.246 2.81e-12 ***
RushingYards    0.0019981  0.0005706   3.502 0.000522 ***
Fumbles        -0.0547601  0.0215481  -2.541 0.011480 *
---
Residual standard error: 2.249 on 346 degrees of freedom
Multiple R-squared:  0.4741,Adjusted R-squared:  0.4665
```

This model has an $R^2_{complex} = 50.97\%$. Can we eliminate information about field-goal attempts without the model suffering? This simpler model has $R^2_{simple} = 47.41\%$. Thus, information about field goals increases R^2 by about 3.56%. Is this statistically significant?

The p-value of the increase in R^2 turns out to be 7.7×10^{-5} (the number under the `Pr(>F)` column heading in the anova output). There is only about a 0.008% chance (much less than 5%) that adding a set of predictors unrelated to the number of wins would increase R^2 by as much as adding information about field goals. Thus, these four variables should be included in the regression model.

In R

```
M.complex <- lm(Win~.,data=OFFENSE)
M.simple <- lm(Win~FirstDowns+PassingYards+Interceptions+
            RushingYards+Fumbles,data=OFFENSE)
```

```
anova(M.simple,M.complex)

Analysis of Variance Table

Model 1: Win ~ FirstDowns + PassingYards + Interceptions + RushingYards +
    Fumbles
Model 2: Win ~ FirstDowns + PassingYards + Interceptions + RushingYards +
    Fumbles + X1to19FGAttempts + X20to29FGAttempts + X30to39FGAttempts +
    X40to50FGAttempts
  Res.Df    RSS Df Sum of Sq      F    Pr(>F)
1    346 1749.8
2    342 1631.2  4    118.59 6.2161 7.727e-05 ***
```

4.4.3 Significance of individual predictors

The significance of an individual predictor can be found via the partial F test comparing the R^2 (or sum of squared errors) of the model with the predictor to the R^2 of the model without it. However, standard regression output reports the p-value of this test automatically (in R it is the number under the `Pr(>|t|)` column in the row with the name of the predictor), so no extra calculations are required.

> An individual predictor is statistically significant if the reduction in the sum of squared errors *when it is added to a model with all other variables already in it* is "large," i.e., unlikely to have been produced by the addition of a predictor unrelated to y.
>
> A predictor that is not significant in a multiple regression model may contain a good deal of information about y (i.e., has a strong association with y), but the information it contains is redundant with the information about y already provided by the other predictors.

If the p-value is less than 5%, the predictor is significant. The predictor offers information about y *above and beyond* what the other predictors have to offer. If the p-value is 5% or greater, the predictor is not significant. It could be eliminated from the model since any information it may have about y is already provided by the other predictors.

An alternative way of checking significance is finding a 95% confidence interval for β_i. If the interval contains zero (implying that zero is a plausible value for the coefficient), then x_i is not statistically significant.

For example, reconsider the `OFFENSE` dataset, where we predict the number of wins based on a variety of offensive statistics (Aside 4.4).

- `FirstDowns` is statistically significant since its p-value (0.031) is less than 5%. This means that adding `FirstDowns` to a model that already contains the eight other predictors reduces the sum of squared errors by more than the reduction that we'd expect from a predictor unrelated to `Win`. `FirstDowns` contributes information about `Win` above and beyond what the other predictors have to offer. We should keep it in the model.
- `PassingYards` is not statistically significant since its p-value (0.087) is greater than 5%. The implication is that the information about `Win` provided by `PassingYards` is redundant with the information already provided by the other variables. We could eliminate it from the model.

PassingYards not being significant in the multiple regression does *not* mean that it tells us nothing about Win. In fact, the regression predicting Win from only PassingYards is highly statistically significant with a p-value of 6.6×10^{-14}.

```
              Estimate Std. Error t value Pr(>|t|)
(Intercept)  1.4513002  0.8507759   1.706   0.0889 .
PassingYards 0.0019068  0.0002441   7.812 6.61e-14 ***
```

While there is a strong association between PassingYards and Win, the analysis suggests that PassingYards offers no *additional* information about Win above and beyond the information that the other variables offer.

As illustrated with the analysis regarding PassingYards, the p-values of predictors can and will vary from model to model. Adding in, say, x_5 to a model that already contains x_1 and x_2 may yield a significant reduction in the sum of squared errors. However, adding x_5 to a model that already contains x_3 and x_4 may not. The implication is that the information in x_5 is redundant with the information provided by x_3 and x_4, but not by x_1 and x_2. See Aside 4.5 for an illuminating example.

The coefficient, p-value, and statistical significance of a predictor are calculated *with respect to a specific model.* These quantities can and will be different depending on what other predictors are in the model. Fundamentally, this is due to the fact that most predictors contain somewhat redundant information about y.

One final point involving the elimination of predictors needs stressing. Too often, people scroll through the list of p-values and instinctively think that none of the non-significant variables need to be kept in the model. This is not the case.

When the p-value of an individual predictor is at least 5%, you can eliminate it from the model since its inclusion does not significantly reduce the sum of the squared errors. However, you *cannot* eliminate *all* predictors with p-values of at least 5% simultaneously!

Since p-values are model-dependent, eliminating one predictor will change the p-values of every other predictor in the model (the p-values are now calculated with respect to a different model). To determine whether you can eliminate all (or some) of the non-significant predictors, the partial F test must be used (Section 4.4.2).

Even practitioners can make the mistake of looking at a non-significant predictor in a multiple regression model and assuming there is no relationship between it and y. Remember that the p-value is a comment on whether a predictor adds significant additional information about y when included in a model, not whether the predictor has *any* information at all about y.

4.4.4 Important "quirks" regarding p-values, coefficients, and standard errors

Multiple regression coefficients and p-values have a variety of "quirky" behaviors that on the surface seem perplexing and lead to great confusion for someone not well-versed in statistical modeling. In general, these behaviors occur when predictors are correlated and some of their information is redundant. These quirks can always be resolved by reiterating *what* the coefficients and p-values actually mean.

Aside 4.5 — Detailed discussion of statistical significance. Consider predicting the body fat percentage of an individual (BodyFat) from his or her triceps skinfold thickness (Triceps) and thigh and midarm circumferences (Thigh and Midarm). In simple linear regressions, Triceps and Thigh are statistically significant while Midarm is not. However, in a multiple regression, the model is significant (p-value of 7×10^{-6}) but *none* of the individual predictors are significant! Note: these measurements are from the BODYFAT2 dataset, a different collection of individuals and measurements than the ones contained in BODYFAT.

```
Simple linear regressions:
             Estimate Std. Error t value Pr(>|t|)
Triceps        0.8572     0.1288   6.656 3.02e-06 ***

             Estimate Std. Error t value Pr(>|t|)
Thigh          0.8565     0.1100   7.786  3.6e-07 ***

             Estimate Std. Error t value Pr(>|t|)
Midarm         0.1994     0.3266   0.611    0.549

Multiple regression:
             Estimate Std. Error t value Pr(>|t|)
(Intercept)   117.085     99.782   1.173    0.258
Triceps         4.334      3.016   1.437    0.170
Thigh          -2.857      2.582  -1.106    0.285
Midarm         -2.186      1.595  -1.370    0.190
---
F-statistic: 21.52 on 3 and 16 DF,  p-value: 7.343e-06
```

At first glance, this appears to be a contradiction. How can a model be statistically significant yet nothing in the model have significance? The resolution of this paradox comes from remembering that p-values are model-dependent. The fact that Triceps is not significant means that adding it to a model that already has Thigh and Midarm does not yield a significant reduction in the sum of squared errors. Likewise, the fact that Thigh is not significant means that adding it to a model that already has Triceps and Midarm does not yield a significant reduction in sum of squared errors, etc.

Thus, while the *combination* of Triceps, Thigh, and Midarm *does* yield a significant reduction in sum of squared errors (relative to the naive model) since the p-value of the multiple regression model is $< 5\%$, none of the individual variables (when added to a model already containing the other two) yields a significant *further* decrease in sum of squared errors. In other words, once you know any two of the predictors, you don't need to know the third.

If you are able to design your own experiment, you can avoid these quirks by carefully choosing the combinations of x's to minimize correlations between them. However, most datasets in business have already been collected and you are at the mercy of how the variables are naturally related to one another.

Quirk 1: A predictor that is not statistically significant in one model may be statistically significant in another model.

Example: In the SALARY dataset, Experience is not significant in simple linear regression predicting Salary, but it is in a model that also contains Education.

```
Predicting Salary from Experience
            Estimate Std. Error t value Pr(>|t|)
(Intercept) 3525.787     72.945  48.335   <2e-16 ***
Experience    10.423      6.458   1.614     0.11

Predicting Salary from Experience and Education
           Estimate Std. Error t value Pr(>|t|)
(Intercept)  3097.93     113.82  27.218  < 2e-16 ***
Experience     13.17       5.87   2.244   0.0273 *
Education      89.83      19.47   4.613 1.31e-05 ***
```

Resolution: the variation in y attributable to sources other than x is large enough that it "drowns out" the association between y and x. After accounting for this extraneous variation by adding the relevant variables to the model, the association between y and x now stands out.

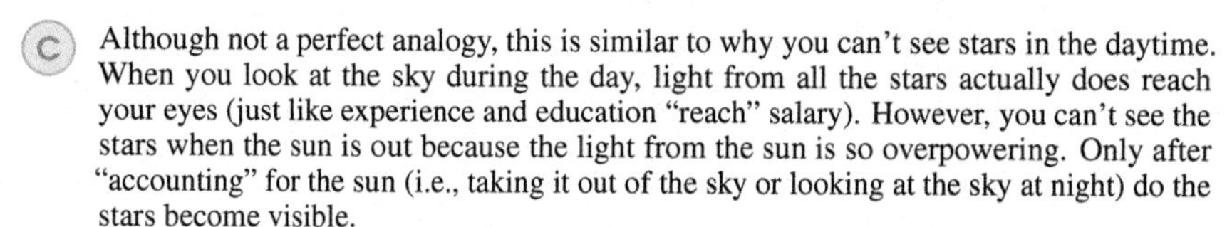

Although not a perfect analogy, this is similar to why you can't see stars in the daytime. When you look at the sky during the day, light from all the stars actually does reach your eyes (just like experience and education "reach" salary). However, you can't see the stars when the sun is out because the light from the sun is so overpowering. Only after "accounting" for the sun (i.e., taking it out of the sky or looking at the sky at night) do the stars become visible.

In fact, during a total solar eclipse, where the moon almost completely blocks out the light from the sun, you can see stars during the daytime. In the salary example, the effect of education is "overpowering" experience. When we account for the variation in salaries attributable to differences in employees' educational levels by putting `Education` into the regression, the relationship between `Salary` and `Experience` emerges.

Quirk 2: A predictor may be statistically significant in one model but not in another model (really an extension of the first quirk).

Example: `BODYFAT` dataset. `Chest` is statistically significant in a simple linear regression but is not significant in a multiple regression model with `Abdomen` and `Neck`.

```
Predicting Body Fat from Chest alone
             Estimate Std. Error t value Pr(>|t|)
(Intercept) -46.21636    4.18460  -11.04   <2e-16 ***
Chest         0.64622    0.04136   15.62   <2e-16 ***

Predicting Body Fat from Chest, Abdomen, and Neck
(Intercept) -13.29745    4.68396  -2.839   0.0049 **
Chest        -0.10232    0.08548  -1.197   0.2325
Abdomen       0.79841    0.06306  12.662  < 2e-16 ***
Neck         -0.82505    0.18125  -4.552 8.33e-06 ***
```

Resolution: while x contains useful information about y, this information is redundant with the information already provided by the other predictors in the model where x lacks significance. With these other predictors in the model, the *additional* information that x provides is no longer significant. In this example, once we know `Abdomen` and `Neck`, `Chest` must not add any significant additional information about someone's body fat percentage.

Quirk 3: A predictor with a positive coefficient in one model may have a negative coefficient in another.

Example: `AUTO` dataset. When predicting the top speed of a car (Figure 2.27), the coefficient of `Weight` is positive in a simple linear regression but negative in a regression including `Horsepower`.

```
Predicting Top Speed from Weight in a simple linear regression
            Estimate Std. Error t value Pr(>|t|)
(Intercept)  76.2457     4.5252  16.849  < 2e-16 ***
Weight        1.1700     0.1416   8.262 2.48e-12 ***

Predicting Top Speed from Weight and Horsepower in a multiple regression
             Estimate Std. Error t value Pr(>|t|)
(Intercept) 96.419959   0.829768  116.20   <2e-16 ***
Weight      -0.705857   0.041801  -16.89   <2e-16 ***
Horsepower   0.322843   0.005987   53.92   <2e-16 ***
```

Resolution: coefficients talk about how y differs *among individuals* in the population, not what happens to a particular individual's value of y when its value of x increases (regression is not a physical law). The sign of b_i may be positive if it is correlated with another variable that itself has a strong, positive correlation with y. After accounting for this correlation by putting the other variable in the model, the coefficient better reflects the association between x and y (which may have the opposite sign).

In this example, laws of physics suggest that cars go slower as they are weighted down. However, the coefficient of `Weight` is *positive* when predicting `TopSpeed` because `Weight` is positively correlated with `Horsepower`, and `Horsepower` has a strong positive correlation with `TopSpeed`. Once we account for `Horsepower` by putting it into the model, the coefficient of weight now describes the expected difference in top speeds of two cars with identical horsepowers that differ in weight by one unit. This coefficient is negative, just as we anticipated.

Quirk 4: The standard error of the coefficient of x may get smaller or may get larger when additional variables are added to the model.

Example: in Quirk 3, the standard error of `Weight` decreases from 0.14 in the simple linear regression to 0.04 in the multiple regression. In Quirk 2, the standard error of `Chest` increases from 0.041 in the simple linear regression to 0.085 in the multiple regression.

Resolution: standard errors get smaller when the amount of correlation between the x's is small and/or the additional predictors significantly improve the model. Standard errors get larger when the amount of correlation between the x's is large (it's hard to disentangle the effect of one predictor from another) or when the additional x's do not improve the model.

4.5 Increasing the flexibility of a model

In any regression model, what we call y and x is arbitrary. They can be the measured variables, e.g., *Salary*, or they can be more complex functions like $\ln Salary$, $Salary^2$, $\sqrt{Salary}$, etc. Transformations of variables was used in simple linear regression to "fix" the model when nonlinearities or unequal vertical spread existed in the scatterplot of the original quantities (Section 3.6). In a multiple regression context, we can include additional polynomial terms

(x, x^2, and x^3, etc.) or even define a predictor to a function of two or more variables, e.g., $Education \times Experience$, $Weight/Height^2$, etc., to capture more complex relationships.

4.5.1 Polynomial models

We have seen that when the relationship between y and x is nonlinear, it may be possible to "straighten out" the stream of points by making a model to predict $1/y$, $\ln y$, $\sqrt{y}$, etc. from $1/x$, $\ln x$, $\sqrt{x}$, etc. An alternative is to use a **polynomial** model.

> A polynomial of degree (or order) m is a weighted sum of the terms $x, x^2, x^3, \ldots, x^m$. If there is noticeable curvature in the scatterplot of y vs. x or residuals vs. x, a polynomial model may be appropriate. While a polynomial model can capture nonlinear (and non-monotonic) relationships, it cannot "fix" unequal vertical spread (which requires a transformation for y).

For example, consider the `BULLDOZER` dataset. The goal is to develop a type of *Kelley Blue Book* (which specializes in giving fair market values for used cars) for bulldozers sold at auctions. We want to predict `Price` based on how many years ago the auction occurred (`YearsAgo`), the model year of the machine (`YearMade`), the level of use of the machine (`Usage`, units are in hours), the blade width (`Blade`, in feet), and tire size (`Tire`, in inches).

Figure 4.8 — Scatterplot matrix of BULLDOZER dataset. Note the obvious curvature between `Price` and `YearMade`.

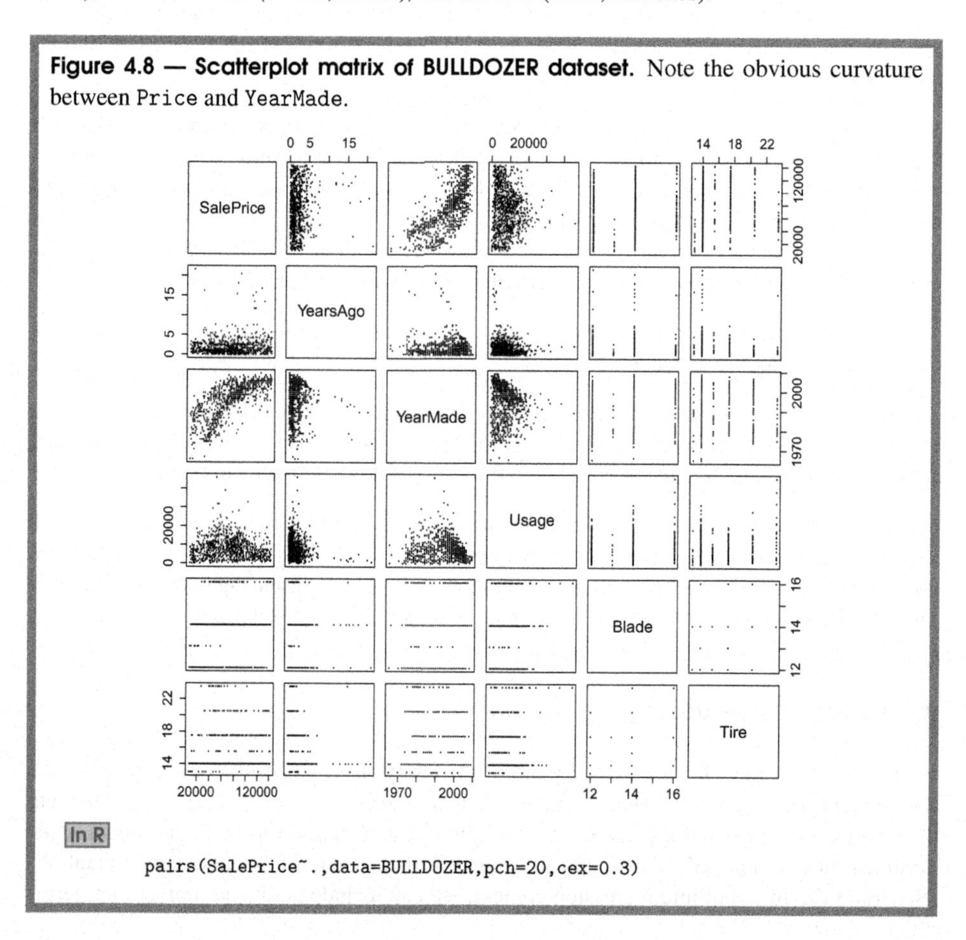

In R

```
pairs(SalePrice~.,data=BULLDOZER,pch=20,cex=0.3)
```

Figure 4.8 shows a scatterplot matrix of the variables. Immediately, we see that there is nonlinearity between `Price` and `YearMade`. In fact, if we fit a multiple regression and look at the residuals plot, we see obvious curvature in the residuals (Figure 4.9). However, once the quantity $\texttt{YearMade}^2$ is added to the model, the curvature goes away.

Choosing the right model is imperative for finding the most appropriate values for the coefficients. For instance, imagine that we are interested in the coefficient of `Tire`. In the (bad) original regression model, the coefficient of `Tire` is 2510—two otherwise identical bulldozers that differ in `Tire` by one inch are expected to differ in `SalePrice` by about $2500 (larger tires tend to have higher selling prices). In the (better) regression with the polynomial in `YearMade`, the coefficient is only $2144, a change of 15%—larger tires are not quite worth as much as we may have originally thought!

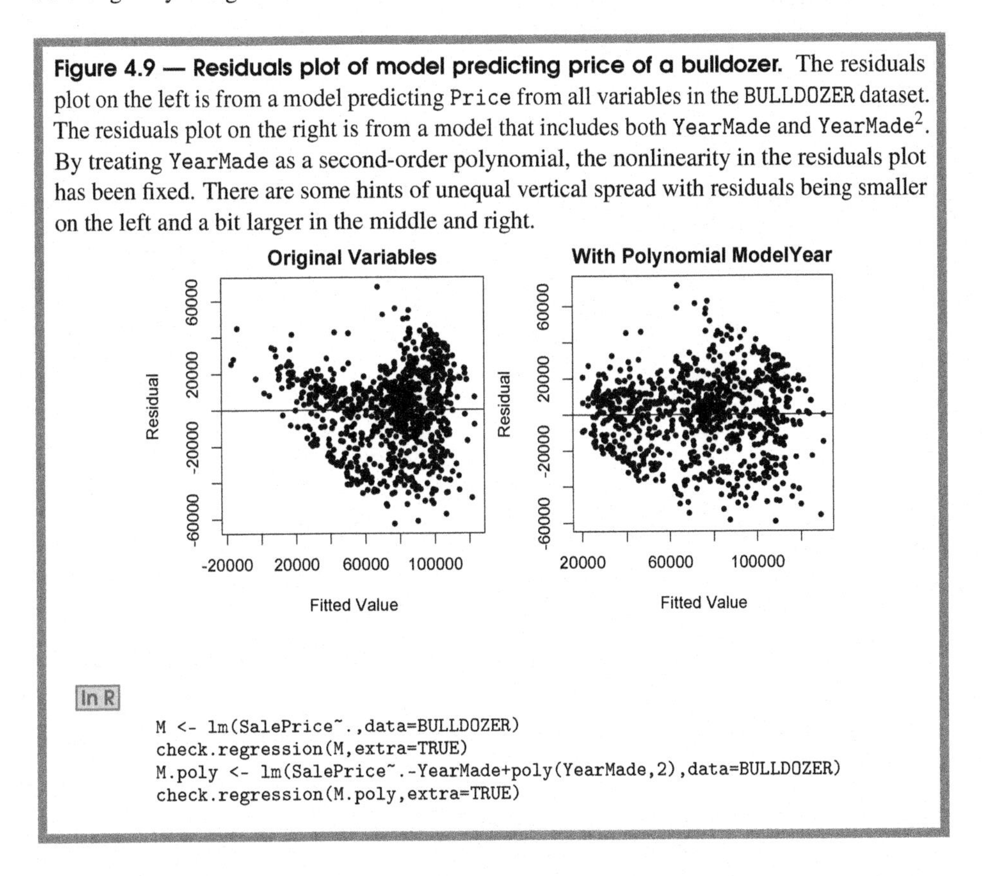

Figure 4.9 — Residuals plot of model predicting price of a bulldozer. The residuals plot on the left is from a model predicting `Price` from all variables in the `BULLDOZER` dataset. The residuals plot on the right is from a model that includes both `YearMade` and $\texttt{YearMade}^2$. By treating `YearMade` as a second-order polynomial, the nonlinearity in the residuals plot has been fixed. There are some hints of unequal vertical spread with residuals being smaller on the left and a bit larger in the middle and right.

In R

```
M <- lm(SalePrice~.,data=BULLDOZER)
check.regression(M,extra=TRUE)
M.poly <- lm(SalePrice~.-YearMade+poly(YearMade,2),data=BULLDOZER)
check.regression(M.poly,extra=TRUE)
```

Adding the quantity $\texttt{YearMade}^2$ to the regression model made the residuals plot look acceptable. Why not try adding the quantities $\texttt{YearMade}^3$, $\texttt{YearMade}^4$, etc.? What order polynomial is the most appropriate for the model?

One strategy to determine the best order is to fit many different polynomial models and to choose the one that is most "reasonable." To compare models with different numbers of predictors, R^2_{adj} is preferable to R^2 since the latter will always increase when an additional power of x is added to the model. With the mantra "simpler is better," there are two ways to make a choice.

Aside 4.6 — Choosing polynomial order in R. The command `choose.order` in package `regclass` provides a tool for choosing a reasonable order of a polynomial model. First, a simple linear regression is fit, then passed to `choose.order`. A table of the orders and the corresponding R^2_{adj} is provided. Typically, the simplest (lowest order) model whose R^2_{adj} is no more than about 0.005 is selected to avoid unneeded complexity. Plots showing the fitted polynomials also aid in the selection—often, higher-order fits do not provide a curve that looks much different from lower-order fits.

In R

```
M <- lm(FuelEfficiency~Horsepower,data=AUTO)
choose.order(M,max.order=4)

order      R2adj      AICc
    1 0.6191715 539.3692
    2 0.8017590 488.9585
    3 0.8292141 479.9017
    4 0.8344025 480.5839
```

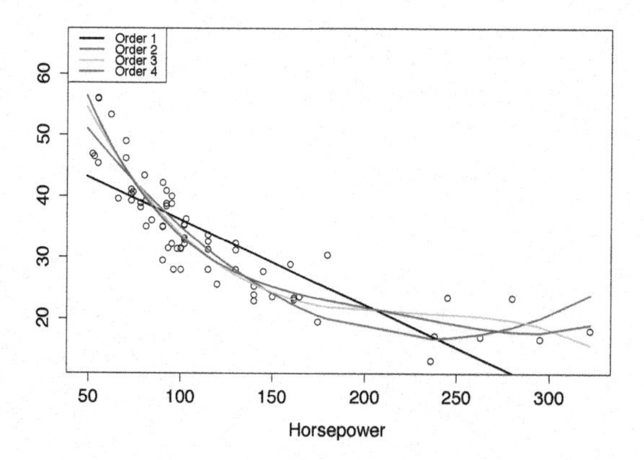

In the example above, the fourth-order polynomial has the highest R^2_{adj}. However, the third-order polynomial has an R^2_{adj} that is only 0.005 lower. Graphically, there looks to be little difference between these curves. Most practitioners would select the third-order polynomial model since it is simpler while providing only a very slightly worse fit.

1. Choose the model with the highest R^2_{adj}.
2. Choose the simplest model with an R^2_{adj} within a "small amount" (e.g., 0.5%) of the highest value.

Consider a table of the model's R^2_{adj} and the degree of `YearMade`.

Degree	1	2	3	4	5
R^2_{adj}	0.5783	0.6172	0.6168	0.6184	0.6183
Degree	6	7	8	9	10
R^2_{adj}	0.6195	0.6195	0.6208	0.6205	0.6203

The model with the largest R^2_{adj} is order $m = 8$, implying that we should have the predictors `YearMade`, `YearMade`^{2}, ..., `YearMade`^{8} in the model. However, such a higher power "feels" needlessly complex. If we choose the simplest model that has an R^2_{adj} within 0.5% (i.e., no smaller than $0.6208 - 0.005 = 0.6158$), then taking a second-order polynomial model ($m = 2$) is sufficient.

One final technique about polynomial models worth noting is *centering*. To make the model more stable from a computational standpoint, it is common to use the variables $(x-\bar{x})^2$, $(x-\bar{x})^3$, etc., instead of x^2, x^3, etc., where $\bar{x}$ is the average value of x in the data. The resulting regression equations are the same with or without centering, but centering decreases the correlation between various powers of x and makes estimating the coefficients easier.

4.5.2 Variable creation

Quite often, some logical combination of the measured variables should be a predictor in the regression model. For example, if you want to model the weight of a tree based on its height, diameter, and density, it makes more sense to fit the model $Weight = \beta_0 + \beta_1 Height \times Diameter^2 \times Density + \varepsilon$ than $Weight = \beta_0 + \beta_1 Height + \beta_2 Diameter + \beta_3 Density + \varepsilon$.

Physically, the weight of an object is equal to its volume times its average density. Assuming that a tree can be treated like a cylinder, the volume is roughly proportional to the area of the tree's base times its height since the volume of a cylinder is $V = \pi \times (Diameter/2)^2 \times Height$.

Since what we call x is arbitrary, we may define x to be any combination or function of the measured variables. However, since the potential number of combinations is infinite, typically we do not create them haphazardly and throw them into the model. Rather, a new variable should have some logical connection to what you are predicting.

For example, consider data regarding the US Census (`CENSUSMLR`). Every 10 years, the government conducts the census by sending survey forms out to all households. By law, these forms must be completed and returned. Workers go door-to-door to manually interview people whose forms have not been returned by the deadline. To intelligently allocate workers, it would be useful to model the response rates of each "block group" using demographic variables.

A block group is on average about 40 blocks, each typically bounded by streets, roads, or water. The number of block groups per county in the US is typically between about 5 and 165 with a median of about 20.

Figure 4.10 gives a scatterplot matrix for some of the demographic variables in the `CENSUSMLR` dataset. For the time being, let us focus on how the number of households that are rural (as opposed to suburban or urban) in a block group is associated with the response rate (`Response`).

One possible model is $Response\% = \beta_0 + \beta_1 Rural + \beta_2 Population + \varepsilon$, with `Population` being the total number of people in the "block group." It is a good idea to have both of these variables in the model because the practical meaning of `Rural` depends on the value of `Population`.

If `Rural` = 1000 and `Population` = 3000, then most people in that block group are rural (remember, each household averages probably about two people), while if instead `Population` = 1,000,000, then very few are rural. We need to account for `Population` if we want to study the association between the response rate and `Rural`.

Figure 4.10 — Scatterplot matrix of CENSUSMLR data. The goal is to predict Response (the percent of households in a block group that mailed in the census form).

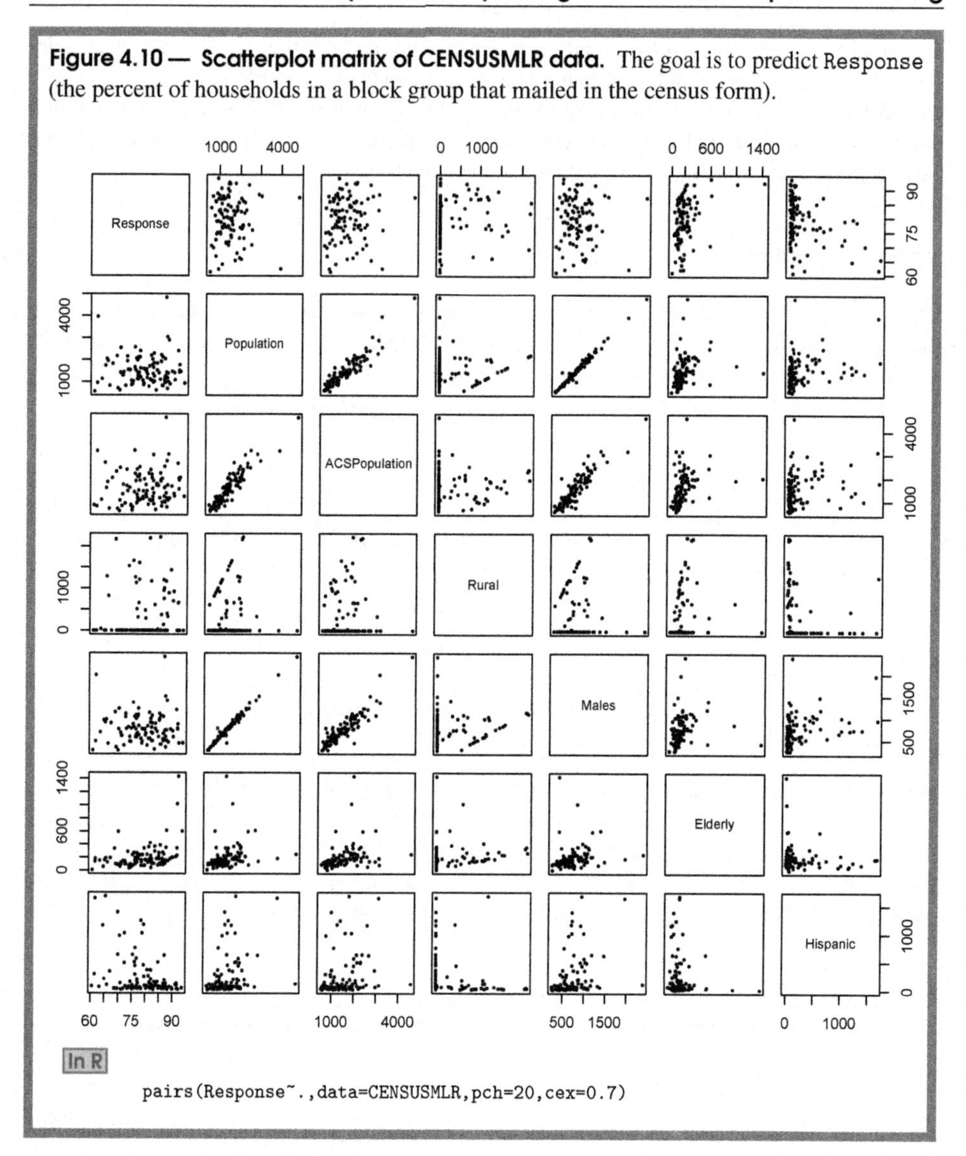

In R

```
pairs(Response~.,data=CENSUSMLR,pch=20,cex=0.7)
```

The output of the regression shows that the model is poor ($R^2_{adj} = 0.019$) and that Population is not significant (i.e., not necessary to include in a model that already has Rural).

In R

```
M <- lm(Response~Rural+Population,data=CENSUSMLR)
summary(M)

                Estimate Std. Error t value Pr(>|t|)
(Intercept) 78.4711149  0.5048926 155.421  < 2e-16 ***
Rural        0.0021410  0.0004643   4.611 4.53e-06 ***
Population  -0.0001249  0.0002836  -0.440     0.66
Multiple R-squared:  0.02088,Adjusted R-squared:  0.01892
```

However, perhaps a more logical approach is to predict the response rate from something akin to the *percentage* of people in the block group who live in rural households. Let us fit the model $Response\% = \beta_0 + \beta_1(Rural/Population) + \varepsilon$. The output shows that it is still a poor model ($R^2_{adj} = 0.028$), but it fits better than the original model.

In R

```
M <- lm(Response~I(Rural/Population),data=CENSUSMLR)
summary(M)

                       Estimate Std. Error t value Pr(>|t|)
(Intercept)             78.1352     0.2935 266.234  < 2e-16 ***
I(Rural/Population)      3.6330     0.6718   5.408 7.97e-08 ***
Multiple R-squared:  0.02847,Adjusted R-squared:  0.0275
```

Note: when including a function of the measured variables in the regression model, it is necessary to wrap that function inside `I()` so that R treats it correctly.

Another piece of information available is a second population estimate for each block group provided by the American Community Survey (ACS). Perhaps the *disagreement* in the populations measured by the census and the ACS could be a predictor of the response rate. Presumably, a large discrepancy indicates a "problem" block, and it would not be surprising if the response rate is lower.

Let us define the disagreement as $|Census - ACS|/Census$, i.e., the absolute percentage difference between the two values. Fitting a regression using only this variable, we see that its coefficient is negative (as anticipated) and statistically significant. Since $R^2_{adj} = 2.1\%$, it performs about as well as the previous model.

In R

```
CENSUSMLR$disagreement <- abs(CENSUSMLR$Population-CENSUSMLR$ACSPopulation)/
                                 CENSUSMLR$Population
M <- lm(Response~disagreement,data=CENSUSMLR)
summary(M)

             Estimate Std. Error t value Pr(>|t|)
(Intercept)   80.3081     0.3908  205.52  < 2e-16 ***
disagreement  -9.8849     2.0856   -4.74 2.45e-06 ***
Multiple R-squared:  0.02201,Adjusted R-squared:  0.02103
```

Best practices in model creation always include thinking about what other variables you can create that may help predict y. Incorporating a new variable can be the key to success. In fact, consider a recent `kaggle.com` competition whose goal was to predict the sales of new products 26 weeks after their release from sales data that was collected during the first 13 weeks. A modified version of the competition data can be found in `SOLD26`.

See `https://www.kaggle.com/c/hack-reduce-dunnhumby-hackathon`. For this example, the number of stores selling the product and the number of items sold on odd-numbered weeks are used as predictor variables (e.g., `StoresSelling1`, `Sold1`). In addition, the planned number of stores that are slated to sell the product on week 26 (`StoresSelling26`) is provided.

Let us first predict `SoldWeek26` with a multiple regression using all predictors. The residuals plot (Figure 4.11) shows that this model is inadequate (though it has a high $R^2_{adj} = 90\%$).

Figure 4.11 — Residuals plot predicting the number of items sold in week 26 from all variables. The regression model is clearly inadequate since there appears to be curvature and unequal spread in the residuals.

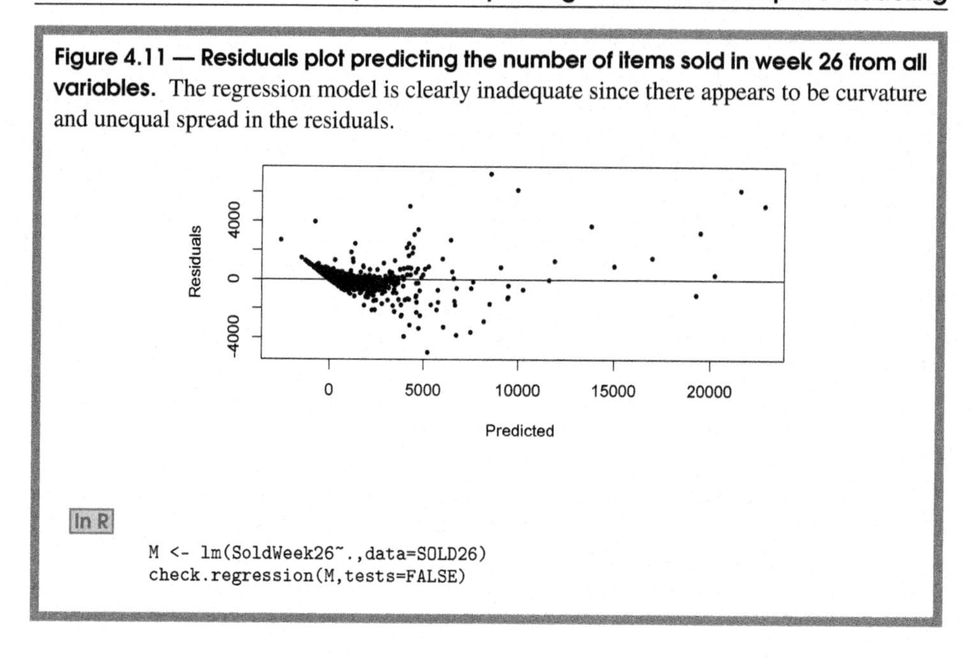

In R

```
M <- lm(SoldWeek26~.,data=SOLD26)
check.regression(M,tests=FALSE)
```

To fix the unequal vertical spread in the residuals plot, we must use a transformation of `SoldWeek26`. The standard transformation for sales data is to take the logarithm. However, there is still extreme curvature in the residuals plot. See Figure 4.12.

Figure 4.12 — Residuals plot when predicting the logarithm of sales in week 26. To fix the unequal vertical spread in the original model, we must have y be a transformation of `SoldWeek26`. A logarithm is a natural choice. However, the resulting model is still clearly inadequate.

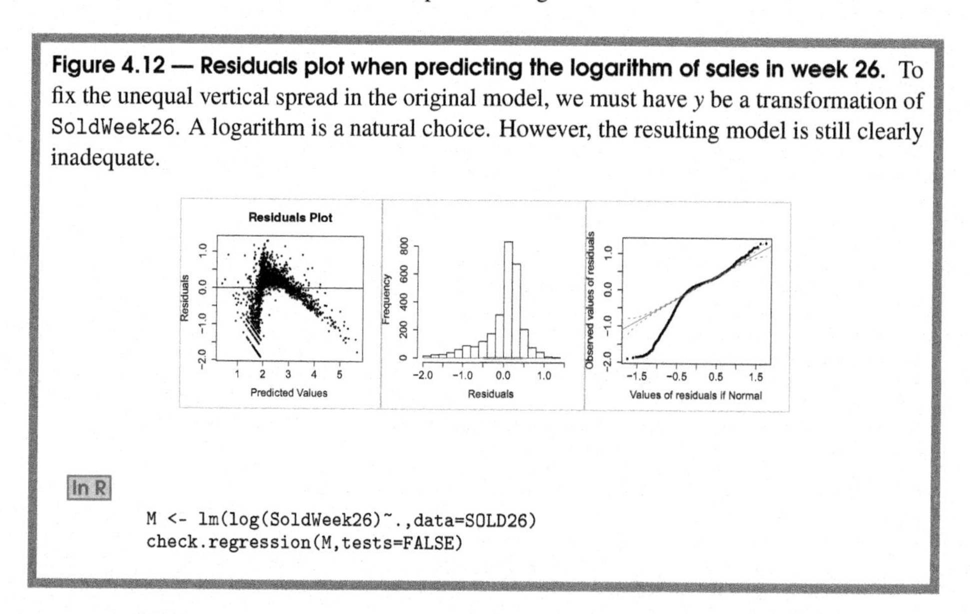

In R

```
M <- lm(log(SoldWeek26)~.,data=SOLD26)
check.regression(M,tests=FALSE)
```

It may be possible to fix the curvature by using additional transformations in the predictor variables. Here, an additional key bit of insight solves the problem. After 13 weeks, any product hype has probably settled down and word of mouth has run its course. It may be reasonable to assume that the *number of items sold per store* should be relatively constant into the future.

Thus, let us define a predictor to be the number of items sold per store in week 13 multiplied by the number of stores expected to sell the product in week 26. The result should be close to the number of items sold in week 26. This model still has curvature in the residuals, so instead, let us use the logarithm of that predictor. The final model is a simple linear regression.

$$\ln Sold26 = \beta_0 + \beta_1 \ln\left(\frac{Sold13}{StoresSelling13} \times StoresSelling26\right)$$

Figure 4.13 shows the residuals plot for this model, and it looks much better. There are strange diagonal bands for small predicted values (this is related to the fact that the minimum number of items a store can sell is zero). Because something interesting is left over after we fit the model, the regression is not a perfect reflection of reality. However, it is highly improved over the previous model (R^2_{adj} is now 98%).

Figure 4.13 — Residuals plot predicting the logarithm of number of items sold in week 26 from custom variable. The simple linear regression using the custom variable has a much-improved residuals plot. The diagonal band on the far left represents residuals when no items were sold in the stores, the second diagonal band represents residuals where only one item was sold in the store, etc. The regression still has issues, but overall, it is not too bad.

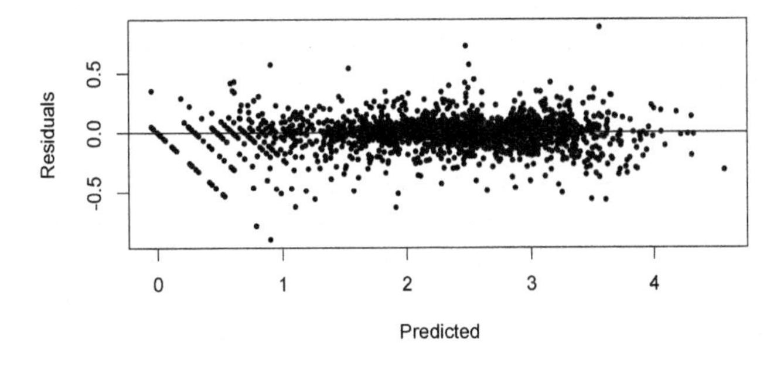

In R

```
M <- lm(log(SoldWeek26)~I(log(Sold13/StoresSelling13*StoresSelling26)),
           data=SOLD26)
check.regression(M,tests=FALSE)
```

4.5.3 Interaction variables

Recall the interpretation of b_i: two otherwise identical individuals (with respect to the other variables in the model) who differ in x_i by one unit are expected to differ in y by b_i units. At face value, this is true *regardless* of the other characteristics of the individuals we are comparing. This is not always realistic.

For example, consider the SALARY dataset and the relationship between someone's monthly salary (Salary) and his or her number of years of education (Education) and years of previous work experience (Experience). A multiple regression model predicting monthly salary from these two variables yields:

- the coefficient of `Education` is about 90. The average difference in salaries when two individuals have equal amounts of prior work experience but differ in educational level by one year is $90. The model assumes this to be true regardless of the amounts of prior work experience of the two individuals we are comparing.
- the coefficient of `Experience` is about 13. The average difference in salaries when two individuals have equal amounts of education but differ in experience by one year is $13. The model assumes this to be true regardless of the amounts of education of the two individuals we are comparing.

The interpretation of the coefficients reveals an overly simplistic approach to the way salary works: an additional year of education is "worth" the same amount regardless of the experience level of the individual. While an additional year of education justifies a boost in salary when an individual has no work experience, does the employer really care about educational level when someone has 10 years of experience?

Based on prior knowledge on how salaries work, we need to incorporate an **interaction** between the amounts of education and experience that an employee has. The average difference in salaries when two employees differ in education by one year *depends* on exactly how much experience the employees have.

> Two predictors x_1 and x_2 have an interaction when the expected difference in y between two otherwise identical individuals who differ in x_1 by one unit *depends* on the exact value of x_2 for the individuals we are comparing (and vice versa).

Another way to think about it is that two variables x_1 and x_2 have an interaction when the *strength* of the relationship between y and x_1 is not a constant but depends on x_2. Here, the relationship between someone's salary and educational level may be strong when the employee has little work experience but relatively weak if the employee has a lot of work experience. In other words, educational level is important only when the employee does not have a proven track record in the industry.

> Two predictors x_1 and x_2 have an interaction when the strength of the relationship between y and x_1 (i.e., its coefficient in the regression model) depends on the exact value of x_2 (and vice versa).

An interaction between x_1 and x_2 can easily be incorporated into a regression model by adding the predictor $(x_1 \times x_2)$. Including this term accomplishes exactly the desired effect. To understand why, let us rearrange terms of the model when an interaction is present.

$$y = \beta_0 + \beta_1 x_1 \beta_2 x_2 + \beta_3 (x_1 \times x_2) = (\beta_0 + \beta_2 x_2) + (\beta_1 + \beta_3 x_2) x_1$$

Thus, *for a particular value of* x_2, the intercept of the line is $\beta_0 + \beta_2 x_2$ and the slope of the line is $(\beta_1 + \beta_3 x_2)$—the slope of the regression and strength of the relationship between y and x_1 depends on x_2! Further, the effective coefficient of x_1 tells us that two individuals who differ in x_1 by one unit are expected to differ in y by $\beta_1 + \beta_3 x_2$ units (which now depends on the exact value of x_2 of the two individuals we are comparing).

Adding the interaction term $x_1 \times x_2$ into the regression allows us to model the *possibility* that the strength of the relationship between y and x_1 might vary based on the value of x_2 (and vice versa). To formally test whether the strength does vary, we look at the p-value of the interaction term. If it is less than 5%, the interaction is statistically significant.

If the interaction is significant, there is strong evidence that:

- the strength of the relationship between y and x_1 depends on x_2 (and vice versa).
- the expected difference in y between two otherwise identical individuals who differ in x_1 by one unit *depends* on the exact value of x_2 of the individuals we are comparing (and vice versa).

Let us revisit the SALARY data with a more sophisticated view of how salaries are determined. Fitting a model predicting Salary from Education and Experience, including the interaction, yields the following output.

In R

```
M <- lm(Salary~Education*Experience,data=SALARY)
summary(M)

                     Estimate Std. Error t value Pr(>|t|)
(Intercept)          2841.525    150.179  18.921  < 2e-16 ***
Education             149.520     30.292   4.936  3.7e-06 ***
Experience             38.234     11.454   3.338  0.00123 **
Education:Experience   -6.175      2.448  -2.523  0.01341 *
```

The interaction term is statistically significant since its p-value is 0.013, so it should be included in the model. The association between Salary and Education is indeed stronger for some values of Experience and weaker for others.

The regression equation is:

$$Salary = 2842 + 150Education + 38Experience - 6(Education \times Experience)$$

To find out how the relationship between Salary and Education changes, we can write out the **implicit regression equations** when Experience = 0 (the smallest value in the data) and when Experience = 20 (one of the larger values).

An implicit regression equation is a multiple regression equation after one or more values for the predictor variables have been "plugged in."

Regression $Salary = 2842 + 150Education + 38Experience - 6(Education \times Experience)$

$Experience = 0$:

$$\begin{aligned} Salary &= 2842 + 150Education + 38 \times 0 - 6(Education \times 0) \\ &= 2842 + 150Education \end{aligned}$$

$Experience = 20$:

$$\begin{aligned} Salary &= 2842 + 150Education + 38 \times 20 - 6(Education \times 20) \\ &= 3602 + 30Education \end{aligned}$$

The implicit regression equations are illuminating.

- Among employees with no experience, it looks like the average starting salary (the intercept, where the educational level is 0) is about $2850. Two individuals with no experience who differ in education by one year are expected to have salaries that differ by $150.
- Among highly experienced (20 years) employees, it looks like the average starting salary is $3600. Two individuals with 20 years of experience who differ in education by one year are expected to have salaries that differ by only $30.
- The relationship between `Salary` and `Education` is strong (slope is far from zero) for small values of `Experience` and weak (slope is close to zero) for larger values of `Experience`.
- The difference in salaries between two employees who differ in education by one year is large when both employees have little experience and small when both employees have a lot of experience.
- `Education` becomes a worse predictor of `Salary` as employees' experience levels increase since the effective slope of `Education` decreases toward zero.

Figure 4.14 — Interaction plots for the SALARY data. To interpret the interaction plots, focus on the relationship that is most important to you. In this case, we are interested in seeing whether the strength of the relationship between `Salary` and `Education` depends on `Experience`, so we look at the plot on the left.

Implicit regression equations for a small value (5th percentile), median value, and large value (95th percentile) of `Experience` are displayed. The slopes of these lines look very different, so there is strong evidence for an interaction. For small values of `Experience`, the relationship between `Salary` and `Education` is strong and positive. As `Experience` increases, the relationship weakens (the slope diminishes toward zero).

An **interaction plot** provides a graphical summary of the interaction between x_1 and x_2 and the implicit regression equations. See Figure 4.14. In the set of interaction plots (one for y vs. x_1 and one for y vs. x_2), three implicit regression equations are displayed: one for a small value (5th percentile), median value, and large value (95th percentile) of the other variable.

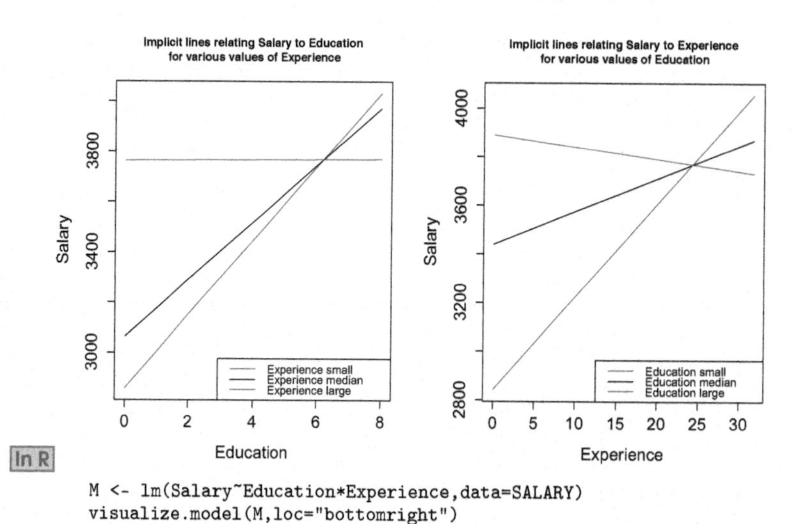

In R

```
M <- lm(Salary~Education*Experience,data=SALARY)
visualize.model(M,loc="bottomright")
```

> An interaction is suspected when the slopes of the implicit regression equations are quite different (especially if they cross). When the lines are nearly parallel, then the strength of the relationship between y and x_1 is nearly a constant and does not depend on x_2 (and vice versa), so any interaction is weak (if it exists at all).

In theory, it is possible to add interactions between three or more variables in the model, e.g., $Experience \times Education \times Months$. Interpreting these higher-order interactions is difficult. They are not typically considered unless there are logical or physical reasons for doing so.

Figure 4.15 shows two sets of interaction plots on simulated data to give you an idea of how different (or similar) the implicit regression lines look when there is and is not an interaction.

Figure 4.15 — More examples of interaction plots. The top pair of plots illustrates a typical example of what interaction plots look like when there is little to no interaction: the slopes of the lines are nearly parallel—the strength of the relationship between y and x_1 does not vary based on x_2 (and vice versa). The bottom pair of plots illustrates a typical example of what interaction plots look like when there is a strong interaction: the slopes of the lines look quite different—the strength of the relationship between y and x_1 varies substantially based on x_2 (and vice versa).

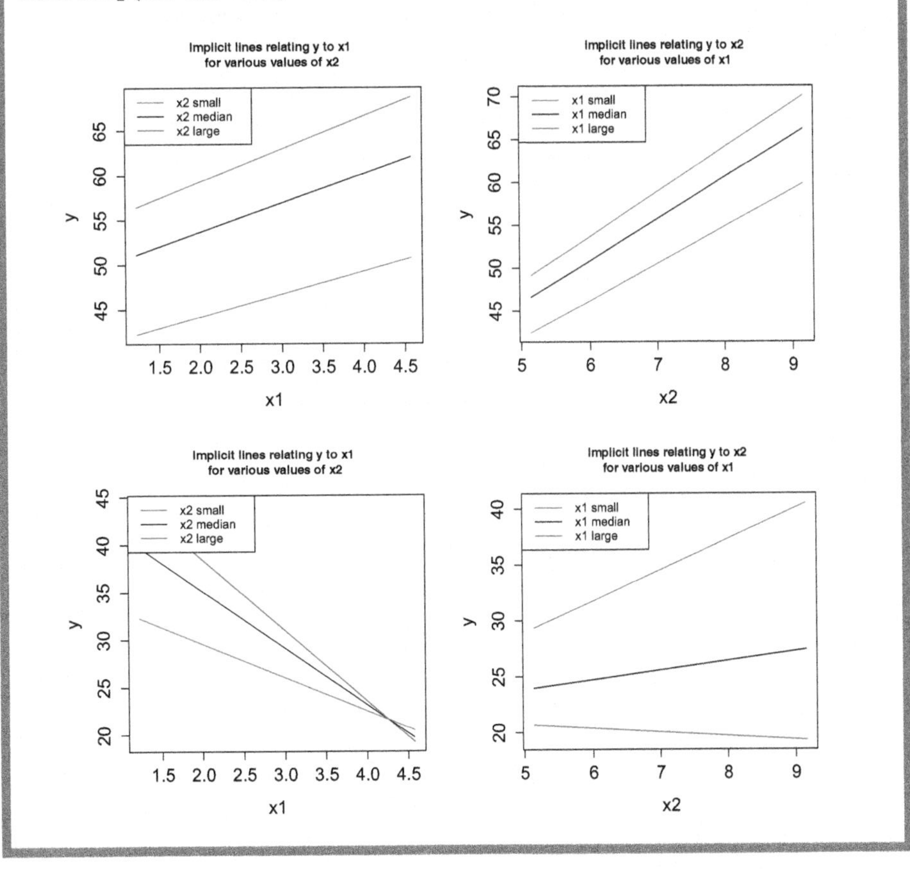

The interpretation of b_i, the coefficient of x_i, needs to be updated.

> If x_i is involved in an interaction, its coefficient (b_i) is not particularly meaningful. To determine the expected difference in y between two otherwise identical individuals who differ in x_i by one unit, it is necessary to know the individuals' exact values for all predictors involved in the interaction.

4.6 Influential points and outliers

In Sections 2.6.4 and 3.2.3, we saw that outliers affect the estimate of Pearson's correlation r and the coefficients of a simple linear regression. Not surprisingly, outliers can heavily influence the values of the coefficients in a multiple regression as well. Not all points in a multiple regression are created equal—some have more influence over the coefficients than others. To complicate matters, there is not necessarily an intuitive visual display that will always identify them.

To understand why visually detecting outliers is difficult, imagine trying to find outliers in the relationship between y and x by only looking at histograms or box plots (which we can think of as univariate "slices" of a bivariate relationship). Figure 4.16 shows that a point can be unusual in the *combination* of x and y while having perfectly typical individual values of x and y. If we rely on histograms and box plots (which consider variables only by themselves), we miss out on unusual pairings.

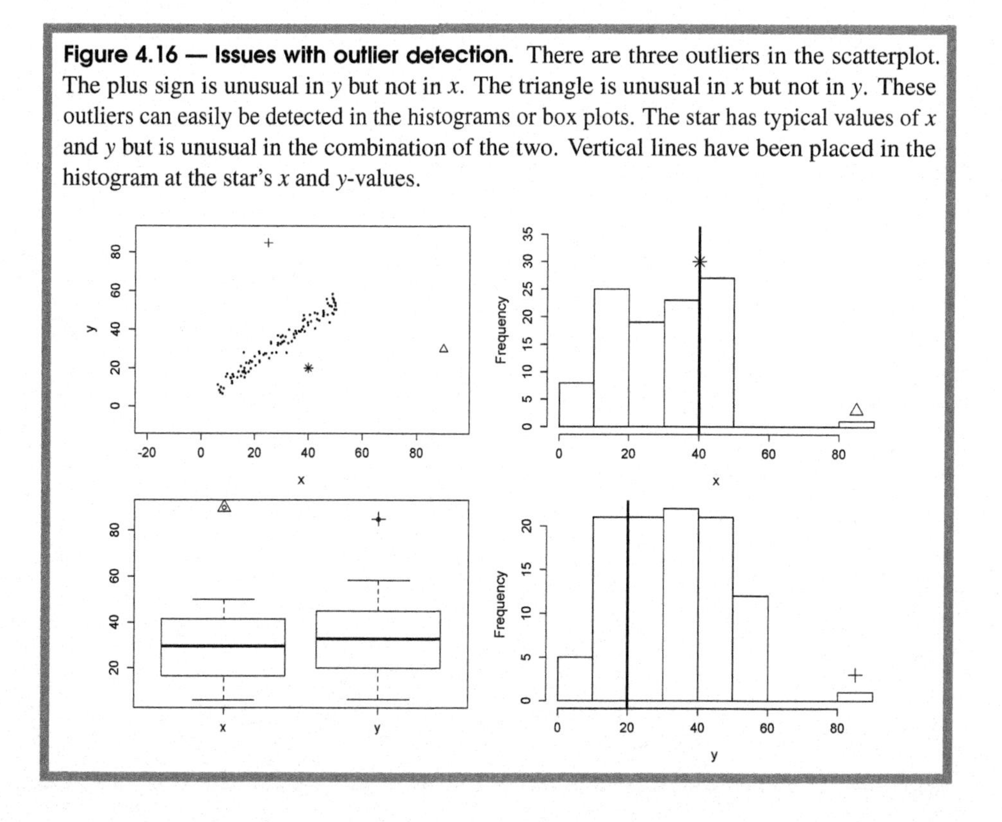

Figure 4.16 — Issues with outlier detection. There are three outliers in the scatterplot. The plus sign is unusual in y but not in x. The triangle is unusual in x but not in y. These outliers can easily be detected in the histograms or box plots. The star has typical values of x and y but is unusual in the combination of the two. Vertical lines have been placed in the histogram at the star's x and y-values.

By extension, the scatterplot matrix can reveal points that are unusual in terms of the individual variables or their pairings. However, it will not reveal points that are unusual in the *combination* of three or more variables.

Often, outliers can be spotted in histograms, box plots, or scatterplots. However, points that have an unusual *combination* of three or more values can remain hidden. Thus, standard graphical displays can miss the presence of outliers.

The good news is that there are *numerical* measures that can identify outliers and other points that may have influenced the regression coefficients.

In general, a point is **influential** when its addition to the dataset causes the coefficients of the regression to change substantially (e.g., Figure 3.5). An **outlier** is a point that is somehow unlike the majority of other observations in the data. While all influential points are outliers, not all outliers are influential points.

The **leverage** of an observation is a measure of the "unusualness" of an individual's combination of x-values. Only points with large leverage have the *potential* to be influential.

In a simple linear regression, a point with a large leverage is one whose x-value is far from the average $\bar{x}$. With two or more x's, the unusualness of a point is measured with respect to the center and shape of the x-datacloud. A point that is "closer" (as measured by a ruler) to the center of the cloud may actually have a *higher* leverage than a point that is "farther away" when the shape of the cloud is considered. See Figure 4.17.

Figure 4.17 — Illustration of leverage. The leverage of a point measures its distance from the center of the x-datacloud. If there is only one predictor variable (left), the leverage of a point is proportional to its distance from the average. A vertical bar is drawn at a value of x that has a high leverage (it is far from the average of $\bar{x} = 0$). If there are two predictor variables (right), the "distance" from the average (the center of the datacloud marked by the large dot) is not what you'd measure from a ruler. Rather, it is measured with respect to the shape of the cloud itself. The two highlighted points are roughly the same (ruler) distance from the center, but the one on the right has a *much* higher leverage because its placement with respect to the elliptical shape of the datacloud is more unusual.

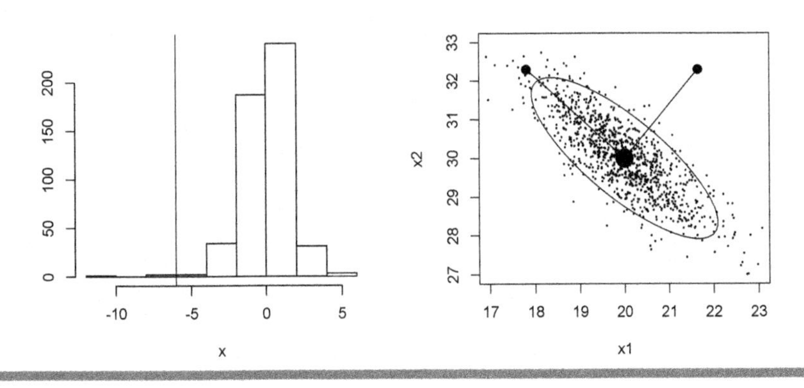

Consider Figure 4.18. Here, the influence of an additional point is studied based on where that point is placed. The lessons from these plots are:

- An outlier with a low leverage is not influential.
- An outlier with a large leverage is not influential if it is where the stream of points is "already going."
- An outlier with a large leverage that is far from the x-datacloud is quite influential.

Leverage alone cannot determine whether a point is influential. We need a secondary measurement that tells us how far the point diverges from where the stream of points is headed. The **deleted studentized residuals** provide insight.

A *deleted studentized* residual is the relative distance between the observed value of y and the value of y predicted by the regression model (i.e., the distance of a point to the line) made on the data *without* that point. Essentially, it measures distance of the point from where the rest of the stream of points is headed.

Figure 4.18 — Illustration of influence. The left panel shows an example of a point with a large leverage (its x-value is well above average) that is not influential. When this point is added to the dataset, the line hardly changes since the point is located where the stream of points was already going. In other words, its deleted studentized residual is small.

The middle panel shows a case where a point with a large leverage is influential. The location of the point is not where the stream was headed (i.e., it has a large deleted studentized residual), so the outlier pulls the line toward it and drastically changes the slope.

The right panel shows a case where an outlier has a large deleted studentized residual but is not influential. This point has a small leverage (its x value is very close to the average), and a point with a low leverage is never influential.

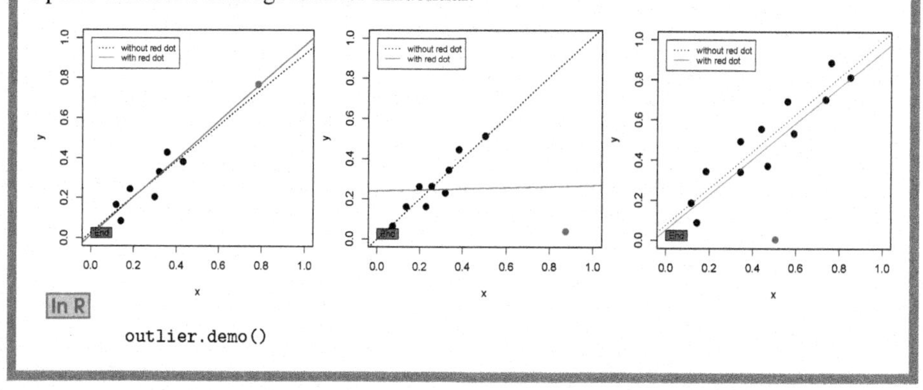

In R

```
outlier.demo()
```

Thus, a point is influential if it has both a large leverage *and* a large deleted studentized residual. The sample size n and the number of predictors in the model k determine the exact cutoff.

An outlier is considered influential if it has both a large leverage (greater than $2(k+1)/n$) and a large studentized residual (larger than 2 or smaller than -2).

Cook's distance measures influence from a slightly different perspective. The Cook's distance of a point is a measure of the discrepancy between the coefficients of the regression with and without that point. While this is a simpler measure of influence to use since it is a single value, there is no consensus on the threshold for a "large" Cook's distance: three times the average Cook's distance, greater than 1.0, greater than $4/n$, etc., have all appeared in the literature.

The **influence plot** is a plot of a point's leverage vs. its deleted studentized residual. The area devoted to a point is proportional to the Cook's distance. Thus, the plot allows simultaneous assessment of both measures of influence. See Figure 4.19 for influence plots for the SALARY, TIPS, and BODYFAT datasets.

Figure 4.19 — Example influence plots. In an influence plot, the areas of the points are proportional to the Cook's distance. The vertical line denotes the threshold for having a high leverage, and the horizontal lines denote the threshold for having a large deleted studentized residual. A point is influential if it has a large Cook's distance (though the threshold for "large" is not very well-defined) and/or a large leverage/residual pair (upper right or lower right rectangles; the center of the point will be marked with an 'X').

The left panel shows the SALARY dataset. There are no influential points according to leverage/residual criteria. The middle panel shows the TIPS dataset. There are three influential points according to leverage/residual criteria. The right panel shows the BODYFAT dataset. There is only one influential point.

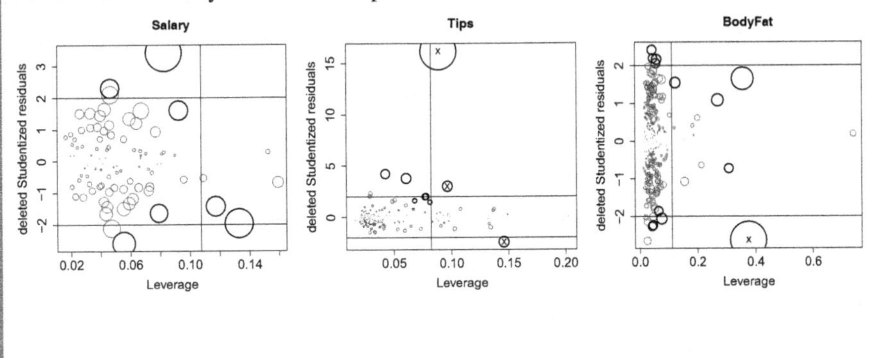

In R

```
M <- lm(Salary~.,data=SALARY)
M <- lm(TipPercentage~.,data=TIPS)
M <- lm(BodyFat~.,data=BODYFAT)
influence.plot(M)
$Cooks
 31  39  81  82  86 128 175 207 216 221 225 231 250
 31  39  81  82  86 128 175 207 216 221 225 231 250

$Leverage
[1] 39
```

In R, once the influence plot is displayed, the row numbers of the influential individuals are printed to the screen.

It is often the case that Cook's distance and the leverage/residual criteria flag different sets of points as influential. This is not a concern since the thresholds that determine whether a point is influential are just heuristics anyway. Once points have been flagged as influential, it is a good idea to review *what* makes these outliers unusual.

In the SALARY dataset, the point with the largest Cook's distance is the person with the highest salary. In the TIPS dataset, the three most influential points are the ones with the largest tip percentages, the two with the largest bills, and the one with the largest tip (one point had the largest bill and tip, which actually was not the largest tip percentage). In the BODYFAT dataset, the single influential point belongs to the heaviest individual. This individual also possesses the largest measurements for many other predictors.

What do we do with the influential points? Are they "bad"? Should they be deleted from the data?

It is only acceptable to remove outliers or influential observations from a dataset when they contain errors in data entry or when they belong to a different group than what you are trying to model (excluding the CEO of the company from the SALARY dataset would be a wise move since the model is for "ordinary" employees). Otherwise, you are stuck with them. You can always fit two models, one with all the data and one with the outliers removed.

Remember that the regression model we are fitting is only an approximation to a more complicated reality. We *expect* there to be outliers since the real world cannot be captured by our simple model. Outliers are often the most interesting cases in the data because they represent "surprises"—individuals who break the mold and stand out for whatever reason.

For example, imagine you are modeling the efficiency of a production center (number of items output per day) based on the number of employees, pay scale, number and length of employee breaks, etc. Influential points are either unusually efficient centers (good or bad) or just have odd combinations of x's. Either way, it is interesting to identify the ones that stand apart.

To summarize, not all points are created equal when it comes to determining the regression coefficients. Since outliers may have a strong effect on the model, it is important to identify them and to validate that they are genuine observations. Usually, you do not delete outliers to obtain a better-fitting model—your model just may not be appropriate. Abandon the model before abandoning the data!

Unfortunately, the influence plot has a major flaw. If extreme outliers are located in a cluster, their deleted studentized residuals will not necessarily be large—the line without one of the outliers is still dragged toward the location of the cluster. Thus, the influence plot is best for detecting the presence of a single outlying individual and is not infallible. How to best identify clusters of outliers is still an open problem.

4.7 Predictions with multiple regression

Making a prediction at some arbitrary combination of predictor variables $x_1, \ldots, x_k$ is as simple as plugging numbers into the regression equation. If b_0, b_1, …, b_k are the estimated coefficients of the regression, then the predicted value $\hat{y}$ is:

$$\hat{y} = b_0 + b_1x_1 + b_2x_2 + \ldots + b_kx_k \tag{4.12}$$

The predicted value $\hat{y}$ is a point estimate, i.e., the best guess of y. Since each coefficient has an associated standard error, $\hat{y}$ has a standard error as well. In Section 3.7, we learned how to construct a confidence interval for the *average* value of y among individuals with some common value of x. We also learned how to make a prediction interval for the y-value of a *particular individual* given his or her value of x.

Fundamentally, nothing really changes when the model has multiple predictors. A review of Section 3.7 may be useful.

- The point estimate for both the average value of y and an individual's value of y is $\hat{y}$.
- The standard error (typical difference between the predicted value and "the truth") for an individual's value is larger than the standard error for the average value—it is uncertain how far the individual will be from the average.
- The standard error of a prediction increases with the distance from $\bar{x}$, the "center" of the x-datacloud (for multiple regression, the "distance from center" is essentially the leverage of the point).
- When the assumptions of the model hold, a point estimate is a predictable amount away from the "truth".
- An approximate 95% confidence interval for $\mu_{y|x}$ (the average value of y among all individuals with a particular combination of the x's) or an approximate 95% prediction interval for an individual's value of y is:

  $$\hat{y} \pm 2 \times SE$$

  Again, the number in front of the standard error may be a little below or above 2 depending on the sample size and the number of predictors. The formulas for the standard errors are different for the average value of y vs. an individual's value of y, with the standard error for an individual being larger (since who knows how far he or she will be away from the average).

One big difference between simple and multiple regression is how to go about determining whether you are extrapolating (predicting at a value outside the range of x-values used to build the model). For simple linear regression, if the x at which you are predicting is much larger or smaller than the maximum or minimum values of x in the data, then you are extrapolating. Such a prediction may be wildly inaccurate if the nature of the relationship changes outside the range of x-values used to build the model.

Detecting extrapolation in multiple regression is not so straightforward. The new point may have typical values for each predictor variable, but it can be very unusual in the *combination* of the predictors. Figure 4.20 shows an example of where a new point (starred) has x_1 and x_2 values that are within the range of x_1 and x_2 used to build the model. However, their combination of values is highly unusual. Predicting at this location would require extrapolation—assuming the nature of the relationship is still the same for values of predictors that have not been seen before.

If there are only two (or maybe three) predictor variables, it is easy to plot the relative location of the new points to see if extrapolation would occur. However, for four or more predictors, the visualization is impossible.

One way to measure how "far away" from the center of the x-datacloud we are making predictions is to calculate the **Mahalanobis distance** of the new points. The Mahalanobis distance is similar to the leverage in that it takes into account the shape of the (presumed elliptically shaped) data-cloud. See Aside 4.7.

Figure 4.20 — Extrapolation in multiple regression. When there is more than one predictor, determining when extrapolation is taking place is more involved than simply checking whether the values for each predictor are within the range used to build the model. Dotted lines are drawn representing the largest and smallest values of x_1 and x_2 in the data. Everything inside the dotted rectangle is naively "in the range" of the x-values used to build the model. The starred point is easily in the rectangle, but making a prediction for it would require extrapolation since its combination of x_1 and x_2 is highly unusual—there is no guarantee that the nature of the relationship between y, x_1, and x_2 is still the same in this region of the x-datacloud.

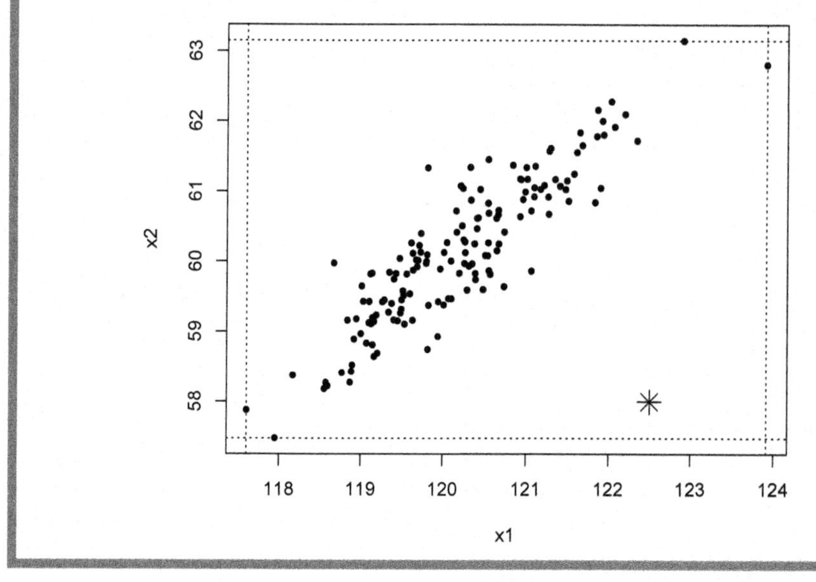

Consider the BODYFAT dataset , where the body fat percentage is predicted from age, weight, height, and circumferences of body parts. Imagine that we want to make a prediction for a person who has values for the first six predictors equal to the 10th percentiles of the respective variables (i.e., small values) and the remaining predictors equal to the 90th percentiles (i.e., large values).

Although each predictor is within the range used to build the model, the *combination* is highly unusual (as we have seen, physical measurements are highly positively correlated, so measurements are typically all large or all small). Indeed, the Mahalanobis distance at this location is larger than 99.6% (all but one) of the individuals used to build the model. This prediction would require extrapolation.

Aside 4.7 — Mahalanobis distance and extrapolating. The Mahalanobis distance of a point is its distance from the center of the x-datacloud with respect to the shape of the stream of points. It is closely related to a point's leverage. Extrapolation occurs when predictions are made at combinations of x that have not been seen before. One way to check for extrapolation is to calculate the new points' Mahalanobis distances to make sure they aren't too large.

In R, `extrapolation.check` will take a data frame containing the locations for predictions and will report the percentiles of their Mahalanobis distances with respect to the distances of the points used to build the model. A large (high percentile) value may indicate extrapolation (though extrapolation may still occur in some unusual cases when the value is low, but this remains undetectable).

In the following example, an extrapolation check is performed on two individuals: one with 2 years of education and 1 year of experience and another with 10 years of education and 12 years of experience. The latter individual requires borderline extrapolation because it is farther away from the center of the x-datacloud than 95.7% of the individuals used to build the model (that pairing of education and experience is highly unusual).

In R

```
M <- lm(Salary~Education*Experience,data=SALARY)
NEWDATA <- data.frame(Education=c(2,10),Experience=c(1,12))
extrapolation.check(M,NEWDATA)

Percentiles are the fraction of observations used in model that are
CLOSER to the center than the point(s) in question.  If Percentile
is about 99% or higher you may be extrapolating.
 Observation Percentile
           1       73.1
           2       95.7
```

4.8 Summary

The multiple regression model gives a phenomenally flexible framework for capturing simultaneous relationships between variables. Fundamentally, the model states that an individual's value of y is essentially a weighted sum of predictor variables plus a random disturbance (whose possible values have the same Normal distribution regardless of the characteristics of the individual).

$$y = \beta_0 + \beta_1 x_1 + \beta_2 x_2 + \ldots + \beta_k x_k + \varepsilon$$

While multiple regression is a powerful tool, there are nuances and complexities that make misinterpreting the model easy to do. Some key insights of a multiple regression model are as follows:

- The coefficient β_i of a predictor variable x_i in a multiple regression (that is not involved in an interaction) has a very precise interpretation: two otherwise identical individuals who differ in x_i by one unit are expected to differ in y by b_i units. If $b_i > 0$, the individual with the larger value of x_i is expected to have a larger value of y. Here, "otherwise identical" is with respect to the other predictors in the model.

- Regarding the significance and p-value of a model or of predictors:
  - A regression model is statistically significant if it predicts y "better" than a model containing only predictors that are unrelated to y. In other words, the reduction in sum of squared errors (compared to the naive model, where y is predicted as the overall average value of y in the data) when using the regression model is "large."
  - The p-value of the model is the probability that a reduction in SSE at least as large as the one obtained by your model would happen by chance (when no predictors have any relationship with y). A p-value less than 5% indicates statistical significance.
  - A predictor variable x is statistically significant if the amount of *additional* information it provides about y (above and beyond the information already offered by the other predictors) is "large."
  - The p-value of x is the probability that adding a predictor (unrelated to y) to a model would reduce the SSE by at least as much the reduction accomplished by adding x.
  - A non-significant predictor can be dropped from a model. To determine if more than one predictor can be dropped, the partial F test must be performed.
- The coefficient, p-value, and significance of x is calculated with respect to a particular model. These numbers will most likely be different when x is in a different model.
- A predictor being statistically significant does *not* mean that x and y are causally linked. A multiple regression is not a physical law and does not tell us what happens to an individual when his or her x value changes.
- To check whether the regression model is an adequate reflection of reality, check the statistical tests of the assumptions. If any are failed and n is less than about 25, the model must be abandoned. Otherwise, check the residuals plots to make sure any statistical violations are minor.
- R^2_{adj} measures how well the model fits the data better than R^2. R^2 has the undesirable property of always increasing when a new predictor is added to a model, even when that predictor is unrelated to y. R^2_{adj} penalizes the goodness of fit by the complexity (number of predictors) of the model.
- Polynomial models, where x, x^2, x^3, etc., are added to the equation, can model nonlinear and non-monotonic relationships between y and x. A rule of thumb is to choose the simplest polynomial model whose R^2_{adj} is no more than 0.005 below the model with the highest R^2_{adj}.
- Since x and y do not have to correspond to the original measurements in the data, you are free to create new variables that are transformations of the original ones or even functions of one or more predictors.
- Interactions between variables often play an important role. Always consider including them in a model.
  - An interaction between x_1 and x_2 exists if the strength of the relationship between y and x_1 (i.e., coefficient of x_1) depends on x_2 and vice versa.
  - An interaction between x_1 and x_2 exists if the expected difference in y between two otherwise identical individuals who differ in x_1 by one unit depends on the specific x_2-value of the individuals we are comparing.
  - If x_1 and x_2 are involved in an interaction, then the coefficient of x_1 by itself is no longer particularly meaningful. To determined the expected difference in y between two individuals who differ in x_1 by one unit, it is necessary to know exactly what value of x_2 the individuals have in common.
- Some points have more influence over the values of the coefficients than others. Checking to make sure any influential points (as identified with an influence plot) are valid is important for checking the validity of a regression model.

4.9 Multiple Regression in R

For the sake of discussion, assume that the data is contained in the data frame `DATA`, `y` is the variable that we want to predict, and `x1`, `x2`, etc., are the predictor variables. By convention, the regression model is saved as `M`.

Scatterplot and correlation matrix

The first step in regression modeling is to visualize the relationships between *y* and the predictors as well as between the predictors themselves. Use `pairs` to see plots. Note: for larger datasets, setting `pch=20` and `cex=0.3` will make the points very small dots so that you can see the streams better.

In R

```
#With all variables
pairs(y~.,data=DATA,pch=20,cex=0.3)

#With all variables except x2
pairs(y~.-x2,data=DATA)

#With just x1 and x5
pairs(y~x1+x5,data=DATA)
```

Correlation matrices are available using `cor.matrix()` and `all.correlations()` as discussed in Chapter 2.

Model Formulation

Model formulation (specifying what variables, transformations, and functions go in the model) has a few shortcuts.

- All variables in `DATA`

  `M <- lm(y~.,data=DATA)`

- Only variables `x1` and `x3`

  `M <- lm(y~x1+x3,data=DATA)`

- All variables except `x1` and `x3`

  `M <- lm(y~.-x1-x3,data=DATA)`

- Two variables (`x1` and `x3`) and their interaction

  `M <- lm(y~x1*x3,data=DATA)`

- All variables as well as the interaction between `x1` and `x3`

  `M <- lm(y~.+x1*x3,data=DATA)`

- All two-way interactions between `x1`, `x2`, and `x3` (along with the variables themselves)

  `M <- lm(y~x1*x2*x3,data=DATA)`

- All two-way interactions between x1, x2, and x3 (as well as x4 and x5)

```
M <- lm(y~x1*x2*x3+x4+x5,data=DATA)
```

- All variables and all two-way interactions

```
M <- lm(y~.^2,data=DATA)
```

- Including logarithms or square roots

```
M <- lm(y~log(x1),data=DATA)
M <- lm(log(y)~log(x1),data=DATA)
M <- lm(sqrt(y)~x1,data=DATA)
```

- A fourth-order polynomial in x1

```
M <- lm(y~poly(x1,4),data=DATA)
```

- All variables including a third-order polynomial model in x5. Note: to find a reasonable order for a polynomial model, fit a simple linear regression first, then run `choose.order` on the model.

```
M <- lm(y~.-x5+poly(x5,3),data=DATA)
```

- Including arbitrary functions (surround function by `I()`)

$$y = \beta_0 + \beta_1 \frac{1}{x_1} + \beta_2 \frac{x_2}{x_3}$$

```
M <- lm( y ~ I(1/x1) + I(x2/x3),data=DATA)
```

$$\frac{y}{1-y} = \beta_0 + \beta_1 x_1 + \beta_2 x_2 (1+x_4)^{0.8}$$

```
M <- lm( I(y/(1-y)) ~ x1 + I(x2*(1+x4)^(0.8)),data=DATA)
```

Model Output

Once the model has been fit, use summary to find the coefficients, standard errors, and p-values. For example:

In R

```
M <- lm(Salary~.,data=SALARY)
summary(M)

Coefficients:
            Estimate Std. Error t value Pr(>|t|)
(Intercept) 2831.079    108.207  26.163  < 2e-16 ***
Education     60.014     16.463   3.645 0.000451 ***
Experience    10.149      4.702   2.158 0.033618 *
Months        15.604      3.467   4.500 2.07e-05 ***
GenderMale   481.633     78.549   6.132 2.41e-08 ***
---
Signif. codes:  0 '***' 0.001 '**' 0.01 '*' 0.05 '.' 0.1 ' ' 1

Residual standard error: 338.3 on 88 degrees of freedom
Multiple R-squared:  0.5109,Adjusted R-squared:  0.4886
F-statistic: 22.98 on 4 and 88 DF,  p-value: 5.079e-13
```

- b_0 (the estimated intercept β_0) is the number in the `Estimate` column in the row labeled `(Intercept)`
- b_i (the estimated coefficient β_i) is the number in the `Estimate` column in the row named after x_i, e.g., the coefficient of `Months` is 15.604.
- The standard errors of the coefficients is in the column `Std. Error`
- The p-values of individual predictors are located in the relevant row under the `Pr(>|t|)` column.
- R^2 is labeled `Multiple R-squared`
- R^2_{adj} is labeled `Adjusted R-squared`
- The root mean squared error (RMSE) is labeled as the first number after `Residual standard error:`
- The p-value of the model itself is the last number of the output after `p-value`.

Checking assumptions

To see the statistical tests of the assumptions behind the regression and to visually evaluate the residuals plot, use `check.regression` with the added option `extra=TRUE` to see the residual vs. predictor plots. If the dataset is large, the results of the statistical tests may take a long time to compute (and are not necessary anyway). Adding the option `tests=FALSE` omits the statistical tests.

```
check.regression(M,extra=TRUE)
```

Confidence/prediction intervals and extrapolation

The procedure for obtaining confidence intervals for the coefficients is identical to that for simple linear regression. The first column of numbers are the lower values in the confidence interval, and the second column of numbers are the upper values.

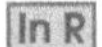

```
confint(M,level=0.95)
```

To make predictions, it is necessary to make (or read in) a data frame containing the x-values where predictions are to be made. The column names of this data frame must match up exactly to the column names in `DATA` used to build the model.

For example, consider predicting `Salary` for three individuals from `Education`, `Experience`, and their interaction, as well as `Months` in the `SALARY` dataset.

In R

```
TO.PREDICT <- data.frame(
  Education=c(0,4,8),
  Experience=c(10,4,2),
  Months=c(0,0,0)
  )
```

When defining the data frame, it is often useful to split up the command like what is displayed above and put the values for each variable on a separate line.

Once the `TO.PREDICT` data frame has been set up, the `predict()` command can be used.

In R

```
M <- lm(Salary~Experience*Education+Months,data=SALARY)

#Predicting average salaries
predict(M,newdata=TO.PREDICT,interval="confidence",level=0.95)
       fit      lwr      upr
1 2996.574 2766.483 3226.666
2 3287.240 3124.589 3449.892
3 3797.689 3550.887 4044.490


#Predicting individual salaries
predict(M,newdata=TO.PREDICT,interval="prediction",level=0.90)
       fit      lwr      upr
1 2996.574 2766.483 3226.666
2 3287.240 3124.589 3449.892
3 3797.689 3550.887 4044.490
```

- The `interval=` argument must be either `"confidence"` (confidence interval for the average) or `"prediction"` (prediction interval for an individual's value).
- The `level=` argument is optional and specifies the level of confidence (if omitted, the default is 0.95).
- The values under the column `fit` give the point estimates (i.e., the values had you plugged those values of x into the regression equation) of each value in the `TO.PREDICT` data frame in order.
- The values under the `lwr` and `upr` give the lower and upper limits of the desired confidence or prediction interval.

It is important to check whether a prediction requires extrapolation. If it does, the predictions may not be trustworthy. Once `TO.PREDICT` has been defined, use `extrapolation.check(M)`.

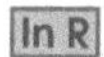

```
extrapolation.check(M,TO.PREDICT)

Note:  analysis assumes the predictor datacloud is roughly elliptical.

Percentiles are the fraction of observations used in model that are CLOSER to
the center than the point(s) in question.  If Percentile is about 99% or higher
you may be extrapolating.
 Observation Percentile
           1       95.7
           2       61.3
           3       77.4
```

Interactions

Visualizing interactions is easier than writing out the implicit regression equations. If your regression model consists of two predictors and their interaction, then `visualize.model(M)` will show the interaction plots. If the model contains many interactions, `see.interactions(M)` will let you scan through a series of interaction plots.

- Both commands can have the extra argument `loc=` to specify the location of the legend. Possible values are `"top"`, `"topleft"`, `"topright"`, `"left"`, `"center"`, `"right"`, `"bottomleft"`, `"bottom"`, `"bottomright"`.
- By default, "small" and "large" are the 5th and 95th percentiles of the distribution. If you want to change this, add in the `level=` argument. Note: `level=0.95` gives the default, `level=0.90` would consider "small" to be the 10th percentile and "large" to be the 90th percentile.

Influential points

An influence plot is made using `influence.plot(M)`. If there are no influential points, the output will be `integer(0)`. The row numbers of influential points are output otherwise.

Partial F test

The partial F test is a test of the significance of a set of a predictors (i.e., does adding the set to a model containing the other variables significantly reduce the sum of squared errors). Two models must be fit and `anova()` must be run. By convention, let `M.simple` be the model without the set of predictors and `M.complex` be the model with the set of predictors.

For example, to test the significance of the set of variables x_2, x_3, and x_5 in the full model:

In R

```
M.simple <- lm(y~.-x2-x3-x5,data=DATA)
M.complex <- lm(y~.,data=DATA)
anova(M.simple,M.complex)
  Res.Df    RSS Df Sum of Sq      F    Pr(>F)
1    107 66862
2    105 45683  2     21179 24.339 2.066e-09 ***
```

The relevant p-value is the number under `Pr(>F)`. If the p-value is less than 5%, the set of variables is statistically significant (adding them to the simpler model significantly reduces the error).

Variance inflation factors

Use the command `VIF(M)` to obtain the variance inflation factors of a model. One useful guideline is to compare the VIF to $1/(1-R^2)$, where R^2 is the `Multiple R-Squared` of the model. If the VIF exceeds this number, the other predictors do a better job predicting x than they do predicting y.

4.10 Exercises

1: Use `EX4.BIKE`. This is a modified version of part of the `kaggle.com` competition data where we are interested in predicting demand at bicycle kiosks in DC.

a) Make the scatterplot matrix. Let us predict `Demand` from `AvgTemp`, `EffectiveAvgTemp`, `AvgHumidity`, and `AvgWindspeed`.

b) Do you believe the relationships between `Demand` and these four predictors are linear enough for multiple regression to be a good model? Explain.

c) Fit the four simple linear regressions. Complete the following table. Report the coefficients to the nearest integer and p-values (keep three digits after the decimal; if a p-value is less than 0.001, record it as 0), along with whether it is statistically significant.

Predictor	Coefficient	p-value	Significant?
AvgTemp	138	0	Yes
EffectiveAvgTemp			
AvgHumidity			
AvgWindspeed			

d) Fit the multiple regression model using these four predictors. Examine the results of `summary()`.

1) Is the model itself statistically significant? Quote the relevant p-value.
2) Report the value of R^2 and interpret this number.
3) Report the value of R^2_{adj} and discuss why we use it rather then R^2 to assess how well the model fits the data.
4) Report the typical error made by the regression.
5) In your opinion, is this a useful model for predicting `Demand`?

e) Write out the fitted regression equation (round coefficients to the nearest integer).

f) Precisely interpret the coefficient of `AvgWindspeed` (the average for the day in MPH).

g) Report a 95% confidence interval for the coefficient of `AvgTemp`. Explain why this, as well as the p-value, implies that `AvgTemp` is not significant in the multiple regression.

h) `AvgTemp` is not significant in the multiple regression model, but it is in the simple linear regression. By carefully explaining what it means for a variable to be significant in a multiple regression model, comment on whether `AvgTemp` does or does not have useful information for predicting `Demand`.

i) Explain why we would be justified in dropping `AvgTemp` from the model, but not BOTH `AvgTemp` AND `EffectiveAvgTemp` (even though they are both non-significant).

j) Perform a partial F test and determine whether we can drop both `AvgTemp` and `EffectiveAvgTemp`.

k) Run `check.regression`. Which statistical tests are failed? Based on the diagnostic plots, are the violations severe enough for the model to be invalidated?

2: Use `EX4.STOCKS`. The first column is the closing price of Alcoa stock (AA), while the remaining columns are the closing prices of other stocks and commodities from two days prior. If we could use the information in the market today to predict the price of Alcoa two days from now, we could make a killing.

a) Fit a model predicting AA from ALL of the other variables using the "dot" shortcut. Run `check.regression` and see whether the assumptions of the model hold up well. Report the value of R^2_{adj} and comment on whether this model may be useful.

b) As a whole, stock and commodity prices are often strongly correlated with each other, so there may be a large amount of redundant information in the predictors. Calculate the cutoff for a "large" variance inflation factor and comment on whether multicollinearity is a problem in this model.

c) Your boss asks what it means to have multicollinearity present in a model. Explain. Does it mean the model is invalid?

d) What is the standard error of the coefficient of `IBMlag2` (closing price of IBM two days prior), and what does this number tell us? The VIF is 17. What does the value of the VIF tell us?

ce its p-value is 0.0001. Does this mean this
bout the closing price of Alcoa? If not, explain

ince its p-value is 0.6633. Does this mean that
nation about the closing price of Alcoa? If not,
y tells us.
ata in EX4.STOCKPREDICT. Using predict(),
osing price of Alcoa stock. How wide (to the
believe these intervals are useful for making
closing price of Alcoa is between \$81 and \$88,
1 from day to day.

dataset on many occasions, and the goal is to
stics (the units of all values are in metric and

les in the dataframe. Do the relationships of
roughly linear? If not, which ones don't?
. Examine summary() as well as
ss at least one issue with the regression that

, so let us try polynomial fits. Fit four simple
run choose.order (max order of 6). Report
on the 0.005 heuristic.
levant polynomial terms and call it M.poly.
compare them to the model in (b). Comment
on whether these extra terms have "significantly" improved the model. Note: your command should look something like (replace the question marks with the selected orders):

```
M.poly <- lm(FuelEfficiency~poly(CabVolume,?)+poly(Horsepower,?)+
            poly(TopSpeed,?)+poly(Weight,?),data=AUTO)
```

e) Run check.regression on the polynomial model (be sure to add extra=TRUE). Comment on whether you think the model's assumptions are satisfied.

4: Use EX4.BIKE.

a) Fit a model predicting Demand from all predictors. Examine the results of summary and the influence plot for this model.
b) There is one extremely influential point in this dataset. Print out the influential row, then explain what makes it so unusual through the use of summary on the dataframe and/or scatterplots with these observations.
c) The influential point represents a data error, so we are justified in removing it. Re-fit the model *without* this point and examine the results of summary. Comment on the change in R^2, $RMSE$, and the significance of predictors using this new model. To do this, run the command (replacing xxx with the offending row to take it out):

```
M.new <- lm(Demand~AvgTemp+EffectiveAvgTemp+AvgHumidity+AvgWindspeed,
              data=EX4.BIKE[-xxx,])
summary(M.new)
```

d) The *strength* of the relationship between Demand and the other predictors may not be a constant. For example, the strength of the relationship between Demand and Temperature may depend on Windspeed (on warm days, wind speed may not matter, but on cold days, wind speed may matter a lot). Fit a model with all two-way interactions (but without that influential point) and use `see.interactions` to scan for possible interactions (note: add the argument `many=TRUE`, or there will be too many plots). Does it look like we should include interactions into the model? Why or why not?

e) Fit a model predicting `Demand` from `AvgTemp` and `AvgWindspeed`, including the interaction (but omitting the offensive row). Examine the results of `summary` and `visualize.model`. Is the interaction statistically significant?

5: Use `TIPS`. The percentage tip left on a bill (`TipPercentage`) has an interesting relationship with the bill amount (`Bill`) and number of people at the table (`PartySize`).

a) Fit a model predicting the tip percentage from the bill amount and size of party, including the interaction. Look at the model using `visualize.model`. You'll see that `PartySize` is not significant. Would we be justified in dropping it from the model? Why or why not?
b) Write out the regression equation. Round each coefficient to two decimal places.
c) Write out the implicit regression equations between tip percentage and bill for parties of size 1 and for parties of size 4.
d) What is the story that the data tells us? In other words, describe how the relationship between tip percentage and bill amount changes as the party size gets bigger. Does it get weaker, stronger? Is it positive, negative?
e) A better predictor of tip percentage may be the bill amount *per person*. Define a variable to be `Bill` divided by `PartySize` (call it `BPP`, the bill per person, and add it to the `TIPS` dataframe). Then fit a simple linear regression predicting tip percentage from it. Examine the `summary` output, and comment on whether this is a better model than predicting tip percentage from bill, party size, and the interaction from (a).

```
BPP <- TIPS$Bill/TIPS$PartySize
TIPS$BPP <- BPP
summary(lm(TipPercentagee~BPP,data=TIPS))
```

Encoding categorical variables
Two levels
Three or more levels
Coefficients of indicator variables
Categorical variables with two levels
Categorical variables with three or more levels
Interactions and categorical variables
Categorical variables with two levels
Categorical variables with three or more levels
Summary
Using R
Exercises

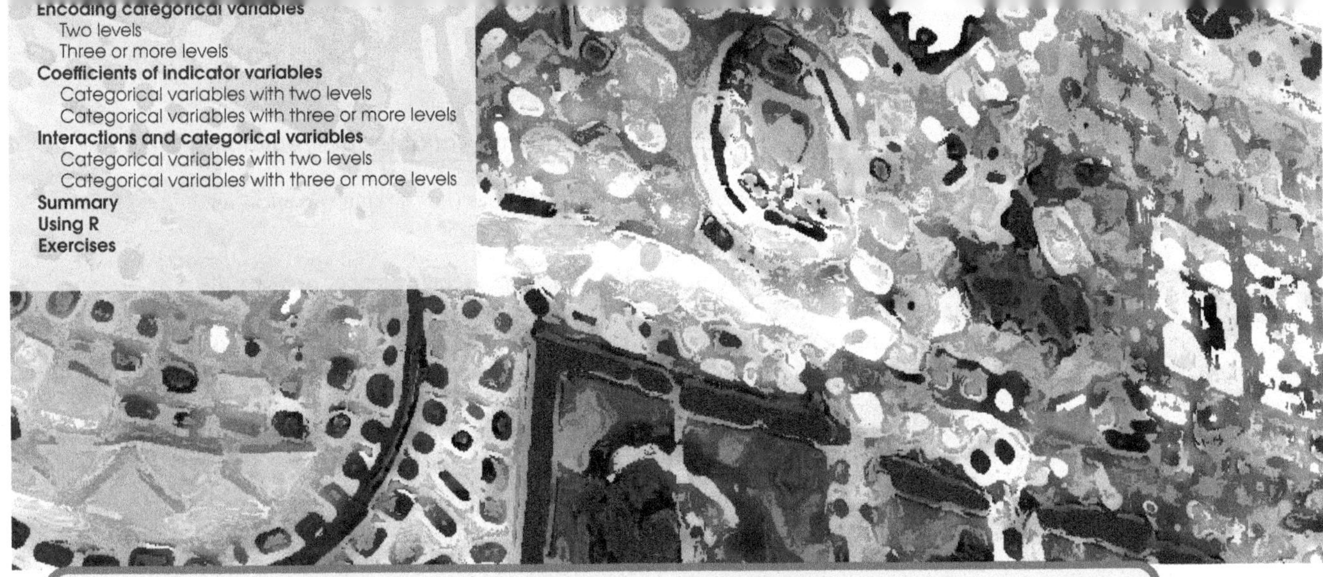

5. Categorical Variables as Predictors

Many interesting potential predictors of y are categorical variables, e.g., gender, homeownership, and relationship status. Since regression models only take numerical variables as input, this poses a problem! Luckily, there are ways to "fool" the regression into thinking that a categorical variable is numerical so that it can be incorporated into the model.

To motivate the discussion, consider the SALARY dataset. This data was originally collected to determine whether there is gender discrimination at a company. At first glance, the evidence is pretty glaring. In the random sample of 93 employees (61 female and 32 male), the average monthly pay is \$545 higher for males. See Figure 5.1. A test for association between pay and gender (Section 2.4) shows this difference is highly statistically significant. Considering the average salary in the company is \$3600, this difference is large and has practical significance.

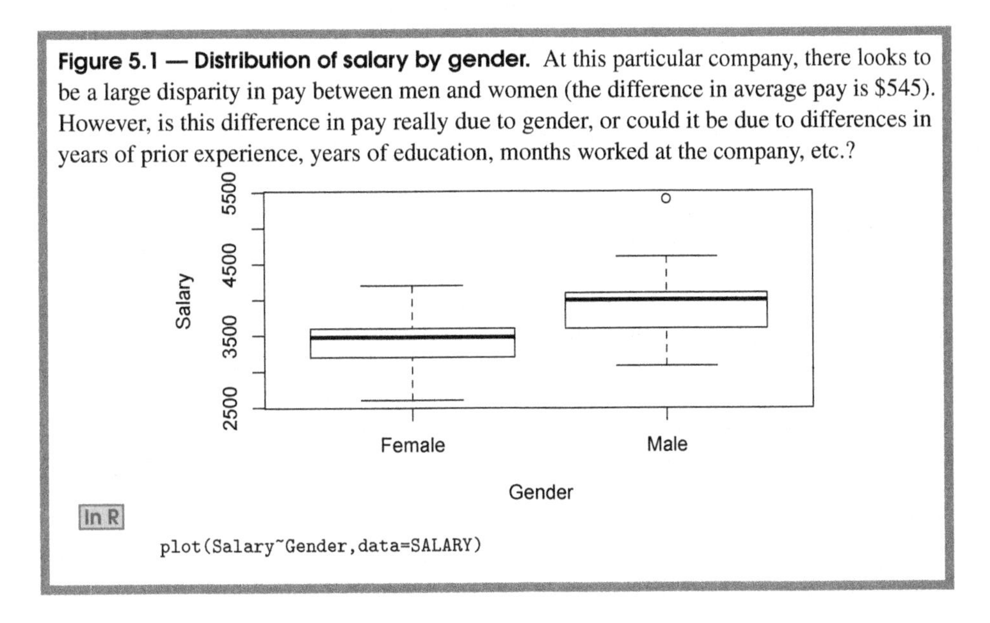

Figure 5.1 — Distribution of salary by gender. At this particular company, there looks to be a large disparity in pay between men and women (the difference in average pay is \$545). However, is this difference in pay really due to gender, or could it be due to differences in years of prior experience, years of education, months worked at the company, etc.?

In R

```
plot(Salary~Gender,data=SALARY)
```

In its defense, the company claims there are alternative explanations (i.e., lurking variables) for the difference in pay.

- Salaries are higher for people with more education. The average number of years of education among its women is 1.5 years smaller than the average among its men.
- Salaries are higher for people with more work experience. The average number of years of experience among its women is 0.3 years smaller than the average among its men.

The company could be correct—the discrepancy in pay *may* be due to differences in these variables rather than due to gender. How can we tell?

Multiple regression provides us with the tools we need to investigate the difference in average pay. To assess the apparent gender disparity, we need to first account for differences in people's experience, education, and months with the company. If we could put `Gender` into a regression model along with `Education`, `Experience`, and `Months`, its coefficient would tell us exactly what we want to know: the typical difference in salary between otherwise identical men and women (i.e., with equal amounts of education, experience, and tenure at the company). So how can we coerce `Gender`, a categorical variable, to be a numerical quantity?

In this chapter, we will learn how to incorporate categorical variables into a regression model through the use of indicator variables. Indicator variables allow us to model the possibility that levels of a categorical variable may have different average values of y and/or the strength of the relationship between y and x may vary between levels.

5.1 Encoding categorical variables

We trick the regression into thinking that a categorical variable is numerical by representing it as a set of numerical variables that take on the values of 0 and 1. These variables are called **indicator variables** (or dummy variables).

5.1.1 Categorical variables with two levels

A variable such as gender has two levels since it typically only takes on two values: female and male. Let us define an indicator variable called *Male* as follows:

$$Male = \begin{cases} 0, & \text{if female} \\ 1, & \text{if male} \end{cases}$$

We could have chosen to represent the levels by different numbers (e.g., 3 and 7), but the choice of 0 and 1 is standard in R and most other software packages.

Another reasonable encoding is to let the values be $+1$ and -1. When this is the case, the interpretation of the coefficients is different than what is presented here. Be very mindful how your software treats categorical variables!

> By convention, the level that comes *last* alphabetically gets assigned a 1, and the variable that comes *first* alphabetically is assigned a 0.

5.1.2 Categorical variables with three or more levels

When a categorical variable has more than two possible values, it is necessary to represent it by a *set* of indicator variables. In fact, if the variable has L levels, then a total of $L-1$ indicator variables are required to fully represent it.

> By convention, the level that comes *first* alphabetically is called the **reference level** and does not have an indicator variable represent it. Each other level is represented by an indicator variable that equals 1 (if the individual has that level) or 0 (if the individual does not).

For example, one of the predictors in the `TIPS` dataset is the day of the week (Thursday-Sunday). Friday comes first alphabetically, so it is the reference level and not represented by an indicator variable. The other levels are represented by the following three indicator variables:

$$Thursday = \begin{cases} 1, & \text{if Thursday} \\ 0, & \text{otherwise} \end{cases} \quad Saturday = \begin{cases} 1, & \text{if Saturday} \\ 0, & \text{otherwise} \end{cases} \quad Sunday = \begin{cases} 1, & \text{if Sunday} \\ 0, & \text{otherwise} \end{cases}$$

The day "Thursday" is represented as $Thursday = 1$, $Saturday = 0$, and $Sunday = 0$, while "Friday" is represented as $Thursday = 0$ (i.e., not Thursday), $Saturday = 0$ (i.e., not Saturday), and $Sunday = 0$ (i.e., not Sunday).

5.2 Coefficients of indicator variables

The net effect of adding a categorical variable with L levels into a regression model (via a set of $L-1$ indicator variables) is that L different regressions are fit, one for each level. These implicit regression equations are allowed to have *different* intercepts, but they are forced to have the *same* coefficients for all other x's.

In other words, the implicit regression lines are all parallel to one another. The distances between them represent the differences in the average value of y between levels after accounting for the other predictors in the model.

Adding a categorical variable to a regression allows us to model the possibility that the average value of y is different for each of its levels among otherwise identical individuals. The coefficients of the indicator variables reveal how the average value of y varies between levels.

> The coefficient of an indicator variable (assuming it is not involved in an interaction) tells us the difference between the average value of y among individuals who possess the level represented by the indicator variable and the average value of y among individuals who possess the reference level after accounting for the other variables in the model (i.e., all individuals have identical values for the other predictors in the model).
>
> If the coefficient is positive, the average value of y is higher for individuals possessing the level represented by the indicator variable . If the coefficient is negative, the average value of y is lower for individuals possessing that level.

> The difference in coefficients of two indicator variables (e.g., $b_i - b_j$) gives the difference in the average value of y between those two levels (level i minus level j) after accounting for the other variables in the model.

The coefficient of an indicator variable can also be interpreted as the expected difference in y between two particular individuals.

> The coefficient of an indicator variable (not involved in an interaction) tells us the expected difference in y between two otherwise identical (with respect to the other predictors in the model) individuals when one possesses the level represented by the indicator variable and the other possesses the reference level.
>
> If the coefficient is positive, the individual with the level represented by the indicator variable is expected to have a larger value of y than the individual with the reference level. If the coefficient is negative, the individual with the level represented by the indicator variable is expected to have a smaller value of y than the individual with the reference level.
>
> The difference in coefficients of two indicator variables (e.g., $b_i - b_j$) gives the expected difference in y between otherwise identical individual when one individual has level i and the other has level j.

Let us walk through a few examples. In this section, we assume that the categorical variable is *not* involved in any interactions. If it is, this discussion does not apply and you must refer to Section 5.3.

5.2.1 Coefficients of indicator variables representing two-level categorical variables

In the `SALARY` dataset, we want to determine whether the average salary between men and women is the same when we compare individuals with equal amounts of education, experience, and tenure at the company. The data shows that the average salary for females is much lower than that of males, but the company has argued that this is because of other factors (e.g., females as a whole at the company have less education, which naturally yields smaller salaries). Let us begin the analysis by incorporating gender into a model with `Education`.

The estimated regression equation will be:

$$Salary = b_0 + b_1 Education + b_2 Male$$

While this looks like a single equation, it is actually two! To see this, let us write the **implicit regression equations** for each level by plugging in the relevant values for the indicator variables. Since "female" comes first alphabetically, we plug in `Male=0`. "Male" comes last alphabetically, so we plug in `Male=1`.

$$\text{Female:} \quad Salary = b_0 + b_1 Education + b_2 \times 0$$
$$= b_0 + b_1 Education$$

$$\text{Male:} \quad Salary = b_0 + b_1 Education + b_2 \times 1$$
$$= (b_0 + b_2) + b_1 Education$$

The implicit regression equations have the same slope (the coefficient of `Education` is b_1 for both genders), but the intercepts differ. Females have the intercept b_0, while males have the intercept $b_0 + b_2$.

Figure 5.2 shows the implicit regression lines on a scatterplot. The two lines are parallel: same slope but different intercepts. The difference in intercepts (and also the constant offset between the regression lines) is b_2. This represents the difference in the average salary between men and women after accounting for `Education`.

The regression output adds more details. The coefficient of `Education` is $53.80 and is the (identical) slope of the implicit regression lines. Two individuals (of the same gender) who differ in education by one year are expected to differ in salary by $53.80 (the person with more education is expected to earn a higher salary).

In R

```
M <- lm(Salary~Education+Gender,data=SALARY)
summary(M)

              Estimate Std. Error t value Pr(>|t|)
(Intercept)   3212.47      88.00  36.505  < 2e-16 ***
Education       53.80      18.45   2.916  0.00447 **
GenderMale     461.21      88.15   5.232 1.09e-06 ***
```

In R, the level that is represented by the indicator variable is appended to the name of the predictor. This variable equals 1 when the individual has that level and is 0 otherwise. Above, `GenderMale` = 1 for men and 0 for women.

The coefficient of `Gender` is $461.21 and is the difference in intercepts of the regression lines (i.e., their separation). Among people with the same value of `Education`, men earn $461.21 more than women on average.

Thus, one of the company's alternative explanations for the difference in salaries appears to be invalid. The company is correct that people with more education do get paid more, and that women at this company typically have fewer years of education than males. However, after taking into account the variation in salary due to differences in education, there is still a $461 average difference. The p-value of the coefficient is about 1 in a million. Chance alone is not a reasonable explanation of the difference in salaries.

The company responds that the analysis is not complete because experience and tenure at the company must also be considered. A more thorough analysis of the `SALARY` data (see Section 7.3.1) shows that a "better" model for predicting `Salary` uses `Education`, `Experience`, `Months` at the company, and the interactions `Education`×`Experience` and `Education`×`Months`. Thus, let us add `Gender` to this model and see if it is statistically significant.

If `Gender` is not statistically significant, then all of the variation in salaries at this company could be attributed to differences in employees' educational levels, prior work experience, and months at the company. If `Gender` is statistically significant, there is strong evidence of there being a real difference in pay based on gender even after accounting for the other variables.

Figure 5.2 — Implicit regression lines for SALARY data. By defining an indicator variable `Male` (1 for males and 0 for females), we have effectively fit two separate regressions, one for women and one for men. These lines have the same slope but different intercepts. The difference in intercepts is the offset between the two lines, which represents the difference in average salary between men and women after accounting for education.

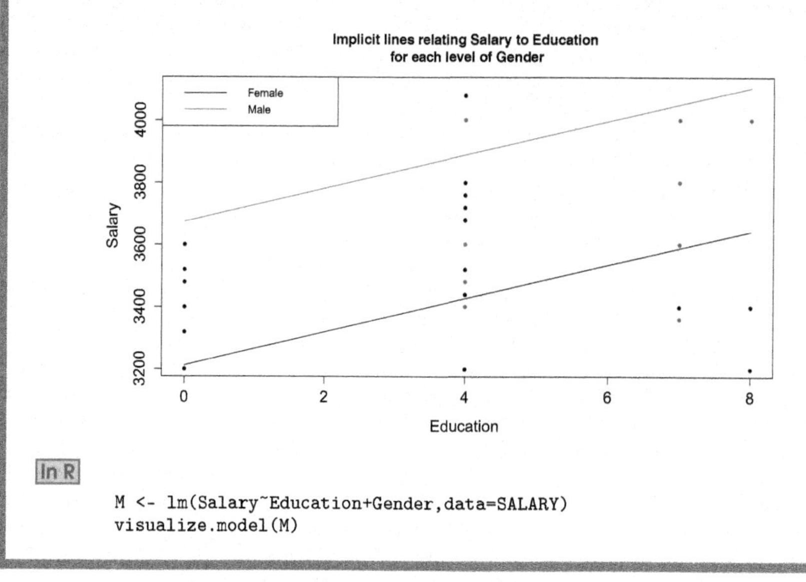

In R

```
M <- lm(Salary~Education+Gender,data=SALARY)
visualize.model(M)
```

In R

```
M <- lm(Salary~.+Education*Experience+Education*Months,data=SALARY)
summary(M)

                     Estimate Std. Error t value Pr(>|t|)
(Intercept)          2831.567    154.631  18.312  < 2e-16 ***
Education              64.847     32.052   2.023   0.0462 *
Months                  6.208      7.276   0.853   0.3959
Experience             26.394     10.096   2.614   0.0106 *
Education:Experience   -3.761      2.137  -1.760   0.0819 .
Education:Months        1.969      1.442   1.365   0.1757
GenderMale            448.657     79.727   5.627 2.24e-07 ***
```

The coefficient of `Gender` reveals the difference in average salaries between otherwise identical (in terms of experience, education, and months) men and women. Men earn an average of $449 more than women, and the difference is statistically significant. Thus, the company's rebuttals have been refuted. We have eliminated `Education`, `Experience`, and `Months` as potential lurking variables and there is still a highly noticeable difference in average pay.

The company still has a few outs. One thing that has not been included in the model is the position of each employee. Differences in job descriptions could explain the differences in salary. Perhaps women in the company have lower-level positions for whatever reason. However, given that the levels of education and experience are not *that* different between men and women, this appears unlikely. It would also raise the question of *why* women tend to have lower-level positions than their male counterparts.

Let us consider the `ATTRACTF` dataset. Recall the data contains the attractiveness ratings of 70 women along with some of their physical characteristics (many of which are categorical). Let us answer the question: "After accounting for other sources of variation in attractiveness score such as fitness, wearing glasses, smiling, etc., is there a statistically significant difference in the average attractiveness scores of women whose pictures were selfies and women whose pictures were taken by someone else?" Figure 5.3 shows side-by-side box plots of the `Score` for both picture types. The difference in averages looks small and may not be statistically significant.

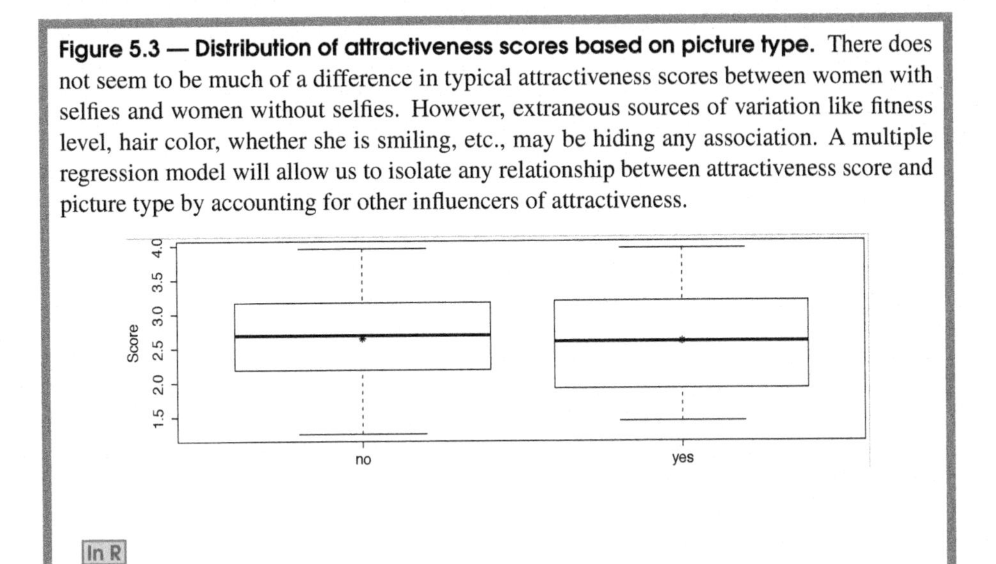

Figure 5.3 — Distribution of attractiveness scores based on picture type. There does not seem to be much of a difference in typical attractiveness scores between women with selfies and women without selfies. However, extraneous sources of variation like fitness level, hair color, whether she is smiling, etc., may be hiding any association. A multiple regression model will allow us to isolate any relationship between attractiveness score and picture type by accounting for other influencers of attractiveness.

In R

```
associate(Score~Selfie,data=ATTRACTF)
```

The two levels of `Selfie` are "yes" and "no." Thus, let us define an indicator variable `Selfie` as

$$Selfie = \begin{cases} 0, & \text{if no} \\ 1, & \text{if yes} \end{cases}$$

Fitting the regression equation $Score = b_0 + b_1 Selfie$ is equivalent to performing a test to see if there is an overall difference in averages between the two levels (Section 2.4.2).

In R

```
M <- lm(Score~Selfie,data=ATTRACTF)
summary(M)
             Estimate Std. Error t value Pr(>|t|)
(Intercept)  2.64266    0.12276  21.528   <2e-16 ***
Selfieyes   -0.04437    0.16884  -0.263    0.794
```

The coefficient of `Selfie` is -0.04, implying that the average rating for women whose pictures are selfies is 0.04 below the average rating for non-selfies. Since the p-value is greater than 5%, this difference is not statistically significant. However, there may be more to the story since many other variables are associated with attraction. The significance may change once more variables are added to the model (Section 4.4.4).

Let us account for differences in the fitness levels of the women and fit the model $Score = \beta_0 + \beta_1 Selfie + \beta_2 Fitness + \varepsilon$. Figure 5.4 shows the two implicit regression lines.

Figure 5.4 — Relating attractiveness level to taking a selfie and fitness score. The model is $Score = \beta_0 + \beta_1 FitnessScore + \beta_2 Selfie + \varepsilon$. By defining an indicator variable $Selfie$ (equals 0 for "no" and 1 for "yes"), we have in effect fit a separate regression for each picture type. The lines are constrained to have the same slope but are allowed to have different intercepts. The difference in intercepts is the offset between the two lines and represents the difference in average attractiveness ratings between the two levels after taking into account fitness level. We see that selfies score higher, but the difference looks minor.

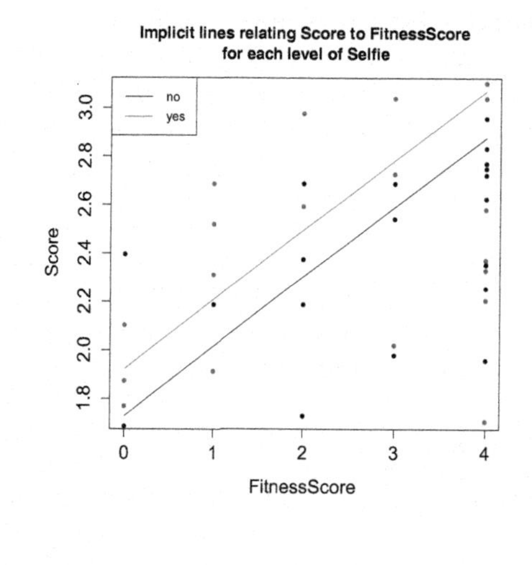

In R

```
M <- lm(Score~FitnessScore+Selfie,data=ATTRACTF)
visualize.model(M)
```

As always, these lines are parallel (same slope) but are allowed to have different intercepts. Unlike the salary example, we see relatively little offset between the lines.

After accounting for fitness, the difference in average attractiveness between selfies and non-selfies is still small. The coefficient of `Selfie` is 0.19, implying that among women with the same fitness level, women with selfies have a higher average attractiveness. However, this difference is still not statistically significant since the p-value is 17%.

In R

```
M <- lm(Score~FitnessScore+Selfie,data=ATTRACTF)
summary(M)

             Estimate Std. Error t value Pr(>|t|)
(Intercept)   1.72954    0.17599   9.827 1.29e-14 ***
FitnessScore  0.28698    0.04589   6.254 3.19e-08 ***
Selfieyes     0.19396    0.14043   1.381    0.172
```

Even in a more sophisticated model for predicting attractiveness score (using information about the woman's fitness, hairstyle, nose, and amount of makeup), the indicator variable representing `Selfie` is not significant. If there is an association between a picture being a selfie and the woman's perceived level of attractiveness, it must be too weak to be detected from this data.

5.2.2 Categorical variables with three or more levels

To add a categorical variable with L levels to a regression, we must define a set of $L-1$ indicator variables. When these variables are added to the model, the effect is that L different regression lines are fit simultaneously, one for each level. These lines will have different intercepts (representing the differences in the average values of y between levels) but identical coefficients for the other predictor variables.

For example, consider the `TIPS` dataset. Is the average tip percentage left on a bill the same across all days of the week, i.e., all levels of the variable `Weekday`? We have seen that tip percentage has a negative association with bill size, and it may be the case that people spend more on the weekend than on weekdays. Thus, we should account for bill size before comparing the average tip percentage between days. Multiple regression is the appropriate tool.

The regression model is

$$Tip\% = \beta_0 + \beta_1 Bill + \beta_2 Thursday + \beta_3 Saturday + \beta_4 Sunday + \varepsilon$$

Dropping the ε term and plugging in the relevant values for each indicator variable, we find the four implicit regression equations are:

$$\begin{aligned}
\text{Thursday:} \quad Tip\% &= \beta_0 + \beta_1 Bill + \beta_2 \times 1 + \beta_3 \times 0 + \beta_4 \times 0 \\
&= (\beta_0 + \beta_2) + \beta_1 Bill \\[1em]
\text{Friday:} \quad Tip\% &= \beta_0 + \beta_1 Bill + \beta_2 \times 0 + \beta_3 \times 0 + \beta_4 \times 0 \\
&= \beta_0 + \beta_1 Bill \\[1em]
\text{Saturday:} \quad Tip\% &= \beta_0 + \beta_1 Bill + \beta_2 \times 0 + \beta_3 \times 1 + \beta_4 \times 0 \\
&= (\beta_0 + \beta_3) + \beta_1 Bill \\[1em]
\text{Sunday:} \quad Tip\% &= \beta_0 + \beta_1 Bill + \beta_2 \times 0 + \beta_3 \times 0 + \beta_4 \times 1 \\
&= (\beta_0 + \beta_4) + \beta_1 Bill
\end{aligned}$$

Thus, β_0 represents the intercept for Friday (the reference level). The value of β_1 represents the difference in intercepts between Thursday and Friday, i.e., the difference in the average tip percentage on Friday vs. Thursday after accounting for any variation in bill sizes.

Fitting the model, we find that

In R

```
M <- lm(TipPercentage~Bill+Weekday,data=TIPS)
summary(M)

                  Estimate Std. Error t value Pr(>|t|)
(Intercept)       21.10638    1.50430  14.031  < 2e-16 ***
Bill              -0.23942    0.04215  -5.680 3.89e-08 ***
WeekdayThursday -0.74686    1.50804  -0.495    0.621
WeekdaySaturday -0.89662    1.46276  -0.613    0.540
WeekdaySunday     0.71099    1.48582   0.479    0.633
```

The four implicit regression lines have the same slope of $b_1 = -0.24$. After accounting for day of the week, two bills that differ by \$1 are expected to differ in their tip percentages by 0.24%, with larger bills having the lower percentage.

The intercept of the implicit regression line for Friday (reference level) is 21.11. The coefficient of the indicator variables for `Weekday` give the difference in intercepts of the implicit regression lines for each day.

- The coefficient of the indicator variable for Thursday is -0.75. Thus, the intercept for the implicit regression line for Thursday is $21.11 - 0.75 = 20.36$.
- The coefficient of the indicator variable for Sunday is 0.71. Thus, the intercept for the implicit regression line for Sunday is $21.11 + 0.71 = 21.82$.

The coefficient also reveals the difference in the average value of y between that level and the reference level after accounting for the other predictors in the model. When comparing bills of the same size, the average tip percentage on Thursday is 0.75% lower when compared to Friday, while the average tip percentage on Sunday is 0.71% higher when compared to Friday.

To obtain the difference in the average values of y between two arbitrary levels, we subtract the coefficients of the relevant indicator variables. When comparing bills of equal sizes, the average tip percentage on Saturday is 1.61% lower when compared to Sunday since $-0.90 - 0.71 = -1.61$.

Although the procedure is tedious, we can write out the implicit regression equations relating the tip percentage to bill amount for each day of the week.

$$Tip\% = 21.11 - 0.24Bill - 0.75Thursday - 0.90Saturday + 0.71Sunday$$

$$\begin{aligned} \text{Thursday:} \quad Tip\% &= 21.1 - 0.24Bill - 0.75 \times 1 - 0.90 \times 0 + 0.71 \times 0 \\ &= 20.36 - 0.24Bill \end{aligned}$$

$$\begin{aligned} \text{Friday:} \quad Tip\% &= 21.1 - 0.24Bill - 0.75 \times 0 - 0.90 \times 0 + 0.71 \times 0 \\ &= 21.11 - 0.24Bill \end{aligned}$$

$$\begin{aligned} \text{Saturday:} \quad Tip\% &= 21.1 - 0.24Bill - 0.75 \times 0 - 0.90 \times 1 + 0.71 \times 0 \\ &= 20.21 - 0.24Bill \end{aligned}$$

$$\begin{aligned} \text{Sunday:} \quad Tip\% &= 21.1 - 0.24Bill - 0.75 \times 0 - 0.90 \times 0 + 0.71 \times 1 \\ &= 21.82 - 0.24Bill \end{aligned}$$

Figure 5.5 shows the four implicit regression lines on a scatterplot. The offsets between lines look minor. Even if the difference in average tip percentages turns out to be statistically significant, this difference is likely not of any practical significance to a waiter.

How can we test whether the categorical variable is statistically significant, i.e., whether there is *some* difference in the average value of y between levels after accounting for the other predictors in the model? We need to check if there is a "large" reduction in the sum of squared errors when the *set* of indicators is added to the model already containing the other predictors.

Figure 5.5 — Tip percentage vs. bill amount for different days of the week. Loosely, the fitted model is $Tip\% = \beta_0 + \beta_1 Bill + Day$. Since Day is a categorical variable with four levels, it is actually represented by three indicator variables. The four implicit regression equations are displayed. They are constrained to be parallel to each other (same slope) but are allowed to have different intercepts. The offset between two lines represents the difference in average tip percentage between those two days when comparing bills of equal size. Since all lines are quite close to one another, there is very little indication that tip percentage varies much with day after accounting for the bill amount.

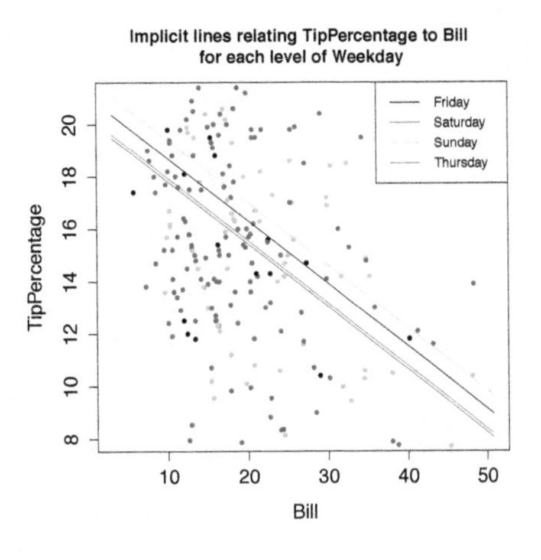

In R

```
M <- lm(TipPercentage~Bill+Weekday,data=TIPS)
visualize.model(M,loc="topright")
```

The procedure for checking the significance of a *set* of predictors has previously been discussed in Section 4.4.2 and is called the partial F test. When the test deals with a categorical variable, we refer to it as an **effect test** instead. To perform an effect test:

- Fit the model without the categorical variable and calculate its sum of squared errors SSE_{simple}
- Fit the model with the categorical variable and calculate its sum of squared errors $SSE_{complex}$
- Calculate the F statistic

$$F_{complex} = \frac{(SSE_{simple} - SSE_{complex})(C-S)}{SSE_{complex}/(n-C-1)} = \frac{(R^2_{complex} - R^2_{simple})/(C-S)}{(1-R^2_{complex})/(n-C-1)}$$

- F values near 1.0 indicate the reduction in sum of squared errors when the set of indicator variables is added to the model could happen "by chance." Large values of F indicate significance of the categorical variable. The p-value can be found via the permutation procedure or with a formula when the assumptions behind regression are valid. In practice, it is read from software.
- If the p-value is less than 5%, then the categorical variable is statistically significant: there is a statistically significant difference in averages between at least two levels after

accounting for the other predictors in the model. Otherwise, the categorical variable is not significant and, for all intents and purposes, each level has the same average value of y. Note: the effect test does not tell us *which* levels have different average values of y, only that there is *some* difference.

The following are the effect tests for both `Weekday` and `Bill` (the p-value of `Bill` is identical to the p-value in the standard regression output).

In R

```
M <- lm(TipPercentage~Bill+Weekday,data=TIPS)
drop1(M,test="F")
        Df Sum of Sq    RSS    AIC F value    Pr(>F)
Bill     1   1067.00 8970.0 887.49 32.2679 3.887e-08 ***
Weekday  3    121.77 8024.7 856.32  1.2275    0.3003
```

The addition of `Weekday` to a model already including `Bill` reduces the sum of squared errors by 121.77. This reduction is not statistically significant since the p-value is greater than 5% (30% from the output)—this reduction could have easily happened "by chance" (i.e., by adding three predictors that are unrelated to tip percentage to the model). Consistent with the visual analysis, we find that there is no solid evidence that tip percentage varies with the day of the week when we compare bills of equal size.

As a final example, consider the timeless debate of which type of pet owner is "smarter": cat people, dog people, people who like both, or people who like neither. A survey of introductory statistics students recorded their current college and final high school GPAs as well as their pet preference (`EDUCATION` dataset). Looking at the regression output, we find that none of the p-values of the indicator variables for `Pet` are statistically significant.

In R

```
M <- lm(CollegeGPA~HSGPA+Pet,data=EDUCATION)
summary(M)

            Estimate Std. Error t value Pr(>|t|)
(Intercept)  1.60462    0.18554   8.649   <2e-16 ***
HSGPA        0.46103    0.04694   9.821   <2e-16 ***
PetCat       0.11568    0.08819   1.312    0.190
PetDog      -0.06230    0.06646  -0.937    0.349
PetNeither  -0.05574    0.07267  -0.767    0.443
```

However, the p-value of the indicator variable `PetCat` is testing whether the average college GPA of "cat people" is different from the average college GPA of people who like both (the reference level) after accounting for any differences in high school GPA. This is not the comparison we are after.

> In standard regression output, the p-values of indicator variables representing a 3+level categorical variable are not important. They test whether the average value of y for that level is different from the average value of y for the reference level (after accounting for the other variables in the model). This is rarely a question that needs answering. The p-value of the *effect test* tells us whether the categorical variable is significant.

Aside 5.1 — Don't bother with p-values of indicator variables when there are three or more levels. This example should convince you that you're probably better off never looking at p-values of indicator variables when they represent a 3+ level categorical variable. Reconsider the `EDUCATION` data. Recode the "Both" category to "Either" so that now "Cat" is the reference level. Further, let us also include `Gender` in the model.

$$CollegeGPA = \beta_0 + \beta_1 HSGPA + \beta_2 Gender + \text{"}Pet\text{"} + \varepsilon$$

Let us look at the summary of the regression output as well as the effect tests.

In R

```
M <- lm(CollegeGPA~HSGPA+Gender+Pet,data=EUDCATION)
summary(M)

Regression output:
             Estimate Std. Error t value Pr(>|t|)
(Intercept)  1.88860    0.19510   9.680  < 2e-16 ***
HSGPA        0.42486    0.04827   8.801  < 2e-16 ***
GenderMale  -0.10223    0.03504  -2.917  0.00366 **
PetDog      -0.16504    0.06498  -2.540  0.01134 *
PetEither   -0.09007    0.08809  -1.023  0.30694
PetNeither  -0.16639    0.07101  -2.343  0.01944 *

drop1(M,test="F")
       Df Sum of Sq    RSS     AIC F value     Pr(>F)
<none>              101.43 -1074.0
HSGPA   1   13.0729 114.50 -1002.4 77.4588 < 2.2e-16 ***
Gender  1    1.4364 102.87 -1067.5  8.5108  0.003662 **
Pet     3    1.2829 102.72 -1072.4  2.5339  0.056032 .
```

The effect test for `Pet` yields a p-value of 5.6%, implying that when we compare individuals with the same gender and same high school GPA, there is no statistically significant difference in averages based on pet preference.

C This does not contradict our previous result where pet preference was significant. Females have higher GPAs than males, and females tend to prefer cats to dogs more often than males. The significant difference in GPAs from pet preference is probably being induced by gender differences.

However, the p-values of `PetDog` and `PetNeither` show that the indicator variables are statistically significant!

This appears to be a contradiction. How can the effect test indicate there is no difference in averages among any of the levels, yet tests comparing individual averages indicate that there is a difference? To resolve this issue, realize that when there are four levels, there are a total of six different pairwise comparisons that can be made (three are displayed in the output, with the others being Cat-Dog, Cat-Neither, and Dog-Neither). By design, each test has a 5% chance of "finding" a statistically significant difference when there really is none. After six comparisons, there is a reasonable chance that at least one of them has "found" a significant result by mistake.

When we perform the effect test, we find that Pet *is* statistically significant since its p-value is less than 5%.

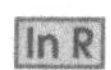

```
drop1(M,test="F")

       Df Sum of Sq    RSS      AIC F value  Pr(>F)
HSGPA   1   16.4815 119.35  -979.27 96.4522 < 2e-16 ***
Pet     3    1.3742 104.24 -1065.42  2.6806 0.04611 *
```

Thus, while the average college GPAs of `cat`, `dog`, and `neither` are not significantly different from `both`, there appears to be *some* difference in the averages among the preferences. Unfortunately, the effect test does not tell us *which* are different! Aside 5.1 illustrates one more example where p-values of individual indicator variables are misleading.

5.3 Interactions and categorical variables

Adding a set of indicator variables to represent a categorical variable allows us to model the possibility that the *average* value of y among otherwise identical individuals may vary between levels. However, what if this difference in averages depends on the characteristics of the individuals being compared? Perhaps the difference is large when the individuals both have the same large value of x, and small when the individuals both have the same small value of x. Further, what if the *strength* of the relationship between y and x also varies between levels?

If either of these characteristics are true, then we say that the categorical variable has an interaction with x. Figure 5.6 illustrates two cases where an interaction may be necessary to fully capture the relationships.

In Section 4.5.3, we said that an interaction between x_1 and x_2 exists if the strength of the relationship between y and x_1 depends on the value of x_2. We modeled the interaction by adding the predictor $(x_1 \times x_2)$ into the model.

> We say that an interaction exists between x and a categorical variable if the strength of the relationship between y and x varies between levels of the categorical variable, i.e., the implicit regression equations relating y and x do not all have the same slope. Without an interaction, the difference in the average value of y between levels is the same regardless of x. With an interaction, the difference in the average value of y between levels is larger for some values of x and smaller for other values of x.

If a categorical variable has two levels, the interaction is represented by the product of its indicator variable times x. When there are L levels, the interaction must be represented with a set of $L-1$ "interaction variables" (x times each of the $L-1$ indicator variables).

> When an interaction is included in the model, the coefficients of the indicator variables tell us how intercepts differ between levels (which is generally not important in this context). The coefficients of interaction variables tell us how slopes differ between levels.

Figure 5.6 — Scatterplots with interactions between a quantitative and categorical variable. Smoking used to be legal in restaurants. On the left, the relationships between the tip percentage and the bill amount are shown for smokers and nonsmokers. There is a noticeable difference in slopes (the lines cross), indicating that the strength of the relationship may vary. On the right, the relationships between tip percentage and bill amount are shown for each day of the week. Again, there is a noticeable difference in slopes.

In both cases, we need to define the model in a way that allows for the *possibility* that the strength of the relationship between y and x varies between levels. We can do this by incorporating interaction variables.

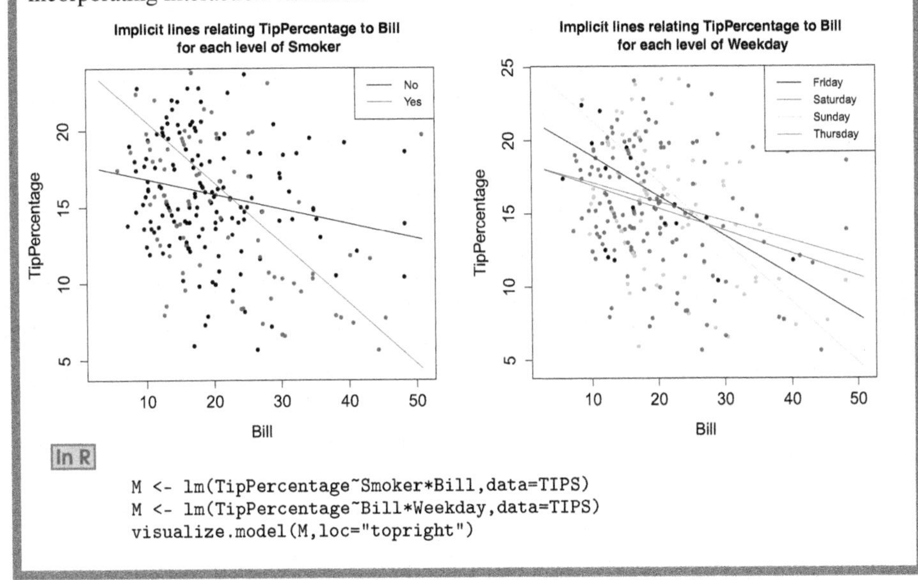

In R

```
M <- lm(TipPercentage~Smoker*Bill,data=TIPS)
M <- lm(TipPercentage~Bill*Weekday,data=TIPS)
visualize.model(M,loc="topright")
```

5.3.1 Interactions with two-level categorical variables

Let us return to the `SALARY` data and investigate whether the strength of the relationship between `Salary` and any of the predictor variables depends on gender. Figure 5.7 shows the scatterplots for `Salary` vs. `Education`, `Experience`, and `Months` for men and for women. The slopes of the implicit regression lines for `Salary` vs. `Education` and `Salary` vs. `Experience` look somewhat different, so an interaction may be present. On the other hand, we do not suspect an interaction between `Gender` and `Months` since the slopes of the two lines are nearly identical.

For the moment, let us focus on the relationship between `Salary`, `Experience`, and `Gender` since the difference in slopes looks to be the largest. The model that includes the interaction is:

$$Salary = \beta_0 + \beta_1 Experience + \beta_2 Male + \beta_3 (Experience \times Male) + \varepsilon$$

To see how this model allows men and women to have different slopes, let us write out the implicit regression equations. Remember that `Male=1` for males (it comes last alphabetically) and `Male=0` for females.

Figure 5.7 — Gauging interactions in the SALARY data. If the slopes of the implicit regression lines are noticeably different between levels, an interaction may be present between x and the categorical variable. In the SALARY data, we suspect an interaction between `Education` and `Gender` as well as between `Experience` and `Gender` because the lines diverge from each other. We do not suspect an interaction between `Months` and `Gender` since the lines are nearly parallel.

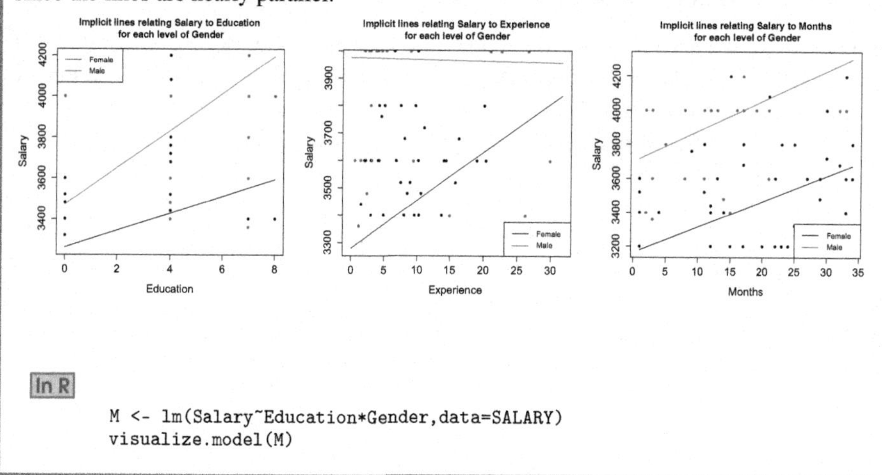

In R

```
M <- lm(Salary~Education*Gender,data=SALARY)
visualize.model(M)
```

$$\text{Female:}\quad Salary = \beta_0 + \beta_1 Experience + \beta_2 \times 0 + \beta_3(Experience \times 0)$$
$$= \beta_0 + \beta_1 Experience$$

$$\text{Male:}\quad Salary = \beta_0 + \beta_1 Experience + \beta_2 \times 1 + \beta_3(Experience \times 1)$$
$$= (\beta_0 + \beta_2) + (\beta_1 + \beta_3) Experience$$

Thus, the slope for females is β_1, while for males it is $\beta_1 + \beta_3$. Let us write out these equations using the following regression output.

In R

```
M <- lm(Salary~Experience*Gender,data=SALARY)
summary(M)

                       Estimate Std. Error t value Pr(>|t|)
(Intercept)            3279.446     76.958  42.613  < 2e-16 ***
Experience               17.579      7.053   2.492   0.0145 *
GenderMale              696.404    124.828   5.579 2.58e-07 ***
Experience:GenderMale   -18.115     10.811  -1.676   0.0973 .
```

$$\text{Female:}\quad Salary = 3279 + 17.6 Experience$$

$$\text{Male:}\quad Salary = 3279 + 17.6 Experience + 696 \times 1 - 18.1 \times Experience \times 1$$
$$Salary = (3279 + 696) + (17.6 - 18.1) Experience$$
$$= 3975 - 0.5 Experience$$

By adding the interaction term, we allow the slopes to be different for men and women.

- Two women who differ in `Experience` by one year are expected to differ in `Salary` by \$18 (more experience is associated with a higher salary).

- Two men who differ in `Experience` by one year are expected to differ in `Salary` by \$0.50 (more experience is associated with a *smaller* salary). For men, salary and experience are nearly unrelated since the slope is very close to zero.

Even though the slopes have different signs (and the slopes looked different in the scatterplot), the difference in slopes is *not* statistically significant since the p-value of the interaction variable `Experience:GenderMale` is 9.7%, greater than the 5% cutoff. Thus, the slope of the relationship between `Salary` and `Experience` can be considered the same for men and women, and there is no need to include the interaction term in the model.

If we repeat this analysis for `Education` and for `Months`, we find that *none* of the interactions are significant. The strengths of the relationships between `Salary` and each of the three variables appear independent of gender. Thus, while we previously discovered that there is a highly significant difference in *average* salaries between men and women (even after accounting for variation in their backgrounds), the *strength* of the relationships between `Salary` and the predictors does not appear to vary based on gender.

> The p-value of the interaction variable tells us whether the strength of the relationship between y and x varies between levels of the categorical variable. If the p-value is less than 5%, then the difference in slopes/strengths is statistically significant. If the p-value is at least 5%, then we can consider both levels to have the same slope (and the interaction term could be dropped from the model).
>
> The p-value of the interaction variable also tells us whether the difference in the average value of y between levels depends on the exact characteristics of the individuals under comparison. If the p-value is less than 5%, then the difference in average value of y between levels is larger for some values of x and smaller for other values. If the p-value is at least 5%, the difference in averages between levels can be considered the same regardless of the x-values of the individuals.

Now let us return to the `ATTRACTM` data and analyze the attractiveness ratings of males. Let us study the relationship between attractiveness (`Score`) and fashionableness (`FashionScore`)—its strength may vary depending on whether the guy has a visible tattoo (`Tattoo`). For example, being fashionable may be important when a tattoo is not visible, but perhaps just having a tattoo is enough for people find him attractive (or unattractive). Figure 5.8 shows the interaction plot for the model:

$$AttractionScore = \beta_0 + \beta_1 FashionScore + \beta_2 Tattoo + \beta_3 (FashionScore \times Tattoo) + \varepsilon$$

The levels of Tattoo are "yes" and "no," so `Tattoo` = 1 if the guy has a tattoo and `Tattoo` = 0 otherwise. Looking at the plot, we suspect an interaction between `FashionScore` and `Tattoo` because the slopes of the implicit regression equations look quite different.

Figure 5.8 — Gauging interactions in the ATTRACTM data. Overall, a male's fashion score and attractiveness score are positively associated. However, the strength of this relationship may vary based on other factors. On the left, men are split into two groups: tattoo/no tattoo. There may be an interaction since the slopes look very different (the difference in average attractiveness is relatively small for men who are not fashionable, with tattooed men being perceived as more attractive, while the difference is relatively large for men who are quite fashionable, with tattooed men being perceived as less attractive). Guys with a tattoo have a fairly strong *negative* association between attractiveness and fashion scores, while the association is positive for guys without a tattoo. There may also be an interaction between `FashionScore` and `Hat` (lines cross). `FashionScore` and `Glasses` do not appear to have an interaction since the slopes look nearly identical.

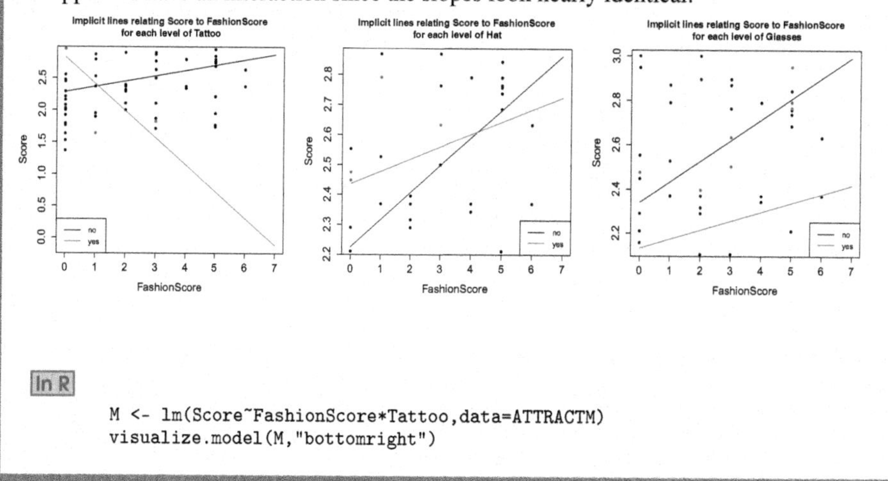

In R

```
M <- lm(Score~FashionScore*Tattoo,data=ATTRACTM)
visualize.model(M,"bottomright")
```

Let us write the implicit regression equations so that we can more easily compare the slopes.

In R

```
M <- lm(Score~FashionScore*Tattoo,data=ATTRACTM)
summary(M)

             Estimate Std. Error t value Pr(>|t|)
                         Estimate Std. Error t value Pr(>|t|)
(Intercept)               2.28386    0.09396  24.307  < 2e-16 ***
FashionScore              0.08314    0.02985   2.785  0.00697 **
Tattooyes                 0.53851    0.33347   1.615  0.11111
FashionScore:Tattooyes -0.50419    0.20455  -2.465  0.01631 *
```

$$AttractionScore = 2.28 + 0.08 FashionScore + 0.54 Tattoo - 0.50(FashionScore \times Tattoo)$$

$$\text{No Tattoo:} \quad Score = 2.28 + 0.08 FashionScore + 0.54 \times 0 - 0.50(FashionScore \times 0)$$
$$= 2.28 + 0.08 FashionScore$$

$$\text{Tattoo:} \quad Score = 2.28 + 0.08 FashionScore + 0.54 \times 1 - 0.50(FashionScore \times 1)$$
$$= 2.82 - 0.42 FashionScore$$

The difference in slopes is large (0.08 vs. -0.42, a difference of 0.5), but is it statistically significant? Only four men had visible tattoos, so with such a small sample size we may expect a large difference just by chance.

The p-value of the interaction variable is 0.016. Since this is less than 5%, the interaction is statistically significant. It is unlikely that we would have observed a difference in slopes of at least 0.5 by chance. For whatever reason, the strength and nature of the relationship between `Score` and `FashionScore` appears to depend on whether the guy has a tattoo. Whether this speaks to the way attraction actually works or whether this difference can be explained by some lurking or "common cause" variable is not known, but the observation is interesting.

Another way to interpret the result is that the typical difference in attractiveness between men with and without tattoos is not a constant but depends on the fashion scores of the men under comparison. Based on the data, the difference in attractiveness is small for unfashionable men and large for fashionable men. In fact, the model suggests that men with tattoos are more attractive than men without tattoos when the men do not appear fashionable, but the reverse is true when men appear very fashionable.

Figure 5.8 also examines the relationship between attractiveness score and fashion score based on whether the guy is wearing a hat or wearing glasses. The p-values for the interactions are 0.65 and 0.47, respectively. Thus, the data suggests that the relationship between `Score` and `FashionScore` is the same regardless of whether a guy wears a hat or wears glasses.

5.3.2 Interactions with categorical variables with three or more levels

Incorporating an interaction that involves a categorical variable with three or more levels into the regression model requires many new variables.

- To represent the categorical variable itself, a set of $L-1$ indicator variables must be added to the equation. The coefficient of an indicator variable represents the difference in intercepts between that level and the reference level (and is typically not of interest).
- To represent the interaction, an additional set of $L-1$ "interaction terms" (each of which is x times an indicator variable) must also be added. A coefficient of an interaction term represents the difference in slopes between that level and the reference level.

While the model now has *many* more terms, it is effectively just longhand for:

$$y = \beta_0 + \beta_1 x + \text{"Categorical Variable"} + \text{"}x \times \text{ Categorical Variable"} + \varepsilon$$

Adding the interaction terms allows *each* level of the categorical variable to get its own regression line, i.e., each level has a different intercept *and* a different slope. Incorporating the interaction between x and a categorical variable allows the strength of the relationship between y and x to vary between levels and allows the difference in average value of y between levels to be larger for some values of x and smaller for others.

For example, in the `BULLDOZER` data, we want to model the selling price of bulldozers at auctions. Imagine we are interested in studying the relationship between `Price` and `Usage` (a measure of how many hours the machine has been in use). The strength of this relationship may vary based on when the bulldozer was made (`YearMade`).

Figure 5.9 — A potential interaction between Usage and Decade when predicting Price. The strength (slope) of the relationship between `Price` and `Usage` does appear to vary based on the manufacturing year. The interaction may be significant.

The plot reveals something surprising. The relationship between `Price` and `Usage` is negative for recently constructed bulldozers. It is common knowledge that used cars sell for less if they have more miles, and the same appears true for bulldozers.

However, the relationship is *positive* for older models. Perhaps a well-used older bulldozer is a sign that it is "good" and has many years of life in it (and thus fetches a higher price). Perhaps the older bulldozers with little use are lightly used for a reason—they are broken down or stopped functioning a while ago. Unfortunately, we can't differentiate between these two options since we have no data on whether the bulldozer is working. If we did, we could put that in the regression model to account for functionality before looking at the relationship between `Price` and `Usage`.

Further, the plot shows that among lightly used bulldozers (points on the left), the selling price varies quite a lot between decades. Among heavily used bulldozers (points on the right), the selling price is much less variable (`Decade` is a "good" predictor of selling price for lightly used bulldozers and a "poor" predictor of selling price for heavily used bulldozers).

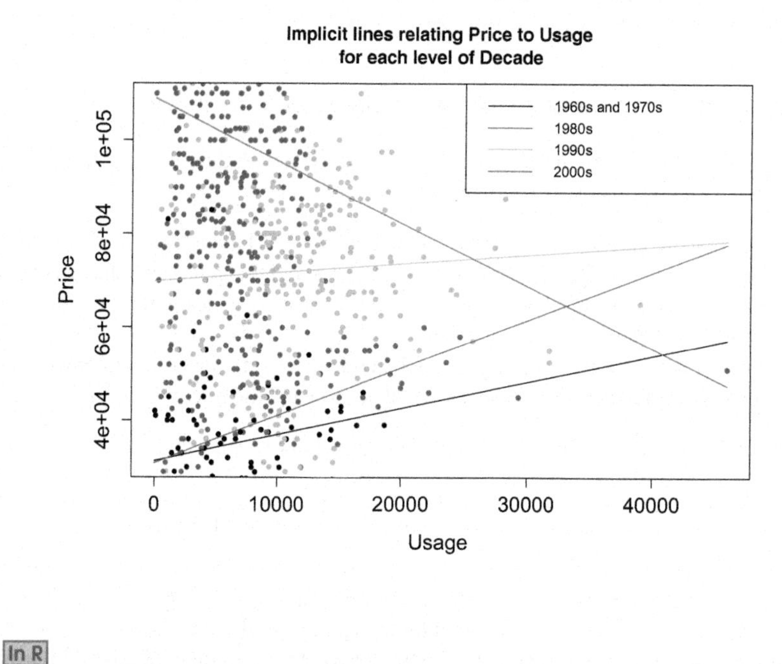

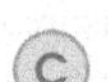

```
M <- lm(Price~Usage*Decade,data=BULLDOZER2)
visualize.model(M,"topright")
```

C You probably would not be interested in buying a brand-new (untested) bulldozer from the 1970s. However, a brand-new bulldozer from 2009 seems acceptable. Thus, the relationship between `Price` and `Usage` may depend on the bulldozer's value of `YearMade`.

Previously, we saw `YearMade` had a quadratic relationship with `Price` (see Section 4.5.1). To make things simpler, let's convert `YearMade` to a categorical variable called `Decade` with four levels by grouping decades together: 1970s and before, 1980s, 1990s, and 2000s (the updated data is in `BULLDOZER2`).

Figure 5.9 shows the relationship between `Price` and `Usage` for each of the four levels of `Decade`. There is some variation in slopes, so the interaction may be significant.

Although the process is tedious, we can write out the regression model and the implicit regression equations. Let "1970s and before" be the reference level. For clarity, each "chunk" of terms will be given its own line.

$$\begin{aligned} Price = \; & \beta_0 + \beta_1 Usage \\ & + \beta_2 1980s + \beta_3 1990s + \beta_4 2000s \\ & + \beta_5 (Usage \times 1980s) + \beta_6 (Usage \times 1990s) + \beta_7 (Usage \times 2000s) \\ & + \varepsilon \end{aligned}$$

The regression output shows

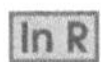

```
M <- lm(Price~Usage*Decade,data=BULLDOZER2)
summary(M)

                     Estimate Std. Error t value Pr(>|t|)
(Intercept)        31361.3627  4219.6808   7.432 2.45e-13 ***
Usage                 0.5625     0.5628    1.000  0.31780
Decade1980s        -458.7509  5308.7276  -0.086  0.93116
Decade1990s       38465.3869  4948.9919   7.772 2.06e-14 ***
Decade2000s       77629.7380  4931.6984  15.741  < 2e-16 ***
Usage:Decade1980s     0.4559     0.6343    0.719  0.47254
Usage:Decade1990s    -0.3778     0.6029   -0.627  0.53109
Usage:Decade2000s    -1.9012     0.6868   -2.768  0.00575 **
```

To recover the implicit regression equations, we will use a shortcut.

- Start with the regression equation for the reference level. This is easy because all indicator variables equal 0.
- Adjust the intercept and the slope for the other levels based on the coefficient of the relevant indicator and interaction variable, respectively.

In this case, the reference level is "1970s and before," and its implicit regression equation is:

$$\text{1970s and before:} \quad Price = 31361 + 0.5625 Usage$$

To get the implicit regression equation for "2000s" we:

- Start with the equation for the reference level. $Price = 31361 + 0.5625 Usage$
- Adjust the intercept by adding the coefficient of the relevant indicator variable (`Decade2000s`). The adjusted intercept is $31361 + 77630 = 108991$.
- Adjust the slope by adding the coefficient of the relevant interaction variable (`Usage:Decade2000s`). The new slope is $0.5625 - 1.9012 = -1.3387$.

$$\text{2000s:} \quad Price = 108991 - 1.3387 Usage$$

Asking "are the interaction terms statistically significant?" is equivalent to asking "are the differences in observed slopes statistically significant?" To answer the question, we must perform an effect test on the set of interaction variables. The procedure is identical to the one presented in Section 5.2.2 except that is applied to the set of interaction variables instead of the set of indicator variables.

In R

```
drop1(M,test="F")

             Df  Sum of Sq        RSS   AIC F value    Pr(>F)
Usage:Decade  3 1.2729e+10 5.0870e+11 18607  7.8363 3.625e-05 ***
```

The p-value of the interaction is much less than 5%, so we can say that it is statistically significant. The difference in strengths of the relationships between `Price` and `Usage` is large and unlikely to occur by chance. In other words:

- the difference in typical selling prices between two bulldozers that differ in `Usage` by one hour is not a constant but depends on the decade in which the machine was manufactured. For bulldozers made in the 2000s, the one with lower usage typically sells for more. For bulldozers made in the 1960s/1970s, the one with the lower usage typically sells for less.
- the difference in average selling prices for different decades is not a constant but varies based on the usage of the bulldozers under comparison. The difference in average selling prices is quite large for bulldozers with little usage (see how far apart the implicit lines are on the scatterplot) and smaller for heavily used bulldozers.

Unfortunately, as with all effect tests, the analysis does not tell us *which* decades have slopes that differ from each other, only that there is *some* difference between decades.

5.4 Summary

Categorical variables can be incorporated as predictors in a regression model by encoding them as numerical variables called indicator variables. If a categorical variable has L levels, a total of $L-1$ indicator variables must be created. Except for the level that comes first alphabetically (called the reference level), each level is represented by an indicator variable that equals 1 if the individual has that level and 0 otherwise.

Many categorical variables only have two levels (Yes/No). In this case, only a single indicator variable is needed. The indicator variable equals 1 for whichever level comes last alphabetically.

When a categorical variable is added to a model via adding the set of indicator variables, in effect separate regression lines are fit for each level. Assuming the categorical variable is not involved in any interactions, these lines are parallel (the coefficients of all other predictors are identical) but may have different intercepts. The difference in intercepts represents both the constant offset between these implicit regression lines and the average difference in y between levels after accounting for the other predictors.

Often, a categorical variable will have an interaction with another predictor x in the model. Interactions are necessary if the strength of the relationship between y and x is different between levels or if the difference in the typical value of y between two individuals that differ in x by one unit is expected to be larger for some levels and smaller for others. In effect, separate lines are fit for each level. These lines will have different slopes and intercepts.

To visually determine if an interaction is present, look at a scatterplot of y vs. x with the superimposed implicit regression lines. If the lines are nearly parallel, an interaction is not needed (the strength of the relationship is the same regardless of the level). If there is a noticeable difference in slopes, interaction variables between x and the categorical variable (i.e., terms consisting of the product of x and the indicator variables) should be added.

A summary of the interpretation of coefficients and statistical significance follows:

- If no interactions are present,
  - the coefficient of an indicator variable representing a categorical variable with two levels gives the difference in the average value of y between levels (after accounting for the other variables in the model).
  - the coefficient of an indicator variable representing a categorical variable with three or more levels gives the difference in the average value of y between that level and the reference level (the one that comes first alphabetically) after accounting for the other variables in the model.
- The significance of a categorical variable with two levels can be gauged from the p-value of its indicator variable.
- The significance of a categorical variable with three or more levels must be gauged from an effect test.
- If interactions *are* present,
  - the coefficient of an indicator variable tells you the difference in intercepts between that level and the reference level.
  - the coefficient of an interaction term (x times the indicator variable) tells you the difference in slopes between that level and the reference level.
- The significance of an interaction involving a categorical variable with two levels can be gauged from the p-value of its interaction term.
- The significance of an interaction involving a categorical variable with three or more levels must be gauged from an effect test.
- A predictor is statistically significant if its p-value is less than 5%.

5.5 Using R

Like most statistical software, R automatically encodes a categorical variable as a set of indicator variables so that you may directly put the predictor into a regression model. R will tell you the level for which the indicator variable equals 1 by appending the name of the level to the name of categorical variable (the indicator variable equals 0 for all other levels).

The following examples use the `EDUCATION` dataset. `Family` is a four-level categorical variable with levels `Middle Child` (the reference), `Oldest Child`, `Only Child`, and `Youngest Child`. `Gender` is a categorical variable with two levels `Female` (the reference) and `Male`. `CollegeGPA`, `HSGPA`, and `ACT` are quantitative variables.

Fitting the model

You may construct all formulas in the typical way. The formula for a model does not depend on whether a variable is quantitative or categorical.

- Checking to see if there is any differences in the average value of y (ACT) between levels (of `Family`). Note: this is equivalent to performing an ANOVA using `associate()` from Chapter 2.

In R

```
M <- lm(ACT~Family,data=EDUCATION)
```

- Adding a categorical variable with no interactions

In R

```
M <- lm(CollegeGPA~HSGPA+ACT+Gender+Family,data=EDUCATION)
```

- Adding a categorical variable with interactions (between `HSGPA` and `Family`)

In R

```
M <- lm(CollegeGPA~ACT + Gender + HSGPA*Family,data=EDUCATION)
```

- Interactions are allowed between categorical variables

In R

```
M <- lm(CollegeGPA~HSGPA + ACT + Gender*Family,data=EDUCATION)
```

Identifying coefficients

R creates indicator variables automatically. You can tell when the indicator variable equals 1 or 0 by checking which level is appended to the name of the categorical variable.

Consider a model with no interactions:

$$CollegeGPA = \beta_0 + \beta_1 HSGPA + \beta_2 ACT + \beta_3 Gender + \text{“}Family\text{”}$$

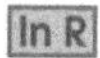

```
M <- lm(CollegeGPA~HSGPA + ACT + Gender + Family,data=EDUCATION)
summary(M)

                     Estimate Std. Error t value Pr(>|t|)
(Intercept)          1.241576   0.204777   6.063 2.36e-09 ***
HSGPA                0.367598   0.049088   7.489 2.50e-13 ***
ACT                  0.025717   0.005489   4.685 3.46e-06 ***
GenderMale          -0.114270   0.034284  -3.333 0.000912 ***
FamilyOldest Child   0.003403   0.046873   0.073 0.942152
FamilyOnly Child    -0.004615   0.066447  -0.069 0.944654
FamilyYoungest Child 0.115120   0.045836   2.512 0.012281 *
```

- `GenderMale` equals 1 for a male and 0 for a female. The estimated coefficient is -0.11, implying that among otherwise identical individuals (same high school GPA, ACT score, and family position), men typically have college GPAs that are 0.11 below women.

- `FamilyYoungest Child` equals 1 for a youngest child and 0 otherwise. The estimated coefficient is 0.12, implying that among otherwise identical individuals (same high school GPA, ACT score, and gender), the youngest children typically have GPAs that are 0.12 higher than middle children (the reference level).
- Among all levels of `Family`, the youngest children have the highest college GPA (most positive coefficient) while only children have the lowest (most negative coefficient). The difference between youngest and only children is $(0.115 - -0.005) = 0.12$.

Consider a model with interactions:

$$CollegeGPA = \beta_0 + \beta_1 HSGPA + \beta_2 ACT + \beta_3 Gender + \text{“}Family\text{”} + \beta_4(Gender \times ACT) + (\text{“}Family\text{”} \times HSGPA)$$

In R

```
M <- lm(CollegeGPA~HSGPA*Family + ACT*Gender,data=EDUCATION)
summary(M)

                            Estimate Std. Error t value Pr(>|t|)
(Intercept)                 1.330217   0.458539   2.901  0.00386 **
HSGPA                       0.326946   0.115231   2.837  0.00470 **
FamilyOldest Child         -0.376634   0.516834  -0.729  0.46645
FamilyOnly Child            0.103926   0.644097   0.161  0.87187
FamilyYoungest Child       -0.012317   0.503942  -0.024  0.98051
ACT                         0.028087   0.007326   3.834  0.00014 ***
GenderMale                  0.033061   0.282935   0.117  0.90702
HSGPA:FamilyOldest Child    0.102684   0.138938   0.739  0.46016
HSGPA:FamilyOnly Child     -0.029748   0.173513  -0.171  0.86393
HSGPA:FamilyYoungest Child  0.034564   0.135482   0.255  0.79872
ACT:GenderMale             -0.005674   0.010700  -0.530  0.59611
```

- `ACT:GenderMale` is an interaction variable between ACT score and gender. The coefficient is -0.006, implying that the difference in slopes between men and women for the relationship `CollegeGPA` vs. `ACT` is -0.006. The effective coefficient of `ACT` is 0.028 for women and $(0.028 - 0.006) = 0.022$ for men. Among otherwise identical individuals (in terms of high school GPA and family position), the strength of the relationship between `CollegeGPA` and `ACT` score is slightly stronger for women than it is for men.
- `HSGPA:FamilyYoungest Child` is an interaction variable between high school GPA and the youngest child level of family position. The coefficient is 0.035, implying that the difference in slopes between youngest children and middle children for the relationship `CollegeGPA` vs. `HSGPA` is 0.035. The effective coefficient of `HSGPA` is 0.327 for middle children and $(0.327 + 0.035) = 0.362$ for youngest children. Among otherwise identical individuals (in terms of ACT score and gender), the strength of the relationship between `CollegeGPA` and `ACT` is slightly stronger for youngest children than it is for middle children.
- `FamilyYoungest Child` equals 1 for a youngest child and 0 otherwise. The estimated coefficient is 0.12, implying that among otherwise identical individuals (same high school GPA, ACT score, and gender), the youngest children typically have GPAs that are 0.12 higher than middle children (the reference level).

Significance Tests

If a categorical variable only has two levels, the p-value for the test of significance can be read directly off of `summary` in the usual location. When it has three or more levels, the effect test must be conducted (which also works for two levels) and individual p-values of indicator variables are ignored.

In R

```
M <- lm(CollegeGPA~HSGPA + ACT + Gender + Family,data=EDUCATION)
drop1(M,test="F")

HSGPA   1    9.1038 106.508 -1044.4 56.0784 2.500e-13 ***
ACT     1    3.5634 100.967 -1076.8 21.9504 3.464e-06 ***
Gender  1    1.8035  99.207 -1087.5 11.1092 0.0009119 ***
Family  3    1.8593  99.263 -1091.1  3.8177 0.0099555 **
```

Here, `Family` is statistically significant since the p-value (0.0099555) is less than 5%. There is some difference (the test does not give specifics) in the average GPAs between the four family positions after accounting for high school GPA, ACT score, and gender. `Gender` is statistically significant as well (note the p-value here is the same as the p-value from `summary`).

Now consider a model with interactions. Note: any variables listed in interactions will *not* be listed individually for the effect tests.

In R

```
M <- lm(CollegeGPA~HSGPA*Family + ACT*Gender,data=EDUCATION)
drop1(M,test="F")

HSGPA:Family  3  0.166628 97.361 -1094.9  0.3406 0.7960
ACT:Gender    1  0.045857 97.241 -1091.6  0.2812 0.5961
```

Here, neither the interaction between high school GPA and `Family` nor the interaction between ACT score and gender are statistically significant since the p-values are greater than 5%. For all intents and purposes, the strength of the relationship between college GPA and high school GPA appears to be the same for each family position (after accounting for ACT score and gender), and the strength of the relationship between college GPA and ACT score appears to be the same for men and women (after accounting for high school GPA and family position).

Visualizing implicit regression lines

If the regression model has a single quantitative predictor and a single categorical predictor, then `visualize.model` will show the implicit regression equations (regardless if the model has an interaction or not).

In R

```
M <- lm(CollegeGPA~HSGPA*Family,data=EDUCATION)
visualize.model(M,loc="bottomright")
```

Note: `loc` is an optional argument that specifies where the legend goes.

If the regression model has many categorical variables or interactions, try `see.interactions`.

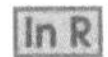

```
M <- lm(CollegeGPA~HSGPA*Family+ACT*Gender,data=EDUCATION)
see.interactions(M,loc="bottomright",many=TRUE)
```

Note: `many` is an optional argument that specifies how many plots are displayed at a time. By default, it is `FALSE` (so it tries to display all plots). If this is too many plots, change it to `TRUE`.

5.6 Exercises

1: Use `EX5.BIKE`. This is a more detailed version of the bicycle demand in DC dataset. There are categorical variables such as day of the week, whether the day was a working day or holiday, and the weather that may help us predict demand. In the last chapter, you saw that row 337 had a data error. This version of the dataset has this row removed, so no modification is necessary. In this set of questions, we will consider inclusion of categorical variables *without* interactions.

a) What is the average demand overall for rainy days and non-rainy days (and the difference between the two)? Is the difference in average demands on rainy vs. non-rainy days statistically significant? Hint: you can use `associate()` on the columns `Demand` and `Weather` to answer this question.
b) If we represent the categorical variable `Weather` (No rain vs. Rain) by an indicator variable, how should it be numerically defined? Which level is the reference level?
c) Let us compare the average demands for rainy and non-rainy days after accounting for the temperature. Fit a regression modeling predicting `Demand` from `EffectiveAvgTemp` and `Weather`. Examine the results of `summary()` as well as `visualize.model()` for this model. Use the regression summary to answer the following questions.
    1) Among days with the same effective temperature, how much smaller is the average demand when it rains than when it does not rain, and is this difference statistically significant? Why or why not?
    2) Compare the above difference in averages to the difference from (1). Are they about the same (i.e., to within 15%) or noticeably different? Sidenote: the difference in (1) is the coefficient of `Weather` in a model predicting `Demand` from that variable alone. We've talked about how coefficients are model-dependent. The coefficient of a predictor can experience large changes when a new variable is added to the model when the new variable is associated with that predictor. Temperature and weather indeed have a significant association in this case (which you can see by running `associate`): in DC, the typical temperature on rainy days is about 23°C, while on non-rainy days it is about 25°C).
    3) Write out the implicit regression equations relating `Demand` to `EffectiveAvgTemp` for rainy and for non-rainy days.
d) Demand for bikes may fluctuate over the course of a week, so let us consider the variable `Day`.
    1) `Day` has seven levels. Behind the scenes, how many indicator variables must be added to the regression to represent `Day`, and which level of `Day` does not have a level named after it?
    2) Include a plot of the implicit regression lines when we predict `Demand` from

EffectiveAvgTemp and Day (use visualize.model()). After accounting for the effective temperature, which days look to have the highest and lowest average demands?

3) Fit the regression model predicting Demand from EffectiveAvgTemp and Day. Examine the results of summary, then write out the implicit regression equations for Friday and for Sunday.
4) On Mondays and Fridays with the same effective temperature, what does the model estimate the difference in average demands to be? Note: this is a single number from the summary output of the model.
5) After accounting for the effective temperature, what is the difference in average demands between Saturday and Sunday? Note: you'll have to subtract two numbers found on the summary output.

e) Now fit a model predicting Demand using all predictors (you can use ~. in your lm() statment). Examine the output of summary().
   1) After accounting for all the information available (i.e., temperature, humidity, windspeed, weather, and if the day was a working day vs. holiday), which day has the highest average demand, and which day has the lowest average demand? Note: these answers are found by scanning the list of coefficients for the indicator variables for Day.
   2) After accounting for all the information available, is there a statistically significant difference in average demands between days? You'll need to run drop1.
   3) All else being equal (i.e., comparing days with identical values for the other predictors), does it look like the demand varies on whether it does or does not rain, i.e., is Weather statistically significant? Justify your answer.

2: In marketing analytics, the relationship between the sales of a product and the amount of money spent on advertising is often studied. What follows is output of a model predicting Sales (thousands of dollars) based on the amount of Internet advertising Ads (thousands of dollars), the Room in which the product would be placed (Kitchen, Bed, Office), and the Size of the product (Small, Large).

```
             Estimate Std. Error t value Pr(>|t|)
(Intercept)  3.24097    0.07193  45.059   <2e-16 ***
Ads          0.96943    0.04335  22.365   <2e-16 ***
RoomKitchen -0.12294    0.05554  -2.213   0.0277 *
RoomOffice  -0.15772    0.08736  -1.806   0.0721 .
SizeSmall    0.01089    0.05593   0.195   0.8457
```

a) Interpret the coefficient of Ads, which you may take to be 0.969.
b) Interpret the coefficient of RoomKitchen, which you may take to be -0.123.
c) What is the implicit regression equation relating Sales to Ads for large products that go in the bedroom?
d) What is the implicit regression equation relating Sales to Ads for small products that go in the office?
e) Among all six type of products (Bed Small, Bed Large, Kitchen Small, Kitchen Large, etc.), which one has the highest average sales (assuming each product has had an equal amount of advertising)?

3: There have been interesting studies that look at the association between someone's income and his or her attractiveness. A recent study found that more attractive real-estate brokers tended to make more money (`http://web.natur.cuni.cz/~houdek3/papers/Salter%20et%20al%202013.pdf`). Imagine predicting the selling price of a house based whether the agent was attractive (treated as a categorical variable Yes/No). Since the selling price of a house depends on many other potential factors, explain how you would isolate the association between selling price and attractiveness. This question is intentionally a little vague and you should not feel the need to give more than a few sentences (you don't need to read either article to answer the question).

4: Use `EX5.DONOR`. This is a modified portion of the `DONOR` data in other parts of the text. It deals with a charity's customer database. Each row represents an individual and whether he or she donated during the last campaign (`Donate`, yes or no), the amount of the donation (`LastAmount`), the age of the account (i.e., number of months since his or her first donation, `AccountAge`), the age of the individual (`Age`), where the customer lives (`Setting`, Urban/Suburban/Rural), etc. Let us model the amount someone donated during the last campaign (`LastAmount`).

a) A logical predictor of someone's last donation amount is the average amount he or she has donated in the last few years (`RecentAvgAmount`). However, the strength of the relationship may depend on various factors, e.g., whether the person owns a home (`Homeowner`).
   1) Include the results of `visualize.model()` for predicting `LastAmount` from `RecentAvgAmount`, `Homeowner`, and their interaction.
   2) Is the strength of the relationship between `LastAmount` and `RecentAvgAmount` stronger for homeowners or non-homeowners? How can you tell?
   3) Is the difference in strengths of the relationships statistically significant? How can you tell?

b) Where someone lives (`Setting`, either Rural, Suburban, or Urban) may also make a difference in the amount someone donates. In fact, the strength of the relationship between `LastAmount` and `RecentAvgAmount` depends strongly on the person's location.
   1) Examine the plot from `visualize.model()` where we predict `LastAmount` from `RecentAvgAmount`, `Setting`, and their interaction. You will use this plot to answer the next two parts.
   2) If we compare households whose *recent* average donation amount is 50, which level of `Setting` has the highest average *last* donation amount?
   3) If we compare households whose *recent* average donation amount is 1, which level of `Setting` has the highest average *last* donation amount? Note: without an interaction, the answer to this part and the last part will always be the same. With an interaction, the answers are allowed to be different.

c) Another strong predictor is `AccountAge` (the number of months since the person's first donation). Fit a model predicting `LastAmount` from `RecentAvgAmount`, `AccountAge`, `Setting`, and the interaction between `RecentAvgAmount` and `Setting`. Examine the coefficient section of `summary()` and the results of `drop1()`.
   1) Write out the implicit regression equation relating `LastAmount` to `RecentAvgAmount` and `AccountAge` for houses in a Rural setting. Feel free to only keep two numbers after the decimal place.
   2) Do the same for houses in an Urban setting.
   3) Is the interaction between `RecentAvgAmount` and `Setting` something we really should be including in our model? Based on the results of `drop1()`, why or why not?

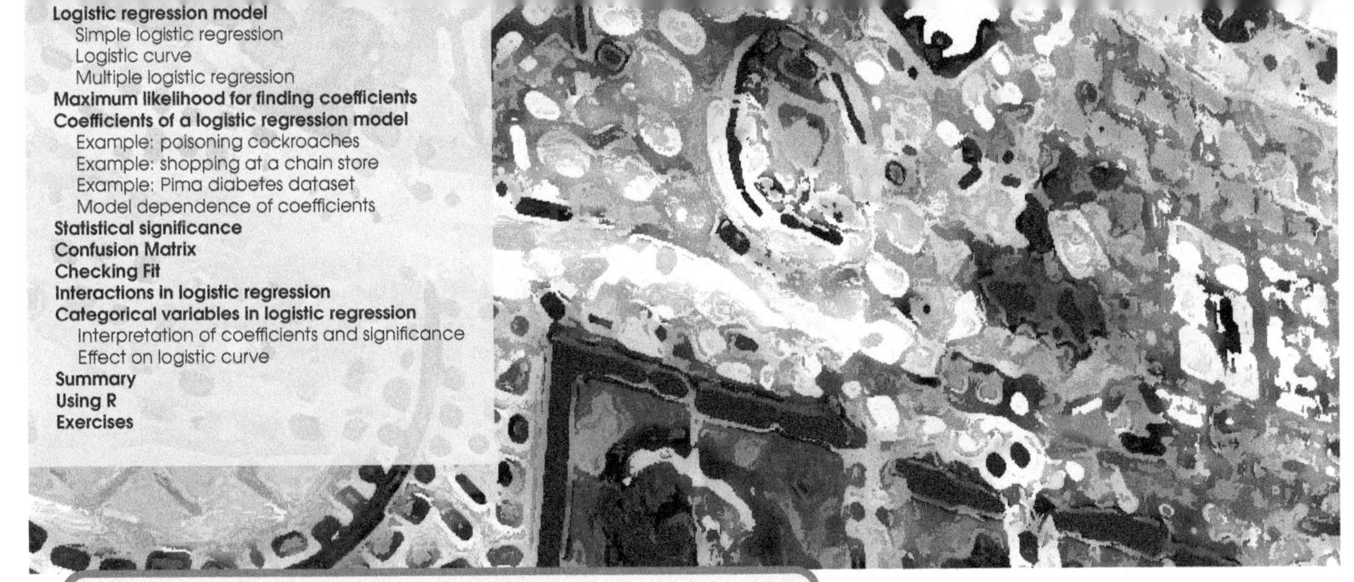

Logistic regression model
- Simple logistic regression
- Logistic curve
- Multiple logistic regression

Maximum likelihood for finding coefficients
Coefficients of a logistic regression model
- Example: poisoning cockroaches
- Example: shopping at a chain store
- Example: Pima diabetes dataset
- Model dependence of coefficients

Statistical significance
Confusion Matrix
Checking Fit
Interactions in logistic regression
Categorical variables in logistic regression
- Interpretation of coefficients and significance
- Effect on logistic curve

Summary
Using R
Exercises

6. Logistic Regression

Until now, the quantity we have tried to model and predict has always been a quantitative variable like price, amount, GPA, sales, score, etc. What if y is a two-level categorical variable like gender (male/female), outcome (buy/not buy), or agreement (yes/no)? When y is not numerical, an entirely different modeling technique is used—logistic regression. Instead of directly predicting whether y is one level or the other, we will predict the *probability* of each level. The level that has the highest probability will be the predicted value for y.

For example, consider a major retailer that is scouting locations for a new store. A model predicting the probability that consumers will make a purchase based on their distance to the store, their income, the number of competing stores in the area, etc., would help guide the decision.

Logistic regression is used extensively in a variety of fields. The medical field uses logistic regression to determine the appropriate dosage for medicines (e.g., the smallest dosage that is 99% effective). Banks want to predict if a customer will pay a loan on time. Service industries want to predict who will "churn" (not renew their contract when it expires). Political pundits want to predict which candidate a person will vote for, etc.

In this chapter, we will discuss the logistic regression model and its assumptions. Just as linear regression assumes that the average value of y is a weighted sum of x's (i.e., the relationship between y and each x is linear), logistic regression assumes something very specific about how the probability of each level of y is related to the predictor variables.

(C) If y is a categorical variable with more than two levels, logistic regression cannot be used. If the possible levels are ordered (small, medium, large), then *ordinal* regression may be useful. Otherwise, *multinomial* regression is an option. These are beyond the scope of this book, but excellent tutorials exist on the web. A Google search or visit to Wikipedia can get you started. Package `VGAM` and function `vglm` are also useful.

6.1 Logistic regression model

Let y be a two-level categorical variable. Let p be the probability that an individual has the level that comes *last* alphabetically. We will call this level the **level of interest**. For example, if we are predicting whether a customer makes a purchase (Yes/No), we will predict the probability that the customer buys (Yes). If we are predicting whether some dosage of a poison kills (Live/Die), we will predict the probability that the individual lives (Live).

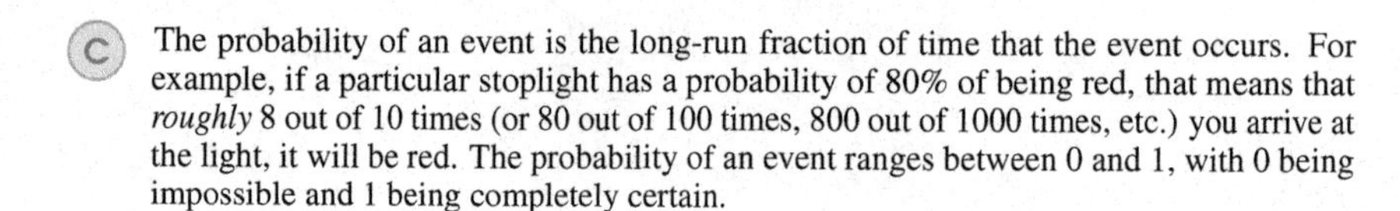

The probability of an event is the long-run fraction of time that the event occurs. For example, if a particular stoplight has a probability of 80% of being red, that means that *roughly* 8 out of 10 times (or 80 out of 100 times, 800 out of 1000 times, etc.) you arrive at the light, it will be red. The probability of an event ranges between 0 and 1, with 0 being impossible and 1 being completely certain.

Predicting the probability of the level that comes last alphabetically (as opposed to the first) is done purely to respect conventions. It is easy enough to switch between the two probabilities since they always sum to one. If A and B are the two levels, then

$$p_A = 1 - p_B \qquad\qquad p_B = 1 - p_A$$

For example, if we predict the probability that someone buys to be 0.8, then the probability that they do not buy is 0.2. If the probability that a dosage will cure an individual is 0.4, the probability it will not cure is 0.6.

To convert a probability into an actual prediction about an individual's level, use the following convention:

- If $p \geq 0.5$, then the individual is predicted to have the level that comes last alphabetically.
- If $p < 0.5$, then the individual is predicted to have the level that comes first alphabetically.

6.1.1 Simple logistic regression

Let x be some predictor variable, e.g., yearly income, dosage, etc. We cannot use a simple linear regression to predict p from x:

$$p \neq \beta_0 + \beta_1 x + \varepsilon$$

Why not? First, probabilities are always between 0 and 1. Depending on the values of x and the coefficients, it is quite possible for the above equation to evaluate to numbers outside these limits. Second, linear regression assumes that the disturbances (ε, the differences between individuals' values and the average) have a Normal distribution. Since probabilities are between 0 and 1, any error made by the above equation has to be between -1.0 and 1.0. Values from a Normal distribution have no restriction and can be 0.5, 1.3, -2.3, etc. Thus, the distribution of ε cannot be Normal.

Instead, the simple logistic regression model predicts a *transformation* of p (called the "logit" of p) from the value of x. The following models are equivalent:

$$logit(p) = \ln\frac{p}{1-p} = \beta_0 + \beta_1 x \quad \Longleftrightarrow \quad p = \frac{e^{\beta_0+\beta_1 x}}{1+e^{\beta_0+\beta_1 x}} \tag{6.1}$$

Regardless of x, the value of p in this equation will *always* evaluate to a number between 0 and 1. Where did the error term ε go? It is not actually necessary to explicitly incorporate the error into the model.

When we collect data, we gather information on whether an individual does or does not have the level of interest—we are not actually recording or measuring p. Since ε represents the numerical difference between an observed and predicted value, it cannot be defined in a logistic regression context. We measure levels, but we predict probabilities. They are not directly comparable.

If numerous individuals with a common value of x are observed, we *could* estimate p for that value of x by finding the proportion of individuals who have the level of interest. Then, we could determine the "residual" by comparing the estimated value of p with the value predicted by the model. While it is possible to set up a model using this framework, we will not pursue it here.

Rather, we assume that an individual's value of x gives the probability p that he or she has the level of interest. The number of individuals (all sharing that common value of x) who have the level of interest is described by a **binomial** distribution. While the details of the binomial distribution are beyond the scope of this book, you are somewhat familiar with it from everyday life. The binomial distribution is used to calculate the probability of observing 45 heads out of 100 coin flips, the probability of having 7 out of 9 green lights on your way to work, or any other calculation that involves looking at the number of "successes" in a fixed number of "trials."

Like simple linear regression, what we call x in the logistic regression model is arbitrary. It can be the measured values, e.g., Income, or it can be any function instead, e.g., Income^2, ln(Income), etc. Further, x can even be a categorical variable, in which case we represent it as a set of indicator variables as in Chapter 5.

6.1.2 Logistic curve

A simple linear regression equation is a straight line and is easy to visualize on a scatterplot. So what does the simple logistic regression equation look like? Refer to Figure 6.1.

In logistic regression, we cannot make a "scatterplot" of p vs. x since p is never actually measured (we observe levels, not probabilities). However, we can plot the equation for p in terms of x once we are given a set of coefficients. This curve is called the **logistic curve**, and varieties of it can be seen in Figure 6.1. The curve illustrates how the logistic regression model assumes p changes with x. The model assumes that p monotonically either increases with x (left) or decreases with x (right).

Just as checking the linearity assumption is critical when using a simple linear regression, checking whether this curve is an adequate description of how the probability changes with x is paramount for simple logistic regression. There will be scenarios where this model is not appropriate.

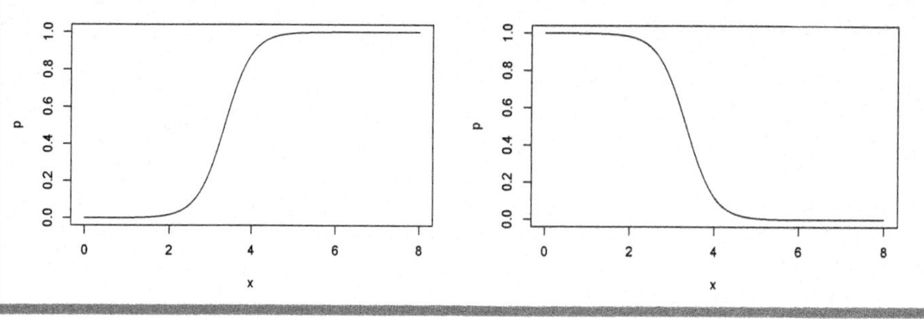

Figure 6.1 — The logistic curve. The logistic regression curve assumes a very specific way for how the probability that an individual has the level of interest changes with x. Either the probability increases with x (left) or it decreases with x (right) according to the S-shape.

For example, consider modeling the probability that someone will like a cake based on how long it is baked in the oven. This probability peaks at the recommended cooking time. For shorter baking times, the cake is not quite done, and there is a smaller chance someone will enjoy it. For longer baking times, the cake will be overcooked or even burnt. The logistic curve would not be a good model for how the probability of enjoying the cake changes with baking time, but a curve similar to the Normal may be a good approximation (Figure 6.2).

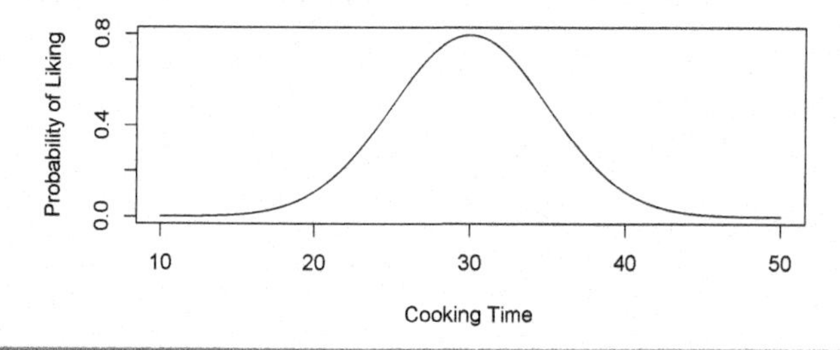

Figure 6.2 — Relationship between cook time and the probability of liking a cake. The probability that someone will like a cake depends on its baking time. If the cake is not baked long enough, it will be runny and unappetizing. If the cake is baked too long, it will burn. Thus, the logistic curve in Figure 6.1 would be a poor model for describing how the probability changes with cook time.

6.1.3 Multiple logistic regression

The simple logistic regression model easily generalizes to the case where there are multiple predictor variables. When there are k predictor variables $x_1, x_2, \ldots, x_k$, then the model is:

$$logit(p) = \ln\frac{p}{1-p} = \beta_0 + \beta_1 x_1 + \ldots + \beta_k x_k \quad \Longleftrightarrow \quad p = \frac{e^{\beta_0+\beta_1 x+\ldots+\beta_k x_k}}{1+e^{\beta_0+\beta_1 x+\ldots+\beta_k x_k}} \qquad (6.2)$$

Once again, what we call x is arbitrary. They can be the values measured in the data, transformations of the original variables, interactions between the variables, sets of indicator variables representing a categorical variable, etc.

In a multiple linear regression, the relationship between y and x_i is always a straight line. Depending on the values of the other predictors, this line shifts up and down, but the slope is b_i (the coefficient of x_i). In a multiple logistic regression, the shape of the logistic curve is always the same. However, depending on the values of the other predictors, the curve shifts left and right.

For example, imagine having two predictors in the model (x_1 and x_2). If the coefficients are $\beta_0 = 2$, $\beta_1 = -1$, $\beta_2 = -2$, then the equation for the probability is:

$$p = \frac{e^{2-x_1-2x_2}}{1+e^{2-x_1-2x_2}}$$

Figure 6.3 shows how the probability p changes as x_1 varies for three different values of x_2. The shapes of the curve are identical, but they are shifted horizontally. This makes the behavior of p with x_1 appear very different depending on the value of x_2. When $x_2 = -5$, the probability hardly changes at all (and stays near 100%) as x_1 varies from -5 to 10. When $x_2 = 1$, the probability quickly drops from near 100% at $x_1 = -5$ to near 0% $x_1 = 5$.

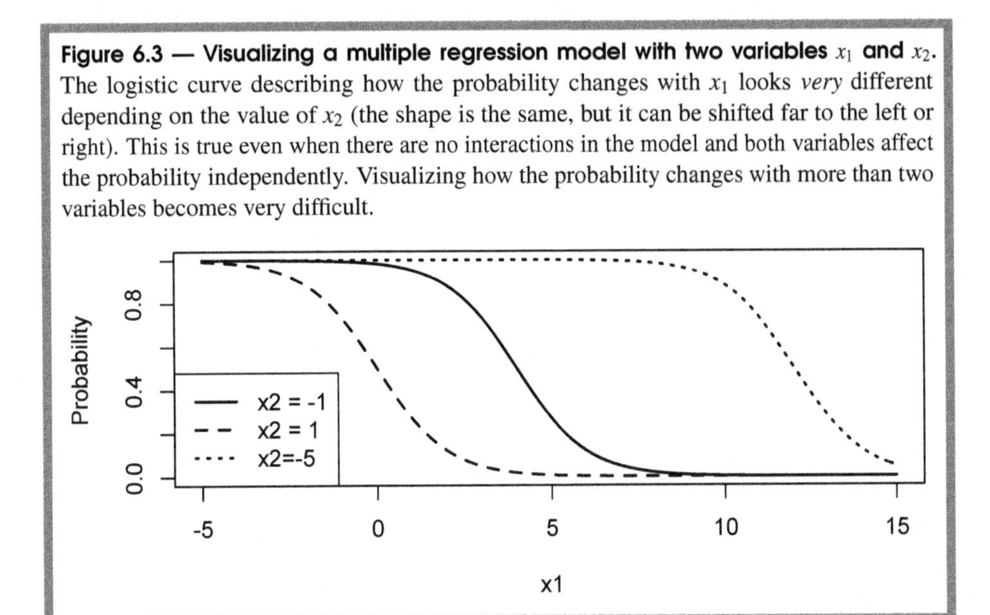

Figure 6.3 — Visualizing a multiple regression model with two variables x_1 and x_2. The logistic curve describing how the probability changes with x_1 looks *very* different depending on the value of x_2 (the shape is the same, but it can be shifted far to the left or right). This is true even when there are no interactions in the model and both variables affect the probability independently. Visualizing how the probability changes with more than two variables becomes very difficult.

6.2 Maximum likelihood for finding coefficients

Unless we have a census, the collected data only provides estimates of β_1, β_2, etc. These estimates are referred to as b_1, b_2, etc. These estimates are found with a procedure called **maximum likelihood estimation**. Essentially, the coefficients are picked so that the resulting model has the highest probability of reproducing the collected data, e.g., individuals 1, 3, and 4 have the level of interest but individuals 2 and 5 do not.

Let us illustrate the procedure with a simple example. Imagine we want to estimate the probability that a stoplight is green when we show up to an intersection. On five different days, we record the color. Assume the colors of the lights on sequential visits are independent. It turns out that the first, second, and fifth lights were green and the third and fourth lights were not green. If p is the unknown probability that the light will be green, then the **likelihood** of the data (defined to be the probability of observing it) is

$$P(data) = P(\text{green on } 1) \times P(\text{green on } 2) \times P(\text{red on } 3) \times P(\text{red on } 4) \times P(\text{green on } 5)$$

$$\text{Likelihood} = p \times p \times (1-p) \times (1-p) \times p = p^3(1-p)^2$$

The maximum likelihood principle assumes the data is typical of what may happen during an experiment and estimates p to be the value that maximizes this probability. After all, why would you choose a value for p that implies your data was a very rare event?

Let us plot the likelihood vs. p to find the maximum. See Figure 6.4. In this case, $p = 0.60$ is where the likelihood peaks. Taking the probability of being green to be 60% best reproduces the data. Intuitively, this choice makes sense. Out of five attempts, the light was green three times (three out of five is 60%).

Figure 6.4 — Likelihood of the stoplight data. The likelihood is the probability of collecting your data for a particular value of p. Depending on p, the probability of collecting the data can be relatively large or small. The maximum likelihood principle says to choose p so the probability of reproducing your data is at its highest. This occurs where the curve is at its peak. In this case, the estimated value of p is 3/5.

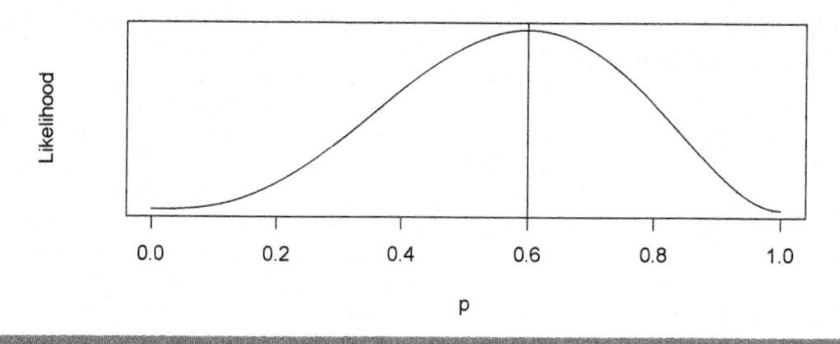

In the stoplight example, we assumed that p has the same value each time we show up at the light. In a logistic regression, the value of p is *not* the same for each individual, but rather depends on the individual's value of x through Equation 6.2.

For illustration (since the math gets very complicated quickly), imagine we want to fit a logistic regression that predicts the probability that someone will shop at Walmart from the distance to their nearest store.

Let p_i be the probability that individual i will shop at Walmart in the next five days. Then $1 - p_i$ is the probability that the individual will not. Let x_i be the distance between an individual's home and the nearest Walmart. Data on five consumers reveals that individuals 1 and 5 ended up shopping at Walmart while the others did not. As a function of the p_i's, the probability of collecting this data (i.e., the likelihood) is

$$P(data) = p_1 \times (1-p_2) \times (1-p_3) \times (1-p_4) \times p_5$$

$$\text{Likelihood} = \frac{e^{b_0+b_1x_1}}{1+e^{b_0+b_1x_1}} \times \left(1 - \frac{e^{b_0+b_1x_2}}{1+e^{b_0+b_1x_2}}\right) \times \left(1 - \frac{e^{b_0+b_1x_3}}{1+e^{b_0+b_1x_3}}\right) \times \left(1 - \frac{e^{b_0+b_1x_4}}{1+e^{b_0+b_1x_4}}\right) \times \frac{e^{b_0+b_1x_5}}{1+e^{b_0+b_1x_5}}$$

The maximum likelihood procedure finds values of b_0 and b_1 so that the probability of collecting your specific set of data is as large as possible. If this equation looks phenomenally complex, it is (and this was for a dataset of size five)! In fact, there are no simple equations that estimate b_0 and b_1 directly (like Equation 3.2 for simple linear regression), and they must be found using smart search procedures on a computer. The good news is that software has efficient routines for finding the estimates. The bad news is that sometimes the search takes a while because the procedure can be computationally intensive.

It turns out that the least squares criterion for linear regression finds the *exact* same values of b_0, b_1, etc., as the ones that are found using maximum likelihood principles. Thus, the underlying procedures for both linear and logistic regression models are fundamentally the same—find the coefficients that maximize the probability of reproducing your data.

6.3 Coefficients of a logistic regression model

In a multiple regression model, b_i (the estimated coefficient of x_i) has a precise and useful interpretation. Two otherwise identical individuals (with respect to the other variables in the model) who differ in x_i by one unit are expected to differ in y by b_i units. Further, this expected difference is the same number regardless of the other characteristics (x-values) of the individuals. Unfortunately, the coefficients of a logistic regression are not easily interpreted.

Since the logistic model is a *curve*, the probability that an individual has the level of interest does not increase or decrease at a fixed rate as x_i changes. Two otherwise identical individuals who differ in x_i by one unit may differ in probabilities by very little for some values of x_i (e.g., 0.001 when their values of x_i are 3 and 4) and a lot for other values of x_i (e.g., 0.2 when their values of x_i are 7 and 8).

What *does* change at a fixed rate as x increases is a quantity called the **log odds** of the level of interest. The **odds** of an event is the ratio of the probability that it occurs to the probability that it does not occur.

In sports betting, odds are presented differently. If the "sports odds" of a team winning is 2 to 1, this means the team has twice the probability of losing than it does of winning: $p_{win} = 1/3$, $p_{lose} = 2/3$. If p represents the probability of losing, then the odds are $p/(1-p) = (2/3)/(1/3) = 2$. Events with higher odds are more likely to occur (but not in a linear way). Working with odds is difficult, and unfortunately, the logistic model makes it less intuitive and uses the logarithm of the odds.

Let b_i be the coefficient of x_i in the fitted model. The interpretation is that two individuals who differ in x_i by one unit (but whose other x's are the same) differ in the log odds of the event of interest by b_i. The previous statement is hard to digest, so we will instead focus on a much simpler interpretation.

Let us concern ourselves with the *sign* of the coefficient and (for simple logistic regression) the ratio of the "intercept" b_0 to the "slope" b_1.

- If the coefficient of x_i is positive, individuals with larger values of x_i (but who are otherwise identical in the other x's) have a *higher* probability of possessing the level of interest.
- If the coefficient of x_i is negative, individuals with larger values of x_i (but who are otherwise identical in the other x's) have a *lower* probability of possessing the level of interest.
- For a simple logistic regression, the quantity $-b_0/b_1$ is the value of x where there is a 50% chance of having either level.

6.3.1 Example: poisoning cockroaches

Consider modeling the amount of poison required to kill a cockroach. Small amounts (10 micrograms, 20 micrograms, etc.) of poison were laced on grains of sugar and served as food. About 60 cockroaches were given each dosage, and the fate of each insect (Live/Die) was recorded. Data is found in the data frame `POISON` with columns `Dose` and `Outcome`. Since "Live" comes last alphabetically, it is the level of interest. The probability that a cockroach lives is represented as p. Let us fit the model:

$$logit(p_{live}) = \ln\frac{p_{live}}{1-p_{live}} = \beta_0 + \beta_1 Dose \Longleftrightarrow p_{live} = \frac{e^{\beta_0+\beta_1 Dose}}{1+e^{\beta_0+\beta_1 Dose}}$$

Figure 6.5 — Cockroach mortality. The model is $logit(p_{live}) = 7.5 - 0.49Dose$. Since the coefficient of `Dose` is negative, the probability of the level of interest (live) gets smaller for larger dosages (this is confirmed by the shape of the curve). The dosage at which there is a 50% chance of living or dying is $-b_0/b_1 = -7.5/(-0.49) = 15.3$.

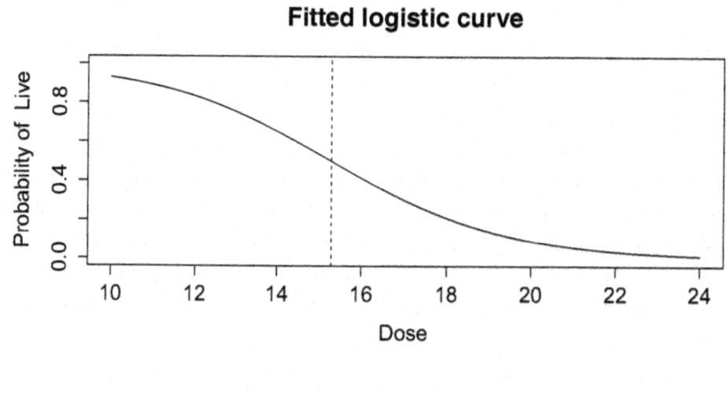

In R

```
M <- glm(Outcome~Dose,data=POISON,family="binomial")
visualize.model(M)
abline(v=-7.47379/-0.48901,lty=2)
summary(M)
             Estimate Std. Error z value Pr(>|z|)
(Intercept)  7.47379    0.66658   11.21   <2e-16 ***
Dose        -0.48901    0.04197  -11.65   <2e-16 ***
```

Figure 6.5 shows the estimated logistic curve. Visually, we see that larger doses are associated with a lower probability that a cockroach lives (and a higher probability that a cockroach dies).

Mathematically, this is confirmed since the coefficient of `Dose` in the model is about -0.49, a negative number.

At what dosage is there a 50% chance of living or dying? From the plot, it looks like somewhere between 15-16. The exact value is $-b_0/b_1 = -(7.474/-0.489) = 15.3$.

6.3.2 Example: shopping at a chain store

Consider predicting the probability that a customer has recently made a purchase at a popular national chain (e.g., Walmart) based on the distance in miles to its closest storefront. The data frame is `PURCHASE`, and the relevant columns are `Purchase` ("Buy" and "No") and `Closest`. The model will predict the probability of *not purchasing* since "No" comes last alphabetically. Figure 6.6 shows the fitted model.

Figure 6.6 — Probability of purchasing. The model is $logit(p_{notbuy}) = 1.03 + 0.01 Closest$. Since the coefficient of `Closest` is positive, the probability of the level of interest (not buy) gets larger as `Closest` (the distance to the closest storefront) increases. The shape of the curve (left) confirms this conclusion. Rephrasing, the probability of making a purchase decreases as the distance to the store increases. You may notice that the fitted curve (left) does not look much like the logistic curve in Figure 6.1. This is because the observed values of x represent only a small section of the curve. The right panel shows the logistic curve drawn from $x = -500$ to $x = 500$ with lines demarcating the range of x used in the model.

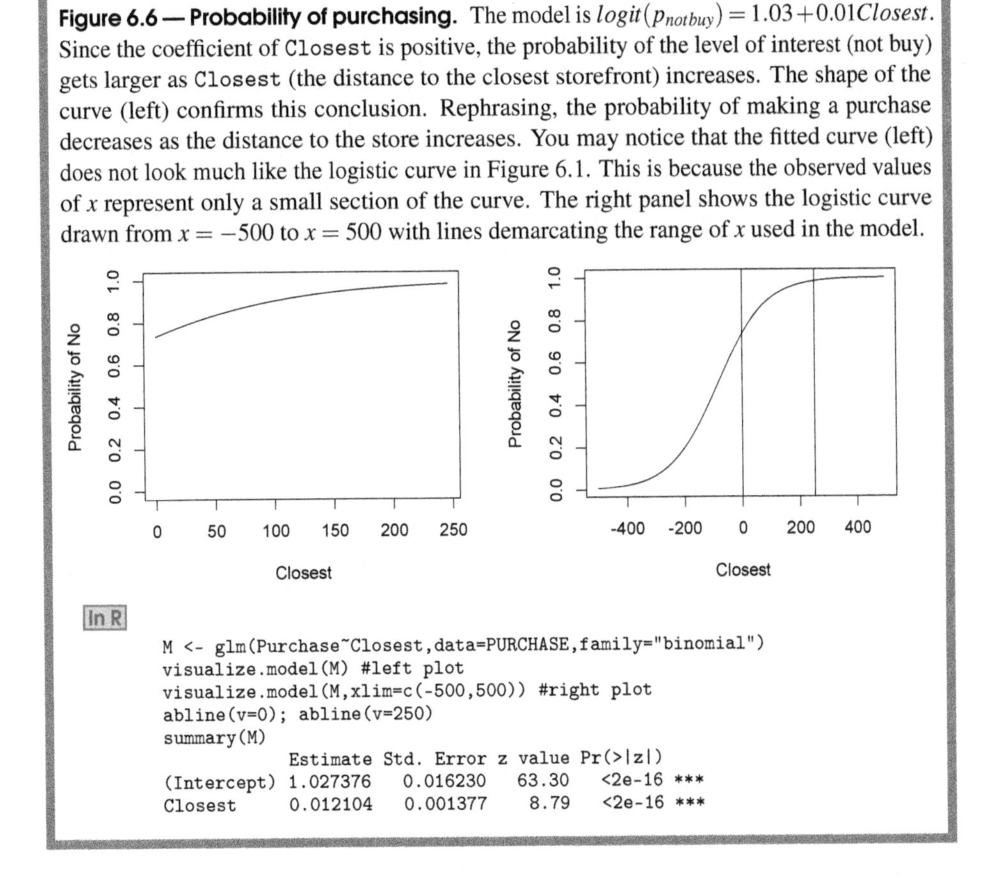

In R

```
M <- glm(Purchase~Closest,data=PURCHASE,family="binomial")
visualize.model(M) #left plot
visualize.model(M,xlim=c(-500,500)) #right plot
abline(v=0); abline(v=250)
summary(M)
            Estimate Std. Error z value Pr(>|z|)
(Intercept) 1.027376   0.016230   63.30   <2e-16 ***
Closest     0.012104   0.001377    8.79   <2e-16 ***
```

The probability of not making a purchase is larger among customers who live farther away (as we may have anticipated), but the probability changes rather slowly. When customers live virtually next door (`Closest` ≈ 0), there is about a 75% chance of not making a purchase (most consumers have not shopped at the chain recently). The probability of not making a purchase slowly increases up to about 100% at around 200 miles. Rephrasing, the probability of making a purchase starts at about 25% and slowly decreases to near zero after a few hundred miles.

The distance at which there is a 50% chance of making a purchase is $-b_0/b_1 = -1.03/0.01 = -103$ miles. This is an impossible value! The implication is that there is *no* distance at which a customer has a 50% chance of making a purchase. From the figure, we see that the smallest probability of not buying (and the largest probability of buying) occurs when `Closest` is zero. The probability of not buying is then about 75%, implying the probability of buying never gets above 25%.

6.3.3 Example: Pima diabetes dataset

Finally, let us consider a multiple logistic regression example. The `PIMA` dataset has records on about 400 women from the Pima tribe. The records indicate whether the woman has diabetes and also contain further information on the number of times the woman has been pregnant (`Pregnant`), her blood glucose level (`Glucose`), blood pressure (`BloodPressure`), insulin level (`Insulin`), body mass index (`BMI`), body fat percentage (`BodyFat`), and age (`Age`).

The Pima tribe is a relatively homogeneous population of people. Diabetes is a complex disease that involves genetic factors. These factors are not entirely known, so we cannot put them into the model to account for their presence. The hope is that the similar genetic pool of women in the Pima tribe will ensure the women in the data are as "identical" as possible without having to record additional variables. A different study using US women in general would most likely be less conclusive since there would be a lot of variation in the probability of having diabetes due to genetic factors that are difficult or impossible to record.

Let us fit a multiple logistic regression model and interpret the coefficients. There are two levels of `Diabetes`: Yes and No. Since "Yes" comes last alphabetically, it is the level of interest, so the model will predict the probability of having diabetes. Consider the output of the model.

In R

```
M <- glm(Diabetes~.,data=PIMA,family="binomial")
summary(M)
                Estimate Std. Error z value Pr(>|z|)
(Intercept)   -9.4590970  1.1733202  -8.062 7.52e-16 ***
Pregnant       0.0671174  0.0541857   1.239   0.2155
Glucose        0.0378649  0.0056951   6.649 2.96e-11 ***
BloodPressure -0.0034573  0.0115081  -0.300   0.7639
BodyFat        0.0151399  0.0168715   0.897   0.3695
Insulin       -0.0006448  0.0012873  -0.501   0.6164
BMI            0.0699113  0.0267260   2.616   0.0089 **
Age            0.0383307  0.0180514   2.123   0.0337 *
```

The actual values of the coefficients are unimportant (their size is arbitrary and based on measurement units), but the signs of the coefficients tell us something interesting. The coefficient of `Glucose` is positive (0.038). This means that among women who differ in `Glucose` but who are otherwise identical (at least in terms of the other variables in the model), those with higher glucose levels are more likely to have diabetes.

The coefficient of `Insulin` is negative (-0.0006). Among women who differ in `Insulin` but who are otherwise identical, women with higher insulin levels are less likely to have diabetes.

6.3.4 Model dependence of coefficients

In a multiple linear regression model, we have seen that both the sign and size of coefficients are model-dependent, e.g., b_i may equal 0.03 in one model and equal -2.7 in another. This phenomenon is due to associations among the predictors. The coefficient reflects the association between y and x after accounting for the other variables in the model, so when this set of "other variables" changes, the coefficient changes as well.

Consider the relationship between a person's weight and number of piercings. The coefficient in the simple linear regression is negative, implying that people with more piercings are expected to be shorter. However, in a multiple regression model with gender as an additional variable, the coefficient is essentially zero. This implies that there is no association between weight and piercings among men or among women. In this case, gender is a lurking variable. The relationship between piercings and weight only exists due to gender differences—girls are typically lighter and have more piercings, while guys are typically heavier and have fewer piercings.

In R

```
M.simple <- lm(Weight~NumBodyPiercings,data=SURVEY10)
summary(M.simple)
                 Estimate Std. Error t value Pr(>|t|)
(Intercept)       169.664      1.649  102.87   <2e-16 ***
NumBodyPiercings   -7.784      0.601  -12.95   <2e-16 ***

M.multi <- lm(Weight~NumBodyPiercings+Gender,data=SURVEY10)
summary(M.multi)
                 Estimate Std. Error t value Pr(>|t|)
(Intercept)      65.48273    0.31544  207.59   <2e-16 ***
NumBodyPiercings   0.1036     0.8213   0.126      0.9
GenderMale        43.4855     3.4049  12.771   <2e-16 ***
```

The sign and size of the coefficients in a multiple logistic regression are also model-dependent for the same reasons. Depending on the degree of association between predictors, the sign of the coefficient in a simple logistic regression may be positive, while the sign may be negative in a model with more variables, etc.

In a multiple logistic regression model, you *cannot* scroll through the list of predictors and say, "The probability of the level of interest increases with x_1 and x_2 but decreases with x_3," etc.

First, the coefficient is interpreted with respect to all other variables remaining fixed. Second, the signs of coefficients may change when new predictors are added to the model or existing predictors are removed. Lastly, the coefficients describe difference in probabilities between two individuals, not what happens to an individual's probability when his or her value of x changes. The implied relationship between a predictor and the probability is not causal. The logistic regression model is not a physical law.

Referring to the `PIMA` dataset, we cannot look at the output and conclude that the probability of having diabetes increases with the number of times the woman has been pregnant, with glucose, etc. These interpretations are overly simplistic because they omit the critical condition that all the other predictors are assumed to remain fixed when interpreting a specific coefficient.

Indeed, a simple logistic regression predicting the probability of having diabetes from BloodPressure (or Insulin) alone results in a coefficient of the opposite sign.

In R

```
M <- glm(Diabetes~BloodPressure,data=PIMA,family="binomial")
summary(M)
                Estimate Std. Error z value Pr(>|z|)
(Intercept)    -3.168012   0.676646  -4.682 2.84e-06 ***
BloodPressure   0.034492   0.009233   3.736 0.000187 ***

M <- glm(Diabetes~Insulin,data=PIMA,family="binomial")
summary(M)
              Estimate Std. Error z value Pr(>|z|)
(Intercept) -1.612947   0.203687  -7.919 2.40e-15 ***
Insulin      0.005653   0.001058   5.345 9.04e-08 ***
```

6.4 Statistical significance in logistic regression

In a linear regression model, a predictor is statistically significant if the (additional) reduction in sum of squared errors, when it is added to a model that already contains the other predictors, is "large," i.e., unlikely to have been produced by chance with a random, unrelated predictor. What does it mean for a variable to be statistically significant in a logistic regression?

Since a logistic regression does not have a well-defined "error" (the model predicts probabilities but the observations are levels), analysis of significance requires a different approach. We will use a different measure known as the **deviance**.

Roughly speaking, the deviance is a measure of how much the model deviates from a model that is a perfect fit to the data. The actual value of the deviance is related to the likelihood of observing the data using a particular model. A "perfect fitting" model is best illustrated with an example. Consider the following small dataset:

x	1	1	1	2	3	3	4
y	Yes	Yes	No	No	No	Yes	Yes

A model with a "perfect fit" would be:

$$p = \begin{cases} 2/3 & when\ x = 1 \\ 0 & when\ x = 2 \\ 1/2 & when\ x = 3 \\ 1 & when\ x = 4 \end{cases}$$

At each value of x, the perfect fitting model gives p to be the proportion of individuals who have the level of interest. The model gives no insight into the behavior of how p changes with x because there is no underlying equation.

Think of the deviance as the "distance" between the logistic regression model and the perfect fitting model. Its mathematical expression does not concern us here, but we can view it as roughly equivalent to the root mean squared error (RMSE) in linear regression (the typical distance of points from the line). Although the actual value of the deviance is not very informative, lower values indicate a better fit.

In the linear regression context, the coefficients that minimize the deviance are the exact same coefficients that minimize the sum of squared errors. In some sense, we can consider the deviance as a generalization of the concept of "error" that works for all models.

Whenever an additional variable is added to a logistic regression model, the deviance decreases (just like the sum of squared errors decreases when a new predictor is added to a linear regression), regardless of whether there is any relationship between it and p. For a predictor to be statistically significant, this reduction in deviance must be "large." "Large" is relative to the reduction expected from a predictor that is unrelated to p.

Calculating the p-value of the reduction in deviation can be done via the permutation procedure, but formulas exist that give good approximations. Software will automatically output these p-values so that you can gauge significance.

For example, the p-values of `Dose` in the `POISON` dataset and of `Closest` in the `PURCHASE` dataset are extremely small (much less than 1 in a trillion), indicating that these predictors are statistically significant. There is a *very* small probability that the reduction in deviance that occurs when the predictor is added would happen by chance. These variables predict p better than a predictor unrelated to p.

In the `PIMA` diabetes example, the p-value of `Age` is 0.0337. Since this is less than 5%, `Age` is a statistically significant predictor of the probability that a woman has diabetes. What this *really* means is that adding `Age` to a model that already contains `Pregnant`, `Glucose`, etc., yields a reduction in the deviance that is much larger than what would be expected "by chance" (i.e., from an unrelated predictor). Knowing a woman's age contributes additional information about the probability of having diabetes above and beyond what the other predictors already offer.

The p-value of `Insulin` is 0.62. Since this is much larger than 5%, it is not a statistically significant predictor. Does this mean that insulin levels are unrelated to the probability of having diabetes? No. Biologically, they are linked. The lack of statistical significance implies that once all the other variables (`Pregnant`, `Glucose`, `BMI`, `Age`, etc.) are known, the *addition* of `Insulin` to the model does not significantly reduce the deviance beyond what we would expect from an unrelated predictor. The information that `Insulin` tells us about the probability of having diabetes must already be contained in the other variables in the model, thus it is redundant.

Most discussions regarding significance focus on individual predictors. Technically, before even considering individual predictors, we need to assess whether the model itself is statistically significant, i.e., if it reduces the deviance by any more than what we would expect from a model full of predictors unrelated to p. However, `R` does not report the p-value of the model by default.

In R

To obtain the p-value of the model itself, you also must fit the naive model (no predictors).

```
M <- glm(Diabetes~.,data=PIMA,family=binomial)
M.naive <- glm(Diabetes~1,data=PIMA,family=binomial)
anova(M.naive,M,test="Chisq")
  Resid. Df Resid. Dev Df Deviance  Pr(>Chi)
1       391     498.10
2       384     351.58  7   146.52 < 2.2e-16 ***
```

The p-value of the model is the number under `Pr(>Chi)`.

> Remember: the p-value of a predictor does not indicate the *strength* of the relationship between p and x. As in other contexts, the p-value is dependent on the sample size, and it is easy for an extremely weak association to be statistically significant when the dataset is large.

6.5 Assessing utility of a logistic regression model with a confusion matrix

In linear regression, R^2 tells us the percentage of the variation in y that can be "explained" by the model. Models with large values of R^2 fit the data well and may be useful. Unfortunately, there is no directly analogous number for a logistic regression model. Rather, the **confusion matrix** yields insight into the percentage of predictions that are correct and what kinds of mistakes the model makes.

To make a confusion matrix, predictions for individuals' levels are made (predict the level of interest if $p \geq 50\%$; otherwise predict the other level) and then cross-tabulated with the actual levels. To illustrate, let us use the `PIMA` diabetes dataset. The two levels are "Yes" and "No" (whether the woman has diabetes or not). "Yes" is the level of interest since it comes last alphabetically.

In R

```
M <- glm(Diabetes~.,data=PIMA,family="binomial")
confusion.matrix(M)
           Predicted No Predicted Yes Total
Actual No           232            30   262
Actual Yes           54            76   130
Total               286           106   392
```

The **misclassification rate** of a model is typically its most useful summary. Here, we see the model misclassifies a total of 84 cases—54 (actual `Yes` but predict `No`) plus 30 (actual `No` but predict `Yes`). The misclassification rate is the percentage of predictions that are wrong, and in this case it is 84/392, or 21.4%. Conversely, the model correctly classifies 78.6% of cases ($232+76=308$ out of 392). The different types of errors are worth analyzing separately.

In total, 130 women have diabetes in the dataset (the total for the row labeled `Actual Yes`). Of these women, the model correctly predicts the status of 76 and misses 54. These errors are **false negatives**, where the model predicts a trait to be absent when in reality it is present. If the model is designed to identify women with the potential to have diabetes (so that preventive measures could be administered), these types of errors are particularly harmful—these women will not receive the care they need.

Further, 262 women do not have diabetes. Of these women, the model correctly predicts the status of 232 and misses 30. These errors are **false positives**, where the model predicts a trait to be present when in reality it is not. For the purposes of preventative care, these errors are not particularly harmful (the woman does not end up with diabetes regardless), but money would have been wasted.

The misclassification rate and number of false positives and negatives are used to gauge the utility of a model. How can we tell if these numbers are "good"? The first step is to compare the predictions with the **naive model**.

In logistic regression, the **naive model** predicts *every* individual to have whatever level of y forms the majority. The misclassification rate of the naive model is the proportion of individuals with the minority level.

The majority of women in the `PIMA` diabetes data do not have diabetes, so the naive model predicts *all* women to not have diabetes. The confusion matrix is below.

In R

```
#Fitting the naive model requires using the formula ~1 (no predictors)
M <- glm(Diabetes~1,data=PIMA,family="binomial")
confusion.matrix(M)
          Predicted No
Actual No          262
Actual Yes         130
```

Let us write out the confusion matrix as an actual table (including the column for predicted `Yes`):

		Predicted		
		No	Yes	Total
Actual	No	262	**0**	262
	Yes	**130**	0	130
	Total	392	0	392

Thus, the misclassification rate of the naive model is $(130+0)/392 = 33.2\%$ since all women who have diabetes would be misclassified. The logistic regression is "good" since it decreases the misclassification rate from 33.2% to 21.7%.

The naive model has no false positives since all women are predicted to not have diabetes. The number of false negatives is 130 since all women who have diabetes are predicted to be healthy.

Now consider the `PURCHASE` dataset. We want to predict if a customer has made a purchase in the last 90 days based on his or her distance to the nearest store. The confusion matrix for this model is:

In R

```
M <- glm(Purchase~Closest,data=PURCHASE,family=binomial)
summary(M)
            Estimate Std. Error z value Pr(>|z|)
(Intercept) 1.027376   0.016230   63.30   <2e-16 ***
Closest     0.012104   0.001377    8.79   <2e-16 ***

confusion.matrix(M)
Predicted levels same as naive model (majority level)
          Predicted No
Actual Buy        6892
Actual No        20831
```

In this case, even though `Closest` is a highly statistically significant predictor of the probability of buying, the model's performance is identical to that of the naive model. Everyone is predicted to not buy! Although it feels like a contradiction to have a statistically significant model perform no better than the naive model, it is not. The predicted probabilities of buying do vary substantially with `Closest`. It is just the case that *all* predicted probabilities are greater than 50%, so all predictions are for "No." See Figure 6.7.

This phenomenon happens quite often when we predict people's behavior. While the x does a better job than an unrelated predictor at describing how the probability changes, it is not useful from a predictive standpoint since it classifies all individuals identically. However, even though the model doesn't make classifications well, it may still be useful for selecting the subset of customers with the highest chance of buying (even if it is not above 50%).

Figure 6.7 — Predicted probabilities of "Not Buying" for the shopper dataset. The model predicting the probability of making a purchase in the last 90 days is highly statistically significant—customers who live further from the store have a lower probability of purchasing than customers who live nearby. However, the chance of a particular customer not buying is so large that all predicted probabilities are much greater than 50%. Thus, the model classifies everyone in the dataset as non-purchasers, the same as the naive model ("not buying" is the majority level). The model may still be useful for selecting the subset of customers with the highest chance of making a purchase.

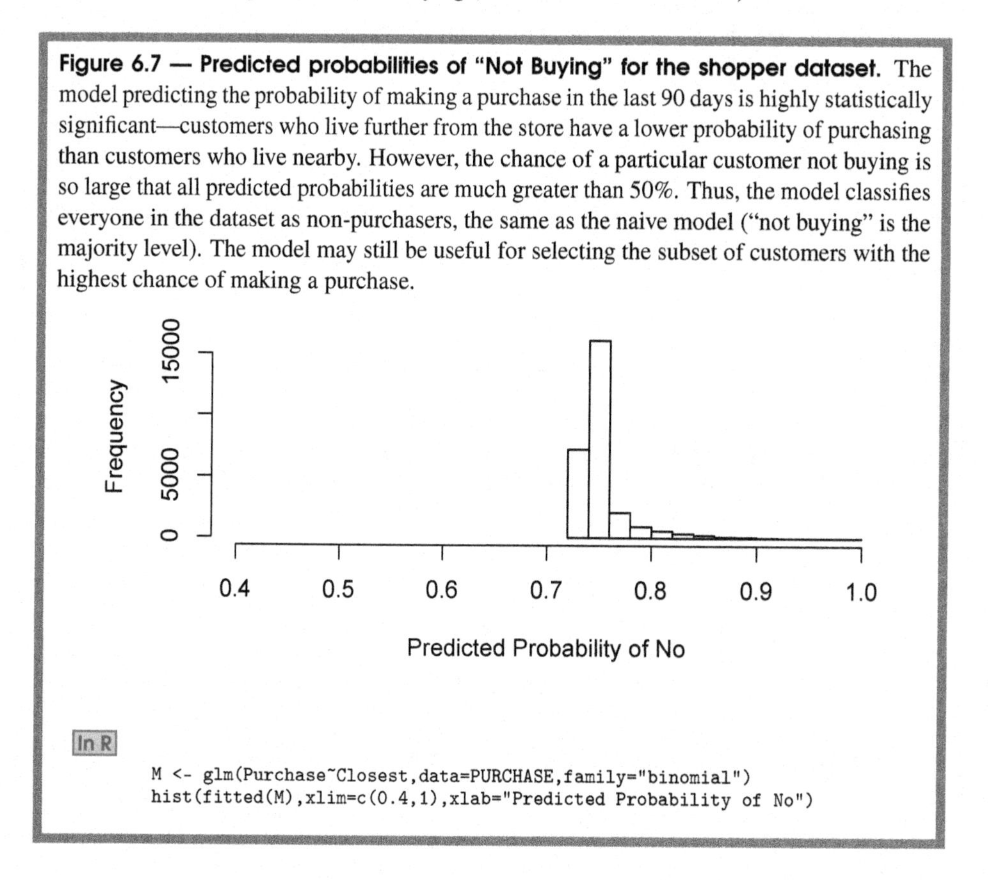


```
M <- glm(Purchase~Closest,data=PURCHASE,family="binomial")
hist(fitted(M),xlim=c(0.4,1),xlab="Predicted Probability of No")
```

6.6 Checking assumptions behind the logistic regression model

We check to see if a linear regression is an adequate reflection of reality by checking residuals plots—if we see any leftover pattern, there is a key component of the relationship between y and the predictors that is missing. This approach will not work for logistic regression since there is no clear definition of a "residual."

Rather, we can rely on the results of a statistical **goodness of fit** test to determine whether the logistic curve is a good description of how the probability changes with the predictors. As we have learned with linear regression, the test can be overly strict when the number of observations is large, but there are no other great options.

To conduct the goodness of fit test, we first split the values of x into categories (e.g., dosage between 10-12, dosage between 14-16, etc.). Next, we compare the number of cases that possess the level of interest with the number predicted by the model. For example, consider the `POISON` data:

Dose	10 or 12	14 or 16	18 or 20	22 or 24
Observed (Live)	100	72	17	1
Expected (Live)	104.8	63.6	18.5	3.1

The observed count is found directly from the data (e.g., 100 cockroaches died when they were given dosages between 10-12). The expected count is the sum of the predicted probabilities of all individuals who fall into the category (e.g., the sum of the predicted values for p for all cockroaches that had dosages of 10-12 is 104.8).

The goodness of fit test finds the "discrepancy" D between the observed and expected counts of this table. The procedure is reminiscent of the test for association between two categorical variables (see Section 2.3.3).

$$D = \text{ sum of } \frac{(Observed - Expected)^2}{Expected} = \frac{(100-104.8)^2}{104.8} + \ldots + \frac{(1-3.1)^2}{3.1} = 2.87$$

Large values of D indicate the model is a bad fit. To determine what value of D is "too large," we can run a simulation.

- Assume the model is correct and create a random sample of outcomes using the predicted probabilities.
- Calculate the discrepancy between the expected counts (which remain the same) and the observed counts (which depend on the results of the random sample). Repeat this procedure many times.
- The p-value of D from the goodness of fit test is the fraction of random samples that exhibited at least as large a value of D.

If the p-value of the goodness of fit test is at least 5%, then the logistic curve provides a statistically valid description of how the probability changes with the predictors. In this case, the discrepancy between observed and expected counts is small enough to arise by chance had the model been correct. If the p-value of the test is less than 5%, then the logistic regression model is not statistically valid.

Package `regclass` provides two ways of assessing the validity of a logistic regression. The first uses `check.regression` and provides two tests.

- Method 1 uses the fitted probabilities to generate an artificial sample. In effect, each individual flips a coin to determine whether he or she has the level of interest (with an appropriately weighted coin so that the probability of having the level of interest is equal to the fitted probability from the model). Then, the levels in the artificial sample are compared to the levels predicted by the model, and the misclassification rate of the model is tabulated.
  The process repeats for many different artificial samples. If the misclassification rate of the model on the observed data is out of line with the misclassification rates of the model on the artificial datasets (where by definition the model is correct), then the goodness of fit test is failed (p-value less than 5%).

- Method 2 uses a Hosmer-Lemeshow test and is the goodness of fit test described in the text. If the p-value of the goodness of fit test is less than 5%, the test is failed and (statistically speaking) the model is not valid.

The second uses `associate` (in the case of a simple logistic regression) and provides a rough visualization of how the probability changes with x. See Aside 6.1.

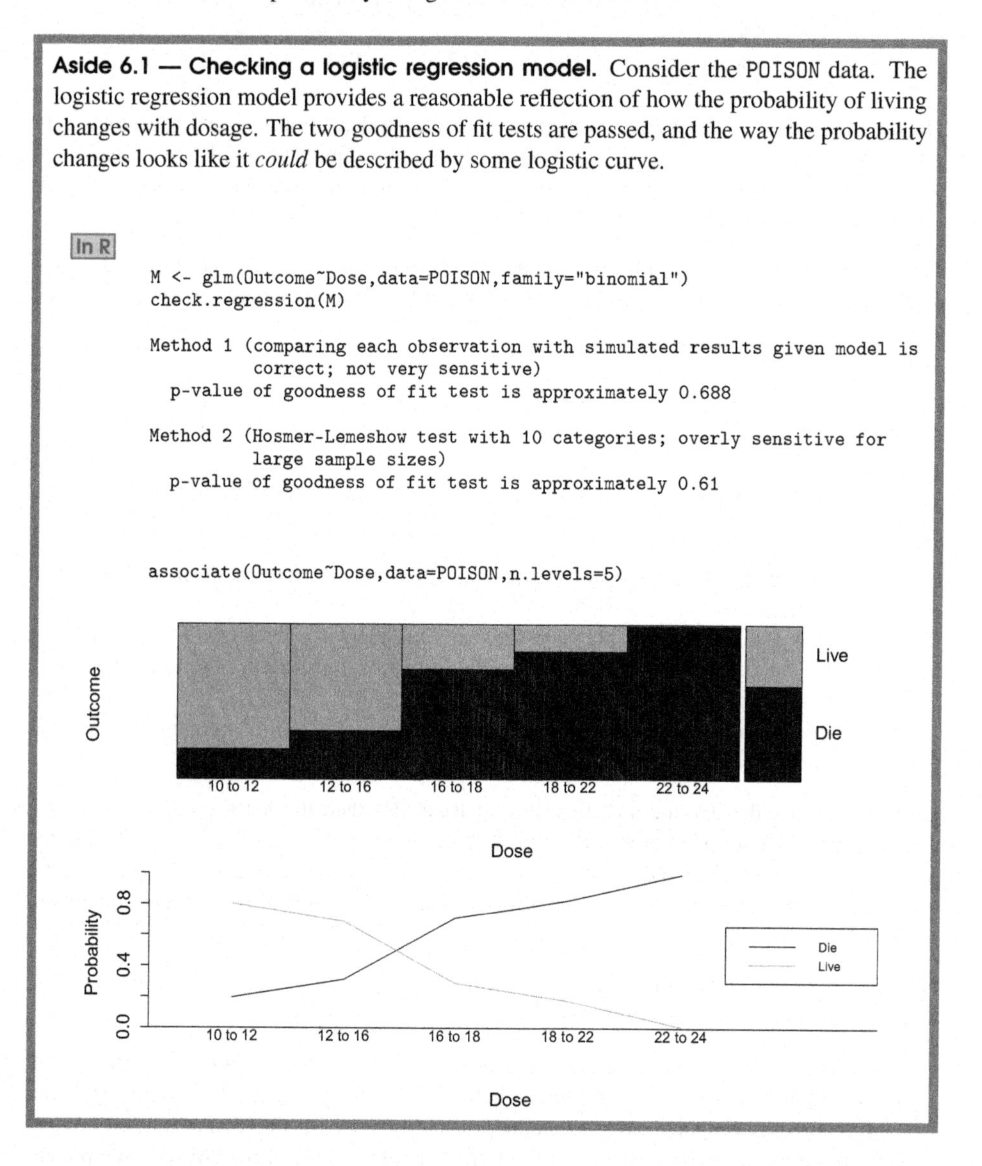

Aside 6.1 — Checking a logistic regression model. Consider the `POISON` data. The logistic regression model provides a reasonable reflection of how the probability of living changes with dosage. The two goodness of fit tests are passed, and the way the probability changes looks like it *could* be described by some logistic curve.

In R

```
M <- glm(Outcome~Dose,data=POISON,family="binomial")
check.regression(M)

Method 1 (comparing each observation with simulated results given model is
          correct; not very sensitive)
  p-value of goodness of fit test is approximately 0.688

Method 2 (Hosmer-Lemeshow test with 10 categories; overly sensitive for
          large sample sizes)
  p-value of goodness of fit test is approximately 0.61


associate(Outcome~Dose,data=POISON,n.levels=5)
```


6.7 Interactions in logistic regression

Interaction variables can provide extra flexibility and can add elements of realism to a linear regression model. The interaction variable $x_1 \times x_2$ allows the strength of the relationship between y and x_1 to vary based on the value of x_2. For example, we saw that educational level and years of experience were decent predictors of someone's monthly salary in the SALARY dataset. However, the strength of the relationship between someone's salary and their educational level was not a constant (review Figure 4.14). The number of years of education was a better predictor of salary among people with little experience than it was among people with lots of experience. Intuitively, this seemed reasonable. When people lack experience, their education is the only indicator of their qualifications. When people are highly experienced, the amount of education is not very important since experience alone indicates their competency.

In a similar vein, the shape of the logistic curve describing how p changes with x_1 may depend on the value of another variable, x_2. For some values of x_2, the probability may change very slowly as x_1 increases. For other values of x_2, the probability may change sharply. The probability may increase with x_1 for some values of x_2 and may decrease with x_1 for other values of x_2.

For example, consider the problem of predicting whether customers churn at the end of their cell-phone contract (churning means not renewing) in the CHURN dataset. Two potential variables to predict the probability of churning (`churn`) are the number of calls made to customer service (`numbercustomerservicecalls`) and the total daytime usage in minutes (`totaldayminutes`). Figure 6.8 explores the model:

$$logit(p_{churn}) = \beta_0 + \beta_1 Calls + \beta_2 DayMinutes + \beta_3 (CustServiceCalls \times DayMinutes)$$

In R

```
M <- glm(churn~numbercustomerservicecalls*totaldayminutes,data=CHURN,
         family="binomial")
summary(M)
                                        Estimate Std. Error z value Pr(>|z|)
(Intercept)                           -9.2419916  0.3693352  -25.02   <2e-16 ***
numbercustomerservicecalls             2.3547377  0.1316621   17.89   <2e-16 ***
totaldayminutes                        0.0328527  0.0016425   20.00   <2e-16 ***
numcustservicecalls:totaldayminutes -0.0096241  0.0006293  -15.29   <2e-16 ***
```

The interaction term is highly statistically significant. The *manner* in which the probability of churning changes with the total daytime minutes depends on how often the customer has called support (and vice versa). See Figure 6.8.

- Among people who have made no calls to customer service, the probability of churning *increases* with daytime usage. We may speculate that perhaps that high-usage customers change plans or carriers at the end of their contract to save money.
- Among people who have made a large number of customer service calls, the probability of churning *decreases* with the number of daytime minutes. This may reflect that customers who have not used their phone much *and* who have experienced many problems are likely to churn (perhaps they experienced problems and switched carriers before the contract ended).
- Customers who do use their phone a lot *and* who have called support many times have a very small probability of churning. This insight is surprising, but that is the story the model tells us.

Figure 6.8 — Effect of interaction variables on the logistic curve. Here, we are predicting the probability that a customer will churn based on the number of calls he or she has made to customer service (left) and the number of daytime minutes he or she has used (right), including the interaction. With the interaction, the shape of the logistic curve describing how the probability varies with daytime minutes is allowed to change based on the number of calls made to customer service (and vice versa). The interaction is highly significant and important. The model suggests that the probability of churning increases with daytime minutes for customers with few calls to customer service, but the probability *decreases* with daytime minutes for customers with many calls to customer service.

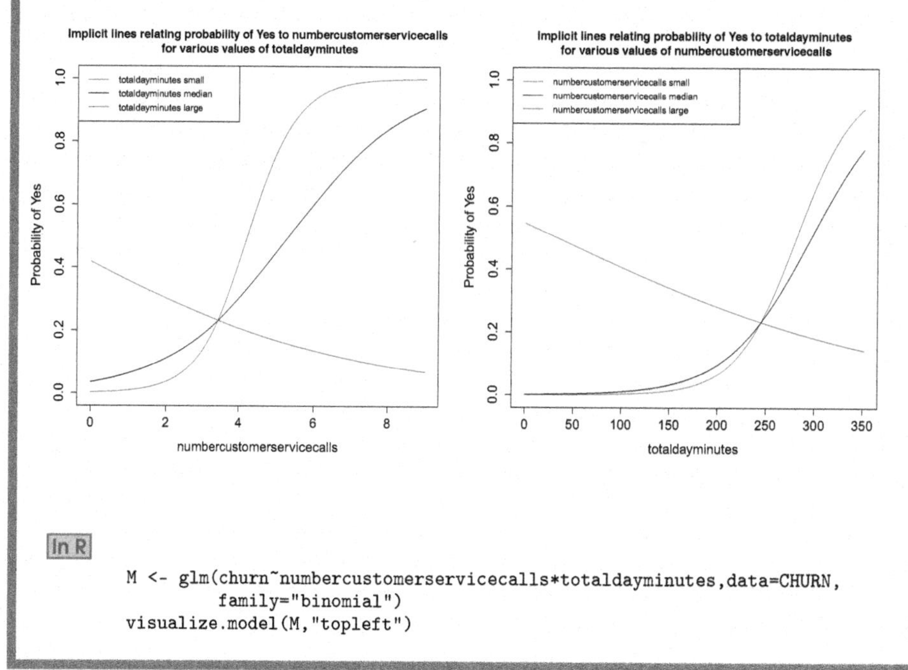


```
M <- glm(churn~numbercustomerservicecalls*totaldayminutes,data=CHURN,
         family="binomial")
visualize.model(M,"topleft")
```

6.8 Categorical variables in logistic regression

Incorporating categorical variables into a logistic regression requires conversion into a set of indicator variables. If the variable has L levels, it is necessary to define $L-1$ indicator variables (review Section 5.1). By convention, the level that comes first alphabetically is not represented by an indicator variable. This level is called the "reference" level.

6.8.1 Interpretation of coefficients and significance

The coefficients of the indicator variables are interpreted with respect to the reference level. The sign of the coefficient (rather than its value) is important.

> If the coefficient of an indicator variable is positive, then p is higher for individuals who have that level than for individuals who have the reference level (assuming the individuals are otherwise identical with respect to the other variables in the model).

If the coefficient is negative, then p is lower for individuals who have that level than for individuals who have the reference level (assuming the individuals are otherwise identical).

The coefficient does *not* tell you the difference in probabilities between levels (this difference is not a constant but depends on the values of the other predictor variables).

For example, consider the problem of predicting whether customers will purchase a new type of account at a bank based on their banking behavior and demographic information. The `ACCOUNT` dataset contains the response variable `Purchase` (Yes/No; "Yes" is the level of interest and the one we predict since it comes last alphabetically) and categorical predictor variables `Homeowner` (Yes/No) and `Area.Classification` (R, S, U for rural, suburban, urban).

Fitting a model with all variables and no interactions, we find that the coefficient of `Homeowner` is -0.01. Since "No" comes first alphabetically, it serves as the reference level (note how there is no indicator variable in the model representing `HomeownerNo`). Thus, among otherwise identical individuals (in terms of checking/savings balances, income, age, and area classification), those who own homes have a smaller probability of purchasing the new account than non-homeowners.

However, the p-value of the coefficient is 70%, implying that once all these other quantities are known about the individual, any additional information gained from knowing his or her homeownership status is redundant. In other words, adding `Homeowner` into the model does not significantly decrease its deviance.

In R

```
M <- glm(Purchase~.,data=ACCOUNT,family="binomial")
summary(M)
                     Estimate Std. Error z value Pr(>|z|)
(Intercept)        -9.164e-01  6.344e-02 -14.444  < 2e-16 ***
Tenure             -7.822e-03  2.339e-03  -3.343 0.000827 ***
CheckingBalance     4.726e-05  3.139e-06  15.057  < 2e-16 ***
SavingBalance       7.638e-05  2.720e-06  28.087  < 2e-16 ***
Income              3.924e-04  5.088e-04   0.771 0.440581
HomeownerYes       -1.091e-02  2.920e-02  -0.373 0.708836
Age                -5.009e-04  1.042e-03  -0.481 0.630835
Area.ClassificationS 9.084e-02  3.639e-02   2.496 0.012552 *
Area.ClassificationU 3.733e-03  3.593e-02   0.104 0.917244
```

The coefficients of the "S" and "U" levels for the area classification are 0.09 and 0.004, respectively. "R" is the reference level because it comes first alphabetically. Among otherwise identical customers, those who live in suburban or urban areas have a higher probability of opening the new account than those who live in rural areas.

Is the difference in probabilities statistically significant? The p-values of these indicator variables do not answer that question. We need to run an **effect test** to see if the addition of the *set* of variables representing `Area.Classification` significantly reduces the deviance.

Similar to multiple linear regression, the p-value of an indicator variable for a 3+level categorical variable comments on whether there is any difference in probabilities between the level represented by the indicator and the reference level. These p-values do not indicate whether the categorical variable as a whole is significant or not. To determine significance, an effect test must be run.

To perform the effect test, we fit the model with and without area classification and look to see if the reduction in the deviance is significant. Below are the results of the effect tests for each variable.

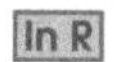

```
M <- glm(Purchase~.,data=ACCOUNT,family="binomial")
drop1(M,test="Chisq")
                    Df Deviance Resid. Df Resid. Dev Pr(>Chi)
Tenure               1     29407 29423     11.70 0.0006237 ***
CheckingBalance      1     29708 29724    313.25 < 2.2e-16 ***
SavingBalance        1     30794 30810   1399.41 < 2.2e-16 ***
Income               1     29396 29412      0.57 0.4507610
Homeowner            1     29395 29411      0.16 0.6932054
Age                  1     29395 29411      0.24 0.6216590
Area.Classification  2     29404 29418      9.17 0.0102010 *
```

The p-value of the effect test for `Area.Classification` is 0.0102, less than the conventional threshold of 5%. We see that adding the set of indicator variables representing `Area.Classification` to a model containing all other predictors yields a statistically significant reduction in the deviance. The implication is that the probabilities of buying a new account are *somehow* different for urban, suburban, and rural customers, though the test does not tell us *which* levels are different.

6.8.2 Effect on logistic curve

When a categorical variable is added to a linear regression model, separate lines are fit to each level. The intercepts of these implicit lines are allowed to differ, but the other coefficients are constrained to be the same. In effect, the lines are shifted up and down relative to each other.

When a categorical variable is added to a logistic regression model, separate logistic curves are fit to each level. The shapes of these implicit curves are constrained to be the same (they rise or fall with the same trajectory), but they are allowed to be offset from each other from left to right. While the probability will always be higher for one level, the difference in probabilities depends on the values of the other x variables.

For instance, consider Figure 6.9, which studies the `CHURN` dataset. The predictors are the calls made to customer service (quantitative) and whether the customer has an international plan (categorical). Implicitly, two logistic curves are fit: one for customers with an international plan and one for customers without. These curves have the same shape, but the curve for customers with an international plan is shifted to the left. The shift represents the fact that they always have a higher probability of churning than customers without an international plan. The difference in probabilities is large among customers who made few calls to customer service and small among customers who made many calls to customer service.

We can include an interaction between a categorical and quantitative variable in the model as well, e.g., we can add the term $ServiceCalls \times IntlPlan$ in the current example. Once again, separate logistic curves are fit for each level of the categorical variable. However, these curves are allowed to have completely different shapes, e.g., the probability may rise quickly with x for one level but slowly with x for another.

Figure 6.9 — Effect of categorical variable on logistic curve. The model:

$$logit(p_{churn}) = \beta_0 + \beta_1 ServiceCalls + \beta_2 IntlPlan$$

has been fit and the two implicit logistic curves (one for each level of international plan) are displayed. When a categorical variable such as international plan (yes/no) is put into a logistic regression model, a separate logistic curve is fit for each level. These curves have the same shape but are allowed to be offset horizontally from each other. The net effect is that the probability for one level will always be higher than the probability for the other. In this case, those customers with an international plan are more likely to churn regardless of the number of calls they have made to customer service.

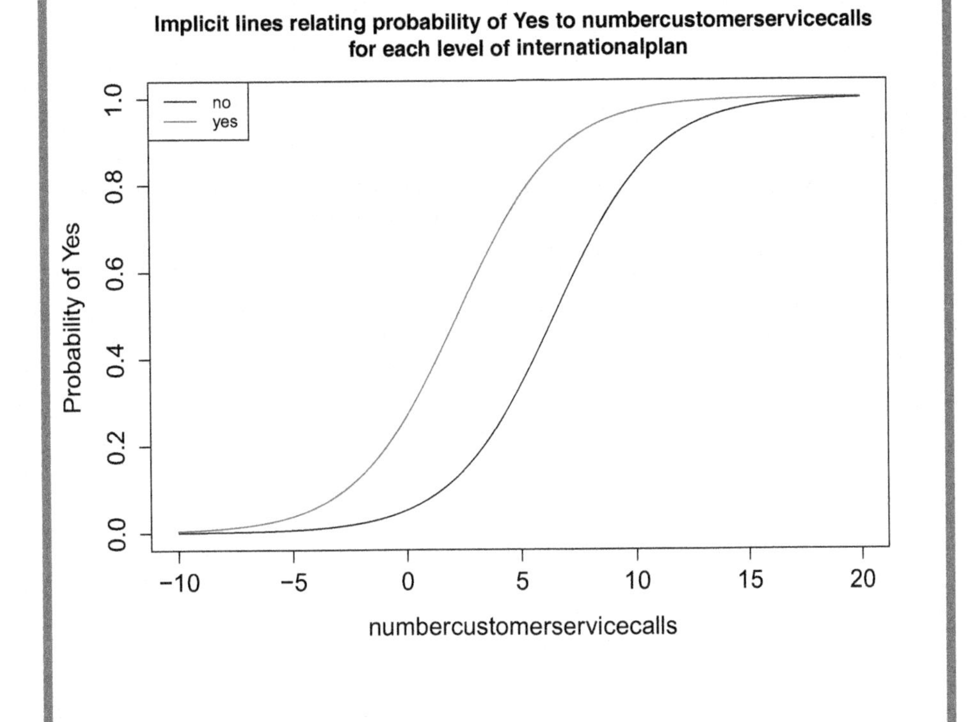

In R

```
M <- glm(churn~internationalplan+numbercustomerservicecalls,
        data=CHURN,family="binomial")
visualize.model(M,xlim=c(-10,20))
```

Adding an interaction offers a greater flexibility in the model since the manner in which the probability changes with x can be quite different across levels. Without the interaction, the logistic curves for each level are constrained to have the same shape. This benefit was also seen when we considered adding an interaction between a categorical variable and a quantitative variable to a linear regression. In that case, the strength of the relationship between y and x was allowed to vary across levels (e.g., the strength of the relationship between the selling price of a bulldozer and its usage depended on the decade the bulldozer was manufactured). Figure 6.10 gives an illustration.

Figure 6.10 — Effect of interaction with a categorical variable on logistic curve. The model:

$$logit(p_{churn}) = \beta_0 + \beta_1 ServiceCalls + \beta_2 IntlPlan + \beta_3 (ServiceCalls \times IntlPlan)$$

has been fit and the two implicit logistic curves (one for each level of international plan) are displayed. With an interaction present, the shapes of the logistic curves are allowed to vary. This allows the probability of churning to be higher for certain customers with international plans and lower for other customers. Indeed, the interaction term is significant in the model, and we can see that when the number of calls to customer service is low, the probability of churning is higher for customers with international plans. When the number of calls to customer service is high, the probability of churning is lower for customers with international plans. Without an interaction, the probability for customers with international plans would either always be above or always be below the probability for customers without international plans.

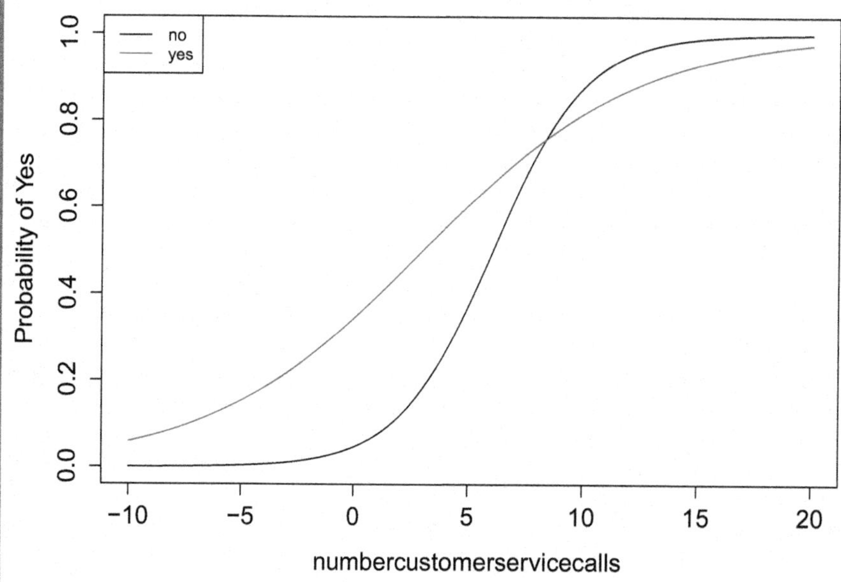

In R

```
M <- glm(churn~internationalplan*numbercustomerservicecalls,data=CHURN,
         family="binomial")
visualize.model(M,xlim=c(-10,20))
```

6.9 Summary

Logistic regression is the cornerstone of business analytics and other fields. To successfully predict y when it is a categorical variable, a mastery of how to interpret coefficients, how to check whether the model adequately describes reality, and how to gauge the significance of predictors is required.

The major highlights of logistic regression are as follows:

- When y is a two-level categorical variable, we use *logistic regression* and predict the *probability* that an individual will possess the level of interest (by convention the one that comes *last* alphabetically). The probability is denoted by p. The probability that an individual possesses the other level is $1 - p$.
- The logistic regression model assumes the probability changes with x according to a very special shape: the logistic curve.

$$logit(p) = \ln \frac{p}{1-p} = \beta_0 + \beta_1 x_1 + \ldots + \beta_k x_k \iff p = \frac{e^{\beta_0+\beta_1 x_1+\ldots+\beta_k x_k}}{1+e^{\beta_0+\beta_1 x_1+\ldots+\beta_k x_k}}$$

- Interpretation of the estimated coefficient b_i when x_i is quantitative: among otherwise identical individuals (i.e., same values for the other predictors) ...
  - $b_i > 0 \Rightarrow$ individuals with larger values of x_i have a higher probability of having the level of interest.
  - $b_i < 0 \Rightarrow$ individuals with larger value of x_i have a lower probability of having the level of interest.
- Interpretation of estimated coefficient b_i when x_i is an indicator variable:
  - $b_i > 0 \Rightarrow$ individuals with the level represented by the indicator variable have a higher probability of possessing the level of interest than individuals with the reference level.
  - $b_i < 0 \Rightarrow$ individuals with the level represented by the indicator variable have a lower probability of possessing the level of interest than individuals with the reference level.
- In simple logistic regression (one predictor x), the quantity $-b_0/b_1$ gives the value of x where each level occurs with a 50% chance.
- In general, we classify y as one level or the other by calculating the probability of the level of interest. If $p \geq 0.5$, then we predict the individual to have the level of interest (last alphabetically). If $p < 0.5$, we predict the individual to have the other level.
- The *deviance* of a model is a measure of how much it deviates from a perfect fitting model. Given a set of predictors, the coefficients are found by minimizing the deviance via the maximum likelihood procedure. This procedure chooses the values of the coefficients that give the highest chance of the model reproducing the data.
- A predictor is statistically significant if, when added to a model with the other predictors already present, it is unlikely that an unrelated predictor would have reduced the deviance by at least as much. If the p-value of the coefficient (or effect test) is 5% or larger, there is no evidence that adding it to the model yields a better fit.
- To assess whether the logistic curve is appropriate for modeling how the probability changes with x, try a goodness of fit test. If the p-value is 5% or greater, the test is passed and it appears that the model provides a reasonable reflection of reality.
- To evaluate the utility of a model, find its confusion matrix. This can be used to find the misclassification rate, false "positives," and false "negatives."
- Interactions between variables allow the shape of the logistic curve to vary based on the values of other variables and can be an important part of a logistic regression model.

6.10 Using R

To fit a logistic regression model, the command glm (as opposed to lm) must be used. The model formulation is identical to linear regression. However, glm does require an additional argument to "turn on" logistic regression, and that is adding family="binomial" (with or without quotes).

In R

```
M <- glm(y~x,data=DATA,family="binomial")
M <- glm(y~x1+x2,data=DATA,family="binomial")
M <- glm(y~x1*x2,data=DATA,family="binomial")
M <- glm(y~.,data=DATA,family="binomial")
M <- glm(y~.^2,data=DATA,family="binomial")
```

Model summary:

In R

```
summary(M)
```

Significance of 3+level categorical variables (effect test):

In R

```
drop1(M,test="Chisq")
```

Checking assumptions:

In R

```
check.regression(M)
associate(y~x,data=DATA) #simple logistic only
```

Visualizing a simple logistic regression or a multiple logistic regression with two variables (one may be categorical, and they may be involved in an interaction):

In R

```
visualize.model(M)
```

Confusion matrix:

In R

```
confusion.matrix(M)
```

Making predictions (assumes that the x-variables are stored in a data frame called TO.PREDICT that has either been read in or defined manually):

In R

```
predict(M,newdata=TO.PREDICT,type="response") #gives probabilities
```

6.11 Exercises

1: Use EX6.DONOR. This is a modified portion of the DONOR data in other parts of the text (it is the same dataset as EX5.DONOR). It deals with a charity's customer database. Each row represents an individual and whether he or she donated during the last campaign (Donate, yes or no), the donation amount (LastAmount), the age of the account (i.e., number months since his or her first donation, AccountAge), the age of the individual (Age), where the customer lives (Setting, Urban/Suburban/Rural), etc. Let us model the amount someone donated during the last campaign (LastAmount). Let us predict whether someone donated during the last campaign (Donate).

a) The levels of Donate are Yes and No. If we fit a logistic regression model, will it be predicting the probability that someone DOES donate or the probability that someone DOES NOT donate?
b) Fit a logistic regression predicting Donate from TotalDonations, which is the total number of donations this person has ever made.
    1) Examine the results of visualize.model(). Does the probability of donating increase or decrease as the total number of donations gets larger?
    2) Examine the results of summary(). What number confirms/justifies your answer to (1) and why?
    3) Calculate the value of TotalDonations where someone has a 50% chance of donating.
    4) Joe Black had donated only once to this charity before the last campaign. What does this model predict for the probability that he DID donate and the probability that he DID NOT donate during the last campaign? Does the model predict him to donate or not? Try doing these calculations by hand.
c) Is the relationship between the probability of donating and the donor's age (Age) statistically significant? Is the relationship strong (i.e., have practical significance)? Take the relationship to be strong if the probability to donate varies by more than 20% over the range of ages in the data. Examine the results of visualize.model() to guide your answer.

2: Use EX6.CLICK. This is a modified part of a kaggle.com competition where the goal is predict whether someone clicked on an ad while using a mobile device. The data is anonymized, so while most of the predictor variables do have meaningful names (e.g., BannerPosition, DeviceModel), the values do not.

Two questions we would like to answer are: "Does the position of the ad matter? If so, where should the ad be placed?" and "Does the probability of clicking on an ad vary based on the device being used, e.g., are iPhone users more likely to click the ad than Galaxy users?" We need multiple logistic regression to answer this question since many factors influence the probability of clicking.

For example, to meaningfully compare the probability of clicking between the two banner positions, we need to make sure the ads/users are as identical as possible in every other regard. Otherwise, any difference in probabilities could alternatively be explained by the other ways in which the ads/users vary. When we fit a multiple logistic regression model predicting Click from all variables and look at the coefficient of BannerPosition, the number is a comment on how the probabilities differ between banner positions among otherwise identical ads/users (at least with respect to the other variables in the model).

a) Fit a multiple logistic regression predicting `Click` from all predictors in the dataset. Look at the `summary()`. You will notice that many values are `NA`. This occurs when there are "singularities" in the model, i.e., some variables (like `SiteCategory`) can be *perfectly* predicted from the other variables. When this happens, R still reports the variables in `summary()`, but it can't give any additional information because it is impossible to estimate their coefficients. Examine the output showing the coefficients, *p*-values, etc., of `BannerPosition` and `DeviceModel`.

b) When we compare ads on the same site, viewed in the same app, on the same device type, etc. (i.e., "otherwise identical ads"), which position (Pos1 or Pos2) has the higher probability of click-thru? Is the difference in probabilities statistically significant? Explain.

c) When we compare ads in the same position, on the same site, viewed in the same app, etc. (i.e., "otherwise identical ads"), which device models (D1-D18; you may ignore D13 since its coefficient is NA) have the highest and lowest probabilities of click-thru? Is the difference in probabilities statistically significant? In other words, all else being equal, is the probability of clicking on an ad genuinely higher for some devices? Explain. Note: you will have to run `drop1(M,test="Chisq")` to comment about significance, and this command will take a while.

d) Is the model any better at predicting clicks than the naive model? Justify your answer by comparing the total number of misclassifications (you can ignore any warnings output from `confusion.matrix()`).

3: Use `EX6.WINE`. This dataset is a slightly modified version of the `WINE` dataset, where one of the predictors is now categorical. We want to predict whether a wine was gauged high or low quality by experts (column `Quality`) based on chemical characteristics of the wine. Having a model to predict whether the wine is "good" would be useful to both ensure quality control and potentially to "design" a new type of wine that people would enjoy.

a) Fit a model predicting `Quality` from `volatile.acidity` and `alcohol` (no interaction). Examine the plot from `visualize.model()` (include `xlim=c(0,20)` and `loc="left"` in the arguments to make it look nice). Focus on the plot with p and `alcohol`.
   1) Which has the larger probability of being *high quality* (careful here): wines with more alcohol or wines with less alcohol (or does the answer depend on the specific value of the wine's volatile acidity)?
   2) Among wines with the same alcohol content, which has the larger probability of being *low quality*: wines with more volatile acidity or wines with less volatile acidity (or does the answer depend on the wine's specific value of alcohol content)?

b) The model in (a) assumes "one curve fits all." In other words, it assumes that the *shape* of the logistic curve describing how p changes with alcohol is the same regardless of the wine's volatile acidity. This may not be the case: the relationship between p and alcohol may be different for different values of volative acidity. Redo the previous model and include the interaction between the two predictors. Examine the results of `summary()` and `visualize.model()` (adding the same arguments as before).
   1) For what types of wine is alcohol a better predictor of quality: wines with low volatile acidity or wines with high volatile acidity? Note: one predictor is better than another when its logistic curve changes more rapidly.
   2) Among wines with the same alcohol content, which has the larger probability of being *low quality*: wines with more volatile acidity or wines with less volatile acidity (or does the answer depend on the wine's specific value of alcohol content)?
   3) Is the interaction between alcohol and volatile acidity something we need to be including in the model? Explain, quoting specific output from `summary()`.

c) Fit a model predicting `Quality` from all variables (no interactions). Does this model provide a statistically valid description of how the probability of being high/low quality changes with the predictors? Examine the results of `check.regression`.
d) Bonus: among wines with the same amount of alcohol, do wines with "Lots" of chlorides or "Little" have a larger chance of being low quality? Does the answer depend on the specific value of the alcohol content of the wines? Justify your answer (note: your model should be predicting the quality from alcohol and chlorides; leave the other predictors out of this).

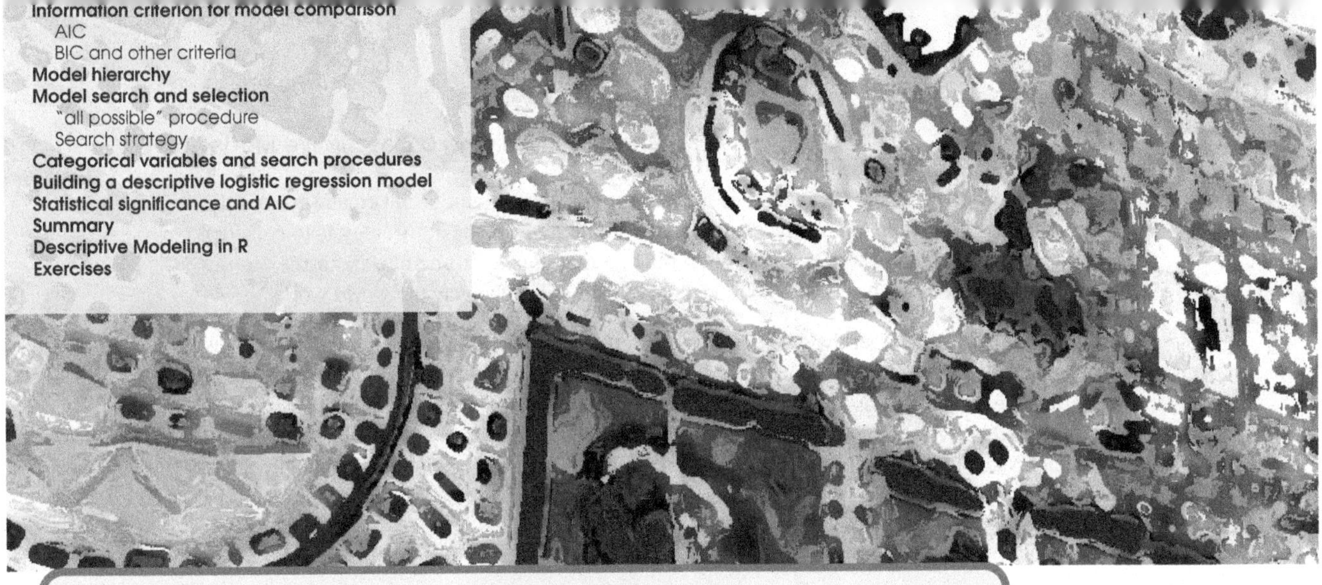

Information criterion for model comparison
AIC
BIC and other criteria
Model hierarchy
Model search and selection
"all possible" procedure
Search strategy
Categorical variables and search procedures
Building a descriptive logistic regression model
Statistical significance and AIC
Summary
Descriptive Modeling in R
Exercises

7. Building a Descriptive Model

The goal of a descriptive model is to come up with an equation that reflects reality as closely as possible. Although we know *a priori* that the real world is more complex than any model, the hope is that it can yield some insight as to *how* variables are related. Often, the coefficient of one particular variable (e.g., the coefficient of gender in a model predicting salary) is of interest. By obtaining as precise an estimate as possible, you may glimpse how y and this predictor are associated after accounting for other extraneous sources of variation (the other x's in the model).

By its very nature, descriptive modeling is a difficult task since "all models are wrong." Variables are related in more subtle ways than our model can possibly hope to capture. However, a "good" model should still be useful and informative.

For example, imagine you wish to study the association between the profit of a new product after its first month of release and the Internet presence of the advertising campaign. A simple linear regression model relating the two quantities may not be sufficient since there may be other factors: TV and radio advertising expenditures, price and color of product, number of stores selling the product, number of competitors products, etc. A multiple regression model allows us to take account of other factors connected to profit, but it is by no means clear ahead of time what other variables must be included in the model.

In the previous chapters, we have focused on interpreting the coefficients, gauging significance, and checking the reasonableness of a *pre-determined* model. We now turn our attention to figuring out *what* model we should be using. Although tests of significance for predictor variables (Section 4.4.2 and 4.4.3) seem like a logical basis for building a model (keep only terms in a model that are statistically significant), they have serious drawbacks.

(C) The results of significance tests do not necessarily provide a guide for making a good model since "statistical significance" is not a direct measure of how far a model is from reality. Further, tests of significance are really only meaningful when they are performed once. Tweaking a model by adding or removing variables based on their p-values is not a good practice because the p-values don't quite mean the same thing after repeated tests.

Modern construction techniques use concepts from *information theory*. Instead of relying on

p-values and statistical significance, they try to minimize the amount of information about the world that is "lost" when using a particular set of predictors. The basic strategy is to consider a vast array of different models and to pick the one that appears to be closest to the "truth." However, we do know *a priori* that no model exactly describes the way the world works.

Before we begin, remember that even after any careful model-building procedure, the variables that appear in the model do not necessarily have a causal relationship with y. Regression equations are not physical laws. The coefficient of a predictor does *not* indicate what will happen to an individual's value of y when his or her x-value increases by one unit. Rather, the coefficient of a predictor is simply a comment on the expected difference in y between individuals who happen to differ in that predictor by one unit (and who have identical values for the other predictors).

7.1 Information criterion for model comparison

The first step in finding the best model is to define what "best" actually means. Historically, the values of R^2_{adj} and the root mean squared error $RMSE$ have been used for model evaluation. One way to select a model is to examine many candidates and choose the one with the highest R^2_{adj} (Section 4.2) or lowest $RMSE$. Of the models under consideration, this one in some sense provides a reasonable balance between how well the model fits the data and the model's complexity (i.e., number of predictors). In fact, we used this criterion for choosing the "best" order of a polynomial model in Section 4.5.1.

Assuming that there is some underlying fundamental relationship (either direct or indirect) going on between y and the x's, a more desirable property of the model is to come as close to this reality as possible. In other words, instead of minimizing the errors the model makes on the data we collected, we try to minimize the difference between our model and "the truth." For a visual motivation, see Figure 7.1.

Figure 7.1 — Distance between models and the truth. Imagine that the "truth" is that the distribution of y is given by the thick solid line. The distribution of y inferred from Model 1 is given by the dashed line, and the distribution of y inferred from Model 2 is given by the dotted line. Clearly, Model 1 is closer to reality than Model 2. A good model-building procedure should be able to gauge the relative distances of models from the truth.

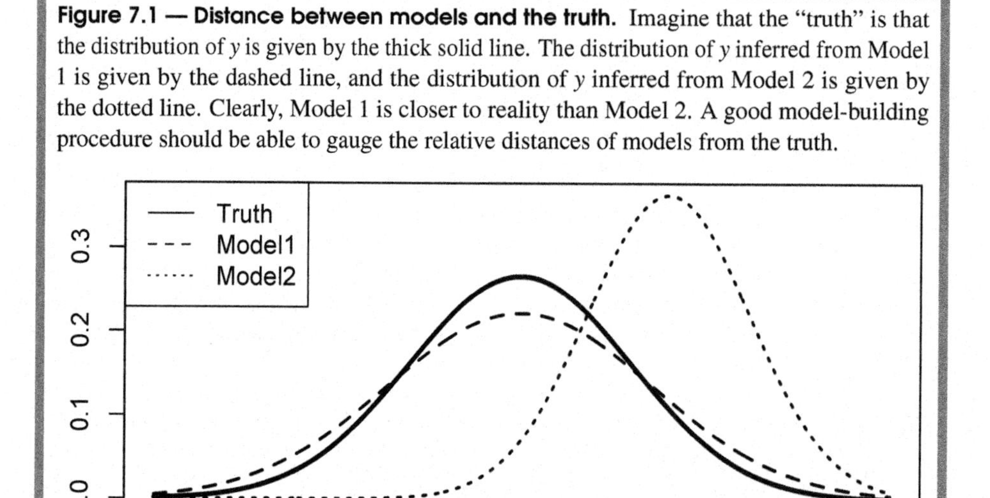

Maximizing R^2_{adj} or minimizing the $RMSE$ may find the model whose distribution of y best matches the distribution of y in the data, but that is not quite what we are after. The **Kullback-Leibler divergence** measures the discrepancy between the distribution of y inferred from the model and the "true" distribution of y. Loosely, the Kullback-Leibler divergence can be thought of as the area between the curves describing the two distributions. Models with smaller values of this quantity are better.

Mathematically, the Kullback-Leibler (KL) divergence of g (the proposed distribution) from f (the truth) is $KL = \int f(y)\log(f(y)/g(y))dy$. Evaluating the quantity requires calculus.

Thinking about model selection in a slightly different way, we want to best separate structural information about the relationship from noise (non-information). In this regard, the term "information" refers to the structure of the relationship (estimates of coefficients). Noise refers to residuals. When we use information criterion to select a model, we are attempting to model the *information* in the data rather than to model the data itself. Such a criterion has a solid statistical foundation, but it begs the question of how we can measure the distance from a model to the truth if we don't *know* the truth.

7.1.1 AIC

Akaike found a remarkable (and simple) approximation to the Kullback-Leibler divergence and the "*relative* distance" between the distribution of y inferred by the model and the true distribution of y. The approximation uses the sum of squared errors (SSE), sample size (n), and number of predictors (k). It is called the AIC, or Akaike Information Criterion, in his honor.

$$AIC = n\log(SSE/n) + 2k \quad (7.1)$$

The AIC can also be thought of as the *relative* amount of information that is lost when a fitted model is used to approximate the full reality. The actual numerical value of the AIC is non-informative since it is the relative distance from the model to the truth (as opposed to an absolute distance), it depends on the units of y, and it can be positive or negative.

> The *difference* between two models' AICs is informative—the model with the lower AIC is "better" since less information is lost about reality and it gets closer to the "truth."

The equation for the AIC has a nice interpretation as well. When a model gets more complex (i.e., more predictors are added to it), the sum of squared errors always decreases, so the first term in the AIC gets smaller. However, this is somewhat offset by an increase in the second term, which serves as a penalty based on the number of predictors. Thus, like R^2_{adj} or the $RMSE$, the AIC balances how well the model fits the data with its complexity, but in a more statistically rigorous and justifiable way.

One small complication arises when the sample size is relatively small. If $n/k < 40$, the formula for the AIC needs to be corrected to give a better approximation to the distance between the model and the truth:

$$AIC_c = n\log(SSE/n) + 2k + \frac{2k(k+1)}{n-k-1} \quad (7.2)$$

When we choose a descriptive model, we select the one with the lowest AIC. However, how large of a difference between AICs matters? If you have fit a large number of models (called the **candidate set**), then some guidelines are:

- A difference in AIC of ≤ 2 is small; models are essentially functionally equivalent
- A difference in AIC between 4 and 7 is fairly large; reasonable evidence that the model with the lower AIC is better
- A difference in AIC of more than 10 is substantial; the model with the lower AIC is almost certainly better

Thus, a model selection strategy consists of fitting a candidate set of models and finding the ones with the lowest AICs. All models with AICs within about 2 of the lowest are essentially equivalent, and statistics alone cannot justify the use of one over the other. Use your favorite (perhaps the simplest).

7.1.2 BIC and other criteria

The BIC (Bayesian Information Criterion) also balances a model's goodness of fit to the data with its complexity, but it puts a higher penalty on the number of predictors.

$$BIC = n\log(SSE/n) + k\log n \tag{7.3}$$

Because of the larger penalty, models selected by BIC tend to be more parsimonious (have fewer variables) than ones selected by AIC. Again, the actual value of the BIC is irrelevant. Only the relative differences between BIC values matter (smaller is better). Note: values of BIC are never compared to values of AIC.

Takeuchi's information criterion (TIC) is defined similarly except with a penalty term that is not a simple function of the number of variables and sample size (in fact, the AIC is an approximation to TIC). Theoretically, it should be more useful in choosing the best approximating model when none of the candidate models are particularly close to the truth. However, in practice, it is difficult to estimate the penalty term from the data without a large number of observations. When there is enough data, this penalty term is very close to AIC's penalty.

Finally, ICOMP (information complexity) is also like AIC or BIC but with a different penalty term. As we have discussed, predictor variables can be correlated and may contain redundant information. While k gives the number of predictors in the model, the "effective" number of predictors is probably smaller. ICOMP takes into account the correlations in the model and uses a more honest penalty term.

7.2 Model hierarchy

Before we discuss strategies for fitting a candidate set of models, one convention should be discussed: **model hierarchy**.

If a model in the candidate set includes an interaction between two variables, it is often *suggested* that each variable involved in the interaction be included in the model as well, regardless of whether its inclusion would increase the AIC.

A model of the form $y = \beta_0 + \beta_1 x_1 x_2$ violates model hierarchy, while the model $y = \beta_0 + \beta_1 x_1 + \beta_2 x_2 + \beta_3 x_1 x_2$ preserves it.

Some examples are:

- The model $Salary = \beta_0 + \beta_1 Education + \beta_2 Experience + \beta_3 Education \times Experience$ preserves hierarchy.
- The model $Salary = \beta_0 + \beta_1 Education + \beta_2 Education \times Experience$ violates model hierarchy (the *Experience* term is missing).

Preserving model hierarchy is more of a suggestion than a rule, and justifications for doing so are mostly philosophical. Some software packages and routines preserve hierarchy; others do not.

7.3 Model search and selection

Choosing which information criterion to use is a matter of personal choice (and there is healthy debate over which one people "should" be using). Our examples will consider the AIC.

There are literally an infinite number of possible models that can be put in the candidate set (the number of transformations and combinations of variables is endless). Thus, some strategy for generating a set of models is required. Unless we have reason to include transformations (e.g., there is curvature present in scatterplots or the distribution of y or the predictors is highly skewed) or complex interactions, we typically consider just the original predictors with perhaps all or a subset of two-way interactions.

7.3.1 "all possible" procedure

The "all possible" procedure generates a candidate set of 2^k models. Any model with an AIC within 2 of the lowest AIC is an acceptable choice for a final model.

To illustrate the procedure, let $k = 3$, i.e., there are three predictors in the data set.

- Fit the naive model (no predictors; y is predicted to be $\bar{y}$, the average value in the data).
- Fit all three simple linear regressions.
- Fit all three regressions that contain 2 predictors: $x_1 \& x_2$, $x_1 \& x_3$, and $x_2 \& x_3$.
- Fit the full model (all predictors).

The "all possible" procedure can be modified to incorporate interactions. However, software typically treats the interaction terms as independent variables and fits models that do not preserve model hierarchy, e.g., $y = \beta_0 + \beta_1 x_1 + \beta_2 x_2 x_3$. It is rare for all interactions to be considered since this increases the number of models in the candidate to 2 raised to the $\frac{1}{2}k(1+k)$ power.

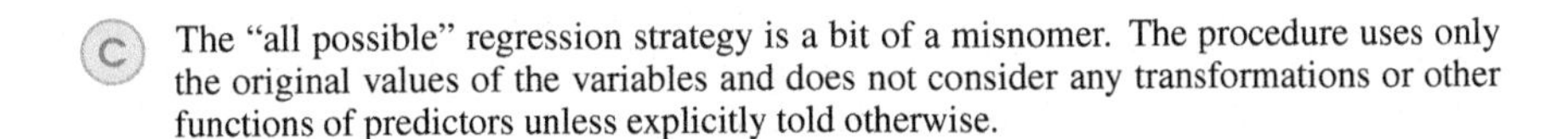

The "all possible" regression strategy is a bit of a misnomer. The procedure uses only the original values of the variables and does not consider any transformations or other functions of predictors unless explicitly told otherwise.

For example, let us consider the SALARY dataset. To determine whether there is gender discrimination at a company, we need to find the difference in average pay between men and women after accounting for differences in educational background, prior experience, and the number of months at the company. Thus, we need a model that fully describes how employees' qualifications are related to their salary.

Let us use the "all possible" procedure that includes two-way interactions. Below are the six models with the lowest AICs. Note: in this case, the AIC turns out to be negative, so -31.5 is indeed lower than -29.5.

In R

```
MODELS <- regsubsets(Salary~(Education+Experience+Months)^2,data=SALARY,
                     nbest=4,method="exhaustive")
see.models(MODELS,report=6)
Reporting the 6 models with the lowest AICs
   AIC NumVars Terms
 -31.5       4  Education Experience Education:Experience Education:Months
 -29.5       5  Education Experience Months Education:Experience
                Education:Months
 -29.5       5  Education Experience Education:Experience Education:Months
                Experience:Months
 -28.7       4  Education Experience Months Education:Experience
 -27.5       6  Education Experience Months Education:Experience
                Education:Months Experience:Months
 -26.9       5  Education Experience Months Education:Experience
                Experience:Months
```

Of the 64 models considered, the one with the lowest AIC has four predictors: Education, Experience, and the interactions between Education&Experience and Education&Months. The AIC is 2 below the next best model, so it is the best choice. Notice that this model violates hierarchy—Months is involved in an interaction but does not appear by itself.

Now consider the BODYFAT data. There are 13 potential predictors of someone's body fat percentage, so a total of $2^{13} = 8192$ models must be considered if we do not allow any interactions. This sounds like a lot, but the computation is very fast with modern technology.

In R

```
MODELS <- regsubsets(BodyFat~.,data=BODYFAT,method="exhaustive")
see.models(MODELS)

Reporting all models with AIC within 4 of the lowest value
    AIC NumVars                                                Terms
 -328.0       8  Age Weight Neck Abdomen Hip Thigh Forearm Wrist
 -327.8       7      Age Weight Neck Abdomen Thigh Forearm Wrist
 -326.4       6           Age Weight Abdomen Thigh Forearm Wrist
 -325.5       5                Weight Neck Abdomen Forearm Wrist
 -324.8       4                     Weight Abdomen Forearm Wrist
```

There are a total of three different models within 2 of the lowest AIC. This is not surprising considering the highly redundant nature of the predictor variables. Statistically, there is no particular reason to prefer one over the other, so we could choose the simplest model. This has six predictors—Age, Weight, Abdomen, Thigh, Forearm, and Wrist.

Interactions often play an important role in the real world, so it would be nice to try them in this model. However, considering all two-way interactions would require fitting nearly $2^{91} = 2.5 \times 10^{27}$ models!

Instead of trying all interactions, one strategy is to consider only the interactions between variables that appear in models with low AICs. For example, let us redo the body fat example but consider two-way interactions between the variables selected in the preliminary model. Below are the top two models (many others have AICs within 2 but are not displayed):

In R

```
MODELS <- regsubsets(BodyFat~(Age+Weight+Abdomen+Thigh+Forearm+Wrist)^2,
          data=BODYFAT,method="exhaustive")
see.models(MODELS)

Reporting all models with AIC within 4 of the lowest value
    AIC NumVars  Terms
 -345.7        7  Age Thigh Forearm Age:Wrist Weight:Abdomen Abdomen:Wrist
                  Thigh:Wrist
 -345.7        8  Thigh Forearm Age:Thigh Age:Wrist Weight:Thigh
                  Weight:Wrist Abdomen:Thigh Forearm:Wrist
 -345.1        6  Thigh Forearm Age:Weight Weight:Abdomen Abdomen:Wrist
                  Thigh:Wrist
 -344.1        5  Thigh Age:Forearm Weight:Abdomen Abdomen:Wrist
                  Thigh:Wrist
 -341.7        4  Thigh Weight:Abdomen Abdomen:Wrist Thigh:Wrist
```

Indeed, considering interactions yields a model with a substantially lower AIC (-346 vs. -328). To make a model predicting body fat percentage that mimics reality as closely as possible, it looks like considering interactions is a must!

As modern computing power increases, running the "all possible" procedure is trivial for datasets with a few hundred data points with up to about $k = 20$ or so predictors if interactions are not included, and about $k = 9$ if interactions are included. However, the size of datasets has been outpacing the speed of computers. Modern datasets may have a few hundred, if not a few thousand, predictors. If $k = 100$, the amount of time to run the "all possible" procedure is staggering—if a billion models could be fit per second, it would take 40 trillion years to complete the computation (and that is for models with no interactions).

For example, one recent data modeling competition on `kaggle.com` looked at online product sales for newly released items (`https://www.kaggle.com/c/online-sales`). This dataset has 419 predictor variables. If we ignore interactions, the "all possible" strategy would need to consider $2^{419} \approx 10^{126}$ models. This is more than the number of particles in the universe. We thus need an intelligent way to *search* for a good model instead of considering every single one.

7.3.2 Search strategy

When it is impractical to perform the "all possible" procedure, we can search through a subset of "reasonably" good models instead. The basic procedure is as follows.

1. Propose a preliminary model that predicts y from a subset of the available predictors.
2. Calculate the AICs of all models that differ from this model by one variable (either one predictor is eliminated or one new predictor added).
3. Update the model by whatever decreases the AIC the most.
4. Repeat until the AIC no longer decreases.

For example, imagine we have predictors x_1, x_2, x_3, and x_4. Our preliminary model may predict y from x_1 and x_2. We then calculate the AICs of models where one predictor has been kicked out (i.e., predict y from x_1 or predict y from x_2) and of models where one predictor has been added (i.e., predict y from x_1, x_2, and x_3 or predict y from x_1, x_2, and x_4). The preliminary model is updated to whichever model gives the biggest decrease in AIC, and the process repeats until nothing can be done to the model to improve it.

The preliminary model is typically taken to be either the naive model (no predictors) or the full model (all predictors) with or without interactions.

Example: Attractiveness

To illustrate the search procedure, let us consider the `ATTRACTF` dataset. Here, the goal is to predict the attractiveness score (average of about 50 ratings, typically from males, on a 1-5 scale) of women using various physical characteristics. For example, `FaceSymmetryScore` is the number of people (in a different statistics class) who agreed the woman's face was roughly symmetric, `FashionScore` is the number of people who agreed that the woman was fashionable, `GayScore` is the number of people who suspected the woman was a lesbian, etc.

In this example, let us only consider the 10 quantitative predictors so that it is trivial to employ the "all possible" strategy and to select the one with the lowest AIC (`FitnessScore`, `GayScore`, `HairstyleUniqueness`, and `MakeupScore` are in this model). Let us see if the search procedure recovers this model.

Let the initial model be one predicting the attractiveness score from `FitnessScore` (the number of people who agreed the woman was fit) and `FashionScore`. This model has an AIC of -79.12. Let us see what happens when we remove or add variables to the model.

```
Start:  AIC=-79.12
AttractionScore ~ FitnessScore + FashionScore

                    Df Sum of Sq    RSS     AIC
+ MakeupScore        1    4.4442 16.305 -93.991
+ HairstyleUniquess  1    3.2999 17.449 -89.244
+ GayScore           1    3.0033 17.746 -88.064
+ GroomedScore       1    1.1810 19.568 -81.221
+ NoseOddScore       1    1.1445 19.605 -81.091
+ HappinessRating    1    1.0000 19.749 -80.577
<none>                          20.749 -79.119
+ FaceSymmetryScore  1    0.0399 20.709 -77.254
+ SkinClearScore     1    0.0108 20.738 -77.156
- FashionScore       1    1.2089 21.958 -77.155
- FitnessScore       1    8.2012 28.950 -57.804
```

It looks like the best move is to add `MakeupScore` to the model, which would decrease the AIC to -94. Notice that taking out `FitnessScore` or `FashionScore` (or adding `FaceSymmetryScore` or `SkinClearScore`) results in worse models.

The process of adding and/or subtracting predictors continues until the model can improve no more. The final model has an AIC of -115 and is identical to the model found using the "all possible" strategy. In this case, the search procedure finds the right answer! For particularly complex problems, this may not always be the case.

Aside 7.1 — Comparing the search to the "all possible" procedure. The "all possible" approach finds that the model with the lowest AIC has four predictors. Notice how instead of typing out all predictors, it is possible to specify their column numbers manually.

In R

```
MODELS <- regsubsets(Score~.,data=ATTRACTF[,c(1,7:10,12,14,15,17,18,20)],
         method="exhaustive")
see.models(MODELS,report=1)

Reporting the 1 models with the lowest AICs
   AIC NumVars                                                     Terms
 -63.8       4  FitnessScore GayScore HairstyleUniquess MakeupScore
```

Now let us conduct the search, starting with a model predicting the score from fitness and fashion scores. Note: the relevant columns of ATTRACTF have been saved to a new dataframe called SMALLATTRACT.

In R

```
SMALLATTRACT <- ATTRACTF[,c(1,7:10,12,14,15,17,18,20)]
M.naive <- lm(Score~1,data=SMALLATTRACT)
M.start <- lm(Score~FitnessScore+FashionScore,data=SMALLATTRACT)
M.complex <- lm(Score~.,data=SMALLATTRACT)
S <- step(M.start,scope=list(lower=M.naive,upper=M.complex),
         direction="both")
summary(S)

                  Estimate Std. Error t value Pr(>|t|)
(Intercept)        1.59910    0.16343   9.784 2.11e-14 ***
FitnessScore       0.30617    0.03492   8.768 1.27e-12 ***
MakeupScore        0.12786    0.02578   4.960 5.34e-06 ***
HairstyleUniquess -0.29048    0.09093  -3.195  0.00216 **
GayScore          -0.03253    0.01495  -2.175  0.03324 *
```

Indeed, the search procedure recovers the model with the lowest AIC.

```
Step:  AIC=-114.68
AttractionScore ~ FitnessScore + MakeupScore + HairstyleUniquess +
    GayScore

                    Df Sum of Sq    RSS      AIC
<none>                           11.791 -114.678
+ NoseOddScore       1    0.2679 11.524 -114.287
+ SkinClearScore     1    0.1643 11.627 -113.661
+ FashionScore       1    0.0754 11.716 -113.127
+ FaceSymmetryScore  1    0.0671 11.724 -113.078
+ HappinessRating    1    0.0238 11.768 -112.820
+ GroomedScore       1    0.0018 11.790 -112.689
- GayScore           1    0.8585 12.650 -111.759
- HairstyleUniquess  1    1.8515 13.643 -106.469
- MakeupScore        1    4.4632 16.255  -94.208
- FitnessScore       1   13.9472 25.739  -62.035
```

In the final model, notice that adding any variable not already in the model, or kicking out a variable in the model, causes the AIC to increase. While kicking out a predictor causes the AIC to increase by more than 2, adding in one additional variable does not. Since models with AICs within 2 of each other are essentially equivalent, we *could* add in another predictor if we so desired. See Aside 7.1 for the fits.

Example: Salary (with interactions)

Let us reconsider the SALARY dataset and conduct a search while considering all two-way interactions. We know the model with the lowest AIC since we previously ran the "all possible" procedure. However, the "all possible" procedure allows models that violate model hierarchy, while the search procedure does not. The selected model may be different.

> The default search procedure step() in R preserves model hierarchy. In order for an interaction to be included in the model, both component terms must be present. For an individual predictor to be removed from the model, it may not be involved in any interaction.

Let us begin with the model predicting Salary from Education and step through the procedure.

```
Start:  AIC=1131.31
Salary ~ Education

             Df Sum of Sq      RSS    AIC
+ Months      1   1992019 15101650 1121.8
+ Experience  1    905830 16187839 1128.2
<none>                    17093669 1131.3
- Education   1   3494460 20588129 1146.6
```

There are three options at the first step above: add in Months, add in Experience, or remove Education. The best move is to add in Months. Now we find the following:

```
Step:  AIC=1121.79
Salary ~ Education + Months
                   Df Sum of Sq      RSS    AIC
+ Experience        1    728669 14372981 1119.2
<none>                          15101650 1121.8
+ Education:Months  1     63037 15038613 1123.4
- Months            1   1992019 17093669 1131.3
- Education         1   3804294 18905945 1140.7
```

The only move that decreases the AIC is to add Experience. Notice, however, that the interaction between Education and Months is considered for addition. To preserve model hierarchy, an interaction is only considered if both components are already in the model. In the first step, when Education was the only predictor in the model, no valid interactions could have been added, so none were considered.

After the procedure runs a few more steps, we come to the final model:

```
Step:  AIC=1115.14
Salary ~ Education + Months + Experience + Education:Experience +
    Education:Months
                       Df Sum of Sq      RSS    AIC
<none>                               13181730 1115.1
- Education:Months      1    394850 13576580 1115.9
+ Experience:Months     1       889 13180841 1117.1
- Education:Experience  1   1065205 14246935 1120.4
```

This is *almost* the same model chosen by the "all possible" procedure. The difference is that this model also includes `Months`. The "all possible" procedure selected a model with the interaction between `Education` and `Months`, but left out `Months` by itself (which violates model hierarchy). It turns out that the model selected by the search is the one with the *second* lowest AIC, so it is still pretty good.

7.4 Categorical variables and search procedures

When a categorical variable has only two levels, it is represented by a single indicator variable and search procedures require no modification. However, categorical variables with three or more levels are represented by a *set* of indicator variables. One could treat each indicator variable separately and add/remove them to/from the model as you would any other variable, but this is generally a bad idea—leaving out an indicator variable *redefines* the reference level.

For example, imagine the categorical variable Class has levels freshman, sophomore, junior, and senior. The reference level is freshman since it comes first alphabetically. If we leave out the indicator variable for junior in a model, then the reference level becomes freshman *or* juniors. There is no logical reason why freshmen and juniors should be grouped together, so this move seems questionable.

The indicator variables are: "sophomore" (equals 1 if the student is a sophomore and 0 otherwise), "junior" (equals 1 if the student is a junior and 0 otherwise), and "senior" (equals 1 if the student is a senior and 0 otherwise). Freshmen are represented by each of these equaling 0 (i.e., not sophomore, not junior, not senior). If we omit the indicator variable "junior," then the combination of sophomore=0 and senior=0 refers to both freshmen and juniors.

While it *may* be true that two or more levels could be combined if they act similarly, leaving out an indicator variable forces the model to treat the level it represents and the reference level as if they are the same. This assumption is typically not warranted.

> Model hierarchy says to treat the set of indicator variables as a whole. When a categorical variable is considered for addition to the model, *all* indicator variables representing it are added simultaneously. The same goes for removing a categorical variable from the model.

There are more advanced procedures that figure out what levels of a categorical variable can be combined ahead of time. Other procedures come up with a scheme where indicator variables *can* be added one at a time by having $+1, 0, and -1$ represent subsets of levels, e.g., a $+1$ for levels A/B and -1 for C/D/E, or $+1$ for levels A/B, -1 for level C, and 0 for levels D/E.

For example, consider the BULLDOZER2 dataset. We want to predict the selling price of a bulldozer at an auction based on its model year, usage, tire and blade size, and when the auction occurred. The model year has been coded as a categorical variable called Decade. It has four levels: 1970s and before, 1980s, 1990s, and 2000s.

Let us use the naive model as the preliminary model. We see that adding in Decade yields the largest decrease in AIC, so its set of indicator variables gets added to the model first. Then, Tire gets added to the model, then YearsAgo.

In R

```
naive.model <- lm(Price~1,data=BULLDOZER2)
complex.model <- lm(Price~.,data=BULLDOZER2)
step(naive.model,scope=list(lower=naive.model,upper=complex.model),
    direction="both")

Start:  AIC=19287.05
Price ~ 1

              Df  Sum of Sq        RSS   AIC
+ Decade       3 5.6166e+11 5.0973e+11 18607
+ BladeSize    1 4.3395e+10 1.0280e+12 19251
+ Usage        1 1.0381e+10 1.0610e+12 19280
+ Tire         1 7.9299e+09 1.0635e+12 19282
+ YearsAgo     1 5.4009e+09 1.0660e+12 19284
<none>                      1.0714e+12 19287

Step:  AIC=18606.67
Price ~ Decade

              Df  Sum of Sq        RSS   AIC
+ Tire         1 2.3483e+10 4.8625e+11 18565
+ BladeSize    1 9.7981e+09 4.9993e+11 18591
+ YearsAgo     1 9.0895e+09 5.0064e+11 18592
<none>                      5.0973e+11 18607
+ Usage        1 1.0248e+09 5.0870e+11 18607
- Decade       3 5.6166e+11 1.0714e+12 19287

Step:  AIC=18565.09
Price ~ Decade + Tire

              Df  Sum of Sq        RSS   AIC
+ YearsAgo     1 1.0423e+10 4.7582e+11 18547
<none>                      4.8625e+11 18565
+ BladeSize    1 1.0513e+09 4.8520e+11 18565
+ Usage        1 5.3472e+07 4.8619e+11 18567
- Tire         1 2.3483e+10 5.0973e+11 18607
- Decade       3 5.7721e+11 1.0635e+12 19282

Step:  AIC=18547.07
Price ~ Decade + Tire + YearsAgo

              Df  Sum of Sq        RSS   AIC
<none>                      4.7582e+11 18547
+ Usage        1 7.8066e+08 4.7504e+11 18548
+ BladeSize    1 7.3369e+08 4.7509e+11 18548
- YearsAgo     1 1.0423e+10 4.8625e+11 18565
- Tire         1 2.4817e+10 5.0064e+11 18592
- Decade       3 5.8171e+11 1.0575e+12 19279
```

If the search procedure considers interactions between a categorical variable and another predictor variable, the same restrictions apply. The set of variables representing the interaction are considered all at once. Either all interaction terms are in the model or they are all excluded. Further, interactions can only be considered for addition to the model if the two individual components are already present. Similarly, a predictor variable cannot be eliminated from the model if it is involved in any interaction terms.

In R, the search procedures respect this restriction on categorical variables. In the "all possible" procedure, this restriction is ignored and model hierarchy is not preserved. Any "missing" indicator variables in the selected model represent levels that behave just like the reference level.

7.5 Building a descriptive logistic regression model

If y is a two-level categorical variable, we use logistic regression to predict the probability of the "level of interest" (the one that comes last alphabetically). Conveniently, model selection criterion and all search procedures operate identically to linear regression.

- The AIC of a logistic regression model equals the deviance (instead of the sum of squared errors) of the model plus two times the number of predictor variables.
- If the "all possible" procedure can be run, choose the model with the lowest AIC (or any model within 2 of the lowest value).
- If a search procedure is used, decrease the AIC of the model by either adding or removing a predictor until no further improvement can be made.

Unfortunately, since estimating the coefficients of a logistic regression model can be computationally intensive, performing the "all possible" procedure (even for a relatively small number of variables) may take too long (considering interactions in this procedure is out of the question), and even search procedures can be slow.

For example, let us consider the `PIMA` dataset, where we try to predict whether a woman has diabetes based on seven different physical characteristics. The naive model (predicting all women to not have diabetes, the majority level) has an AIC of 500 and a misclassification rate of 33.2%. Let us search for the model with the lowest AIC while considering interactions (this takes a while).

In R

```
naive.model <- glm(Diabetes~1,data=PIMA,family="binomial")
full.model <- glm(Diabetes~.^2,data=PIMA,family="binomial")
S <- step(full.model,scope=list(lower=naive.model,upper=full.model),
          direction="both")

Step:  AIC=360.25
Diabetes ~ Glucose + BloodPressure + BodyFat + Insulin + BMI +
    Age + Glucose:BloodPressure + Glucose:BodyFat + Glucose:BMI +
    Glucose:Age + BloodPressure:Insulin + BodyFat:Age + Insulin:Age +
    BMI:Age

confusion.matrix(S)
           Predicted No Predicted Yes Total
Actual No           233            29   262
Actual Yes           47            83   130
Total               280           112   392
```

Many interactions appear in the model with the lowest AIC. The AIC is 360.25, and the misclassification rate turns out to be (47+29)/392 = 19.4%. If we instead omit any consideration of interactions, the selected model has three predictors (Glucose, BMI, and Age). This simpler model has an AIC of 362.37 (slightly less preferable than the model with interactions since the difference in AICs is more than 2) and a misclassification rate of 20.4%.

Occasionally, you may find that a model with a higher AIC has a lower misclassification rate. This is not a contradiction. While we may be personally interested in the misclassification rate, this number (like R^2_{adj} in multiple linear regression) does not necessarily indicate the distance between the model and the "truth". The search procedure tries to minimize the AIC, not the misclassification rate.

7.6 Statistical significance and AIC

When a model is selected via AIC criterion, it is often the case that one or more predictors are not statistically significant. For instance, consider the BODYFAT model and the model with the lowest AIC.

```
                  Estimate Std. Error t value Pr(>|t|)
(Intercept)     -8.024e+01  7.264e+00 -11.046  < 2e-16 ***
Age             -6.053e-01  3.636e-01  -1.665   0.0972 .
Thigh            2.866e+00  3.066e-01   9.348  < 2e-16 ***
Forearm          2.753e-01  1.587e-01   1.735   0.0841 .
Age:Wrist        3.600e-02  1.989e-02   1.810   0.0716 .
Weight:Abdomen -1.016e-03  2.401e-04  -4.231  3.3e-05 ***
Wrist:Abdomen    5.463e-02  5.122e-03  10.666  < 2e-16 ***
Thigh:Wrist     -1.444e-01  1.551e-02  -9.308  < 2e-16 ***
```

Both the variable Forearm and the interaction between Age and Wrist are not statistically significant. Can we eliminate one (or both) of these predictors?

Previously, we said that we are justified in eliminating any one non-significant predictor (it does not significantly decrease the sum of squared errors when it is added to the model already containing the other predictors). However, we are *not* allowed to further modify the model with the lowest AIC, regardless of the significance of the variables.

Remember, our concern when building a descriptive model is to find the best one that models the *information* in the data, not the one that fits the data the best. Do not discard non-significant variables from the model chosen by AIC. Statistical significance is a comment on how well the model fits the data, not how close the model is to the truth.

7.7 Summary

In descriptive modeling, our goal is to model the information contained in the data rather than to model the data itself. The AIC measures the amount of information lost when a given model is used to describe reality. After considering many models, we pick one with a relatively small

AIC. For all intents and purposes, models whose AICs differ by no more than 2 are essentially equivalent, so any model whose AIC is within 2 of the lowest value is acceptable.

Ideally, the "all possible" procedure will be performed, but for a large number of variables this may not be practical. Technically, all interactions and transformations should be considered as well, though this is rarely done.

Instead, search procedures are conducted. The search starts out with some proposed model (usually one with either no predictors or all the predictors in it) and then changes the model in steps. Each step either adds or removes a variable, whichever leads to the largest improvement in AIC. The procedure stops when the model can no longer be improved.

The search procedure may not find the model with the absolute lowest AIC, but it should find a model that is "close" to the optimal model. In many cases, the selected model will have an AIC within 2 of the lowest possible AIC.

Interactions sometimes have special rules when it comes to adding or deleting them from a model. If model hierarchy is preserved, an interaction can only be added to a model if both of its component variables are already in it, while individual variables cannot be removed from the model if it is involved in an interaction.

Categorical variables require special consideration as well. Typically, the set of indicator variables that represent a categorical variable is considered all at once, meaning that either all indicator variables representing a categorical variable are in the model or all of them are excluded.

Descriptive modeling is challenging from a philosophical point of view because we know *a priori* that all models are wrong. The real world is very complex, and it's extremely unlikely that you have collected all the variables that matter or know what correct transformations and/or interactions to incorporate.

We now move on to predictive modeling, which does not pose any of these philosophical problems. As long as the model "works," i.e., makes accurate predictions, we do not care if the model is close to reality. We can pick one among many similarly performing good models.

7.8 Descriptive Modeling in R

There are a variety of tools for choosing a model with a relatively low AIC in R.

All possible procedure

To fit "all possible" linear regression models, use the function `regsubsets` in the package `leaps`. The first argument should be a formula giving the "full" model, i.e., the most complicated model under consideration. Usually, the formulation is `y ~ .` (all predictors, no interactions) or `y ~ .^2` (all predictors, all two-way interactions).

In R

```
MODELS <- regsubsets(y~.^2,data=DATA,method="exhaustive")
see.models(MODELS)
```

- `regsubsets` has optional additional arguments like `nbest` (the number of "best" models at each number of predictors to keep around), `nvmax` (the maximum number of variables to consider in any particular model), `force.in` and `force.out` (which, respectively, specify the variables that *must* be included and *must not* be included in any model), and `method` (which is typically taken to be `exhaustive` but it can be turned into a search procedure with `seqrep`).

- `see.models` in package `regclass` prints out a list of the models with the lowest AICs. It has optional arguments `report` (a number that controls how many models it reports, regardless of how far their AIC is from the lowest value) and `aicc` (which makes the models be sorted by AICc instead of AIC).

Another command in `regclass` that will perform the "all possible" procedure is `build.model` with argument `type="descriptive"`. More details are presented in the following chapter, but this remains the easiest way to perform the "all possible" procedure when y is categorical.

Note: none of the "all possible" procedures respect model hierarchy.

Search procedure

The `step` command performs searches for both linear and logistic regression models. To set this command up, you need to define your initial model (usually the naive or full model), simplest model to be considered (usually the naive model), and most complex model to be considered (usually the full model, with or without interactions). The output at each step is reported by default, and this is usually too much information. To turn that off, use `trace=0`.

In R

```
initial.model <- lm(y~x1+x2,data=DATA)
naive.model <- lm(y~1,data=DATA)
full.model <- lm(y~.^2,data=DATA)
S <- step(initial.model,scope=list(lower=naive.model,upper=full.model),
     direction="both",trace=0)
```

Note: the search procedure does respect model hierarchy.

7.9 Exercises

1: Use `EX7.BIKE`, which is the DC bike demand dataset. The data has been "cleaned" so you do not need to eliminate any rows. Let us build the best descriptive model so that we can compare the average demands between days with particular characteristics.

a) In total, there are 4 quantitative predictors, 3 categorical predictors with 2 levels, and 1 categorical variable with 7 levels. If we run the "all possible" procedure (which ignores hierarchy) without interactions, how many models will be generated?
b) Run `regsubsets()` and `see.models()` to come up with a set of models with "low" AICs (do not put anything for `nvmax` or `nbest` arguments). Do not consider interactions.
   1) What predictors are in the model with the lowest AIC?
   2) How many other models are "equivalent" to the one with the lowest AICc?
   3) In the model with the lowest AIC, you see that the day of the week is in the model, but it is only represented by the indicator variable `DaySunday` (no other indicator variables for `Day` appear). What is the implication? In other words, which days are being treated together and which are being treated separately?

c) Interactions may be important to incorporate into the model, but running `regsubsets()` with interactions would take too much time (k would be 77). Instead, we will run `step()` to search for a model. In `step()`, let's use `direction="both"` so that the procedure is free to add or remove terms from the model as needed. Remember the "full" model in this case includes all two-way interactions, so use `Demand~.^2`!
   1) Use the naive model as the initial model. What predictors are in the selected model and what is the AIC of the model (obtained by using `AIC()`)?
   2) Use the full model as the initial model and consider `direction="both"`. Is the selected model the same as the one above? If not, what is the AIC of this model, and is it "closer to the truth" than the above model?

d) Imagine the goal is to answer: What is the difference in average demands between days that rain and days that don't (column `Weather`)? Based on the "best" model fit so far, is there a simple answer (e.g., 500 bikes) to this question, or is the answer more complex (e.g., the difference depends on the windspeed and specific day of the week, etc.)? If the answer is more complex, be as specific as possible as to what other quantities must be known for us to be able to compare the difference in average demands.

2: Use `EX7.CATALOG`. We want to build a descriptive model that answers the question: "Is the probability of buying an item from a catalog (`Buy`) higher for people who have received more catalogs (`CatalogsReceived`)*a priori* Use `build.model()` to build the best descriptive model (no interactions), then answer the question. For extra practice, use a search procedure to find an even better model using `step`. However, the selected model may include `CatalogsReceived` in an interaction. Thus, the question would have no easy answer since the probability may be higher or lower depending on the other characteristics (whatever is involved in the interaction with `CatalogsReceived`) of the individuals.

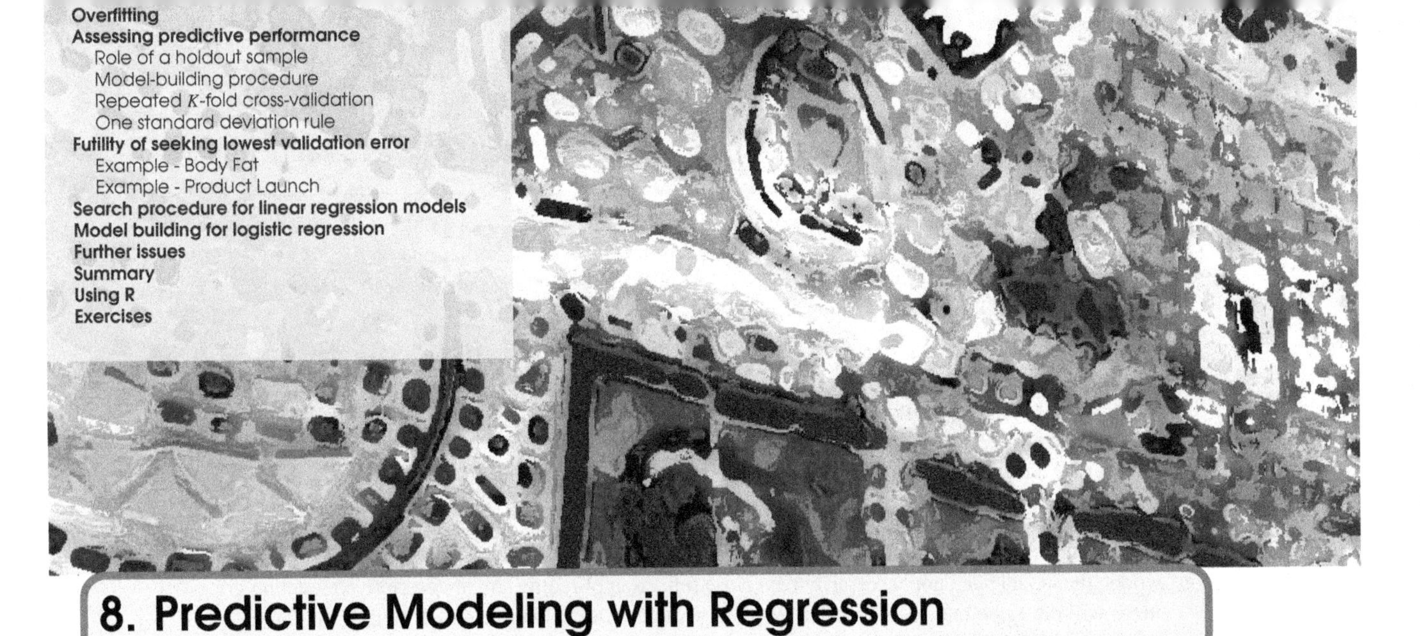

8. Predictive Modeling with Regression

Throughout the book so far, we have mainly concerned ourselves with *describing* the relationships between variables with measures of association or with regression models. The overall goal of a descriptive model is to determine the "right" set of variables to predict y and to estimate coefficients with as much precision as possible. In many arenas, the actual values of the coefficients are unimportant. What is important is the quality of the model's *predictions*.

For example, the US government is required every 10 years to conduct the census. Forms are mailed to each household and must be completed and returned by law. To collect responses from households that do not mail in forms, workers must go door-to-door and manually interview people. To intelligently allocate workers, it would be useful to predict the response rates of each "block group."

A block group is on average about 40 blocks, each typically bounded by streets, roads, or water in cities and sometimes other features in rural areas. The number of block groups per county in the US is typically between 5 and 165 with a median of about 20.

Finding the most precise estimates of coefficients of the predictor variables (demographic information such as a block group's racial, gender, and age makeup, income level, house values, etc.) is of secondary importance to having the model make accurate predictions for the next census.

Further, consider trying to model a consumer's reaction to an emailed promotion (perhaps a $10 off coupon if they spend $40 or more). While it is "nice" to know whether the probability of purchasing increases or decreases with predictor variables such as the yearly income of the family, number of kids and pets in the family, etc., the critical performance metric is the false negative rate (the fraction of consumers the model predicts would not respond but who in reality would have responded had they been given the offer).

Developing a regression equation requires a different approach when the goal is *predictive* rather than *descriptive* modeling.

We do not care how well a predictive model fits the data on hand (we already know the answers for this set of individuals), but rather how well it makes predictions on data *it has not seen before*. In other words, we measure the utility of a predictive model by how well it *generalizes* to new data.

The "all possible" and search procedures for generating potential models (the candidate set) are unchanged in a predictive modeling context. Rather, the criterion for what makes a good model is different. Instead of a low AIC, a small generalization error is valued.

In this chapter, we will discuss the challenges of predictive modeling and the techniques designed to find a good predictive model. At its core, a predictive model is like a "hack" job—as long as it works, the model need not necessarily be a close reflection of reality. As in descriptive modeling, there will rarely be one "best" model. Typically, there will be a *multitude* of models that have more or less the same prediction accuracy, with no solid justification for picking one over the other. Although it sounds a bit fatalistic, the strategy will be to pick one of the seemingly good models and hope for the best.

8.1 Overfitting

Surprisingly, one of the biggest dangers in predictive modeling is putting too *much* information into the model! This phenomenon is called **overfitting**, and it occurs when the model fits the collected data well but predicts poorly on new data.

Why does this happen? Every dataset has its own set of quirks. These peculiarities become "burned in" to a model when a set of variables and their coefficients are chosen. Since these quirks are unlikely to appear in new data, the model's predictions will be biased and inaccurate. In essence, if the model "memorizes" the data and does not generalize well to new cases, it is said to be *overfit*.

For a practical illustration of overfitting, consider two strategies for studying for this year's final exam. One is to review only your notes and the book so that you have a broad understanding of the major topics. Another way is to acquire a copy of last year's exam, only making sure you know the answers to every question on it.

The former technique has the disadvantage of missing out on easy points if the instructor recycles many questions. The latter technique has the disadvantage that your knowledge may be too specific and narrow to answer new questions if this year's exam is very different.

If you choose to only study from last year's exam, you run the risk of "overfitting." You memorize the quirks on the data on hand (last semester's exam), and this may leave you unable to generalize to genuinely new data (this year's exam).

Generally, overfitting occurs when there are too many predictors in the model (i.e., it is overly complex). Adding an additional predictor always decreases the model's sum of squared errors with regard to the data on which it is being built (it may also decrease the *RMSE* and *AIC* as well). However, it could be the case that this decrease is due to the model now doing a better job of fitting some quirk that as-yet-unobserved individuals will not have. Adding an additional variable to a model may cause predictions on new data to become worse.

For example, consider the `LAUNCH` dataset. In this data, the total sales of items over the first four weeks after their release are recorded along with nearly 400 (anonymized) predictor variables (e.g., amount advertising on the Internet, number of stores carrying the item, etc.). For illustration, let us consider only the first 14 predictors in the data along with all two-way interactions. The model with the lowest AIC (i.e., the model "closest" to the process that generated the data) may not necessarily be the model that predicts new cases with the most accuracy.

Figure 8.1 shows the AIC of the model during each step of a search procedure on a random sample of 150 cases. The AIC continually decreases as new variables are added to the model. However, the typical prediction error on a previously unseen set of 150 cases (referred to as $RMSE_{holdout}$) begins to increase after six variables are added to the model. Beyond eight or nine predictors, the model is overfit. Additional predictors make the model memorize quirks that are particular to the data being used to build the model and that are not present in the new data.

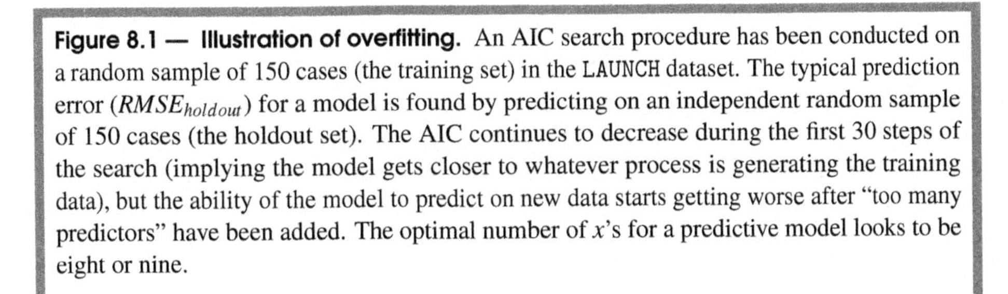

Figure 8.1 — Illustration of overfitting. An AIC search procedure has been conducted on a random sample of 150 cases (the training set) in the `LAUNCH` dataset. The typical prediction error ($RMSE_{holdout}$) for a model is found by predicting on an independent random sample of 150 cases (the holdout set). The AIC continues to decrease during the first 30 steps of the search (implying the model gets closer to whatever process is generating the training data), but the ability of the model to predict on new data starts getting worse after "too many predictors" have been added. The optimal number of x's for a predictive model looks to be eight or nine.

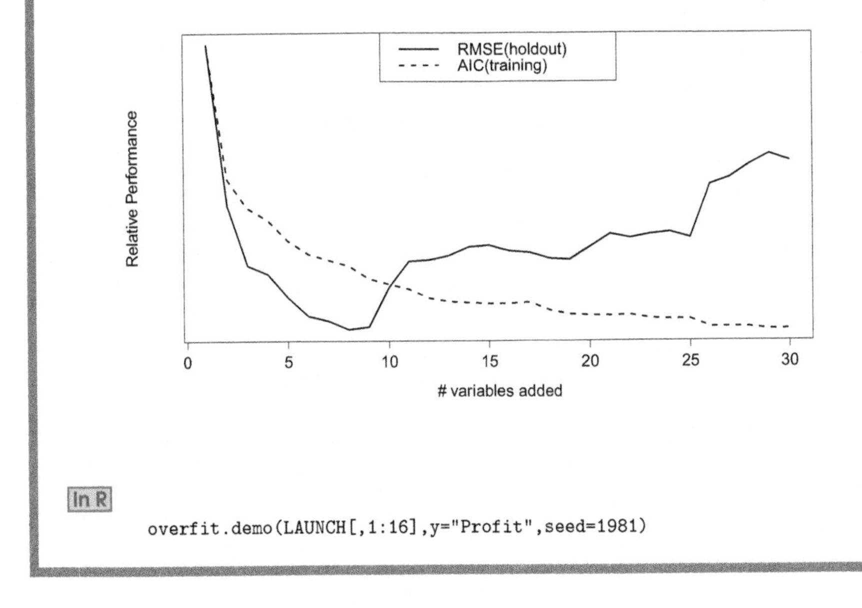

In R

```
overfit.demo(LAUNCH[,1:16],y="Profit",seed=1981)
```

8.2 Assessing predictive performance

The **generalization error** of a model is the typical prediction error it makes on "new data," i.e., data that was not used to build or tune the model. The model that has the smallest generalization error possible is desired.

8.2.1 Estimating generalization error using a holdout sample

Unfortunately, calculating the "real" generalization error is an impossible feat since there are an infinite number of new observations that could *potentially* be collected. However, this error can be *estimated* in one of two ways.

- Wait for new data to arrive and calculate the typical error on this new sample.
- Split the original data into two parts: a **training** and a **holdout** sample. Fit a model using the training data and make predictions on the holdout sample. The typical error on the holdout is a reasonable estimate of the model's generalization error.

$$\text{Generalization Error} = \sqrt{\frac{1}{n_{holdout}} \times \sum_{\text{holdout data}} (Observed - Predicted)^2} \tag{8.1}$$

$$\text{Generalization Error} = RMSE_{holdout}$$

The generalization error on a particular holdout sample will most likely be different from the typical error on a set of genuinely new data or the typical error on some other holdout sample (if the original data is split a different way). The generalization error on a holdout sample is *truly* just an estimate. As we will see, the model with the lowest estimated generalization error in a candidate set is usually *not* the one that ends up predicting the best on new data.

8.2.2 Model-building procedure

How can we develop a model that minimizes generalization error when the model does not have access to the holdout sample? The answer is to reserve a chunk of the training sample to serve as a mock holdout sample. This is referred to as the **validation** sample. See Figure 8.2.

Figure 8.2 — Division into training, validation, and holdout samples. To build a predictive model, the data is split into a training sample (left box) and holdout sample (right box). Part of the training sample is then reserved for validation. Many models are built using the training data, each of which makes predictions on the validation sample. The model with the lowest error on the validation sample is selected, and its predictions on the holdout sample are recorded. If the error on the holdout sample is no more than about 10-20% larger than the error on the validation set, we can say the model generalizes well.

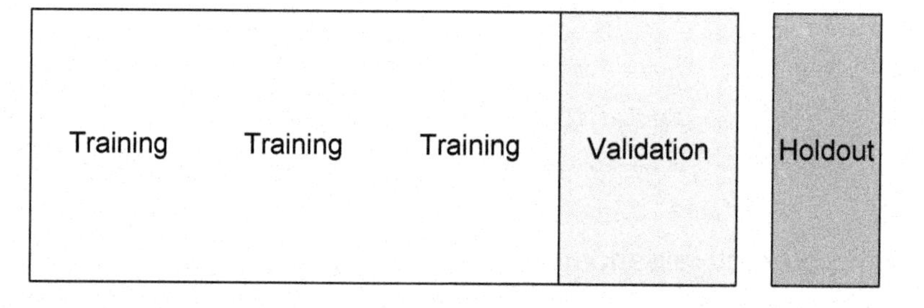

A model-building strategy that should proceed a model that generalizes well to new data is as follows:

- Randomly split the data into training and holdout samples.
- Randomly reserve part of the training data to serve as a validation sample.
- Fit a multitude of different models in the candidate set using the training data and make predictions on the validation sample. The typical prediction error on the validation sample, $RMSE_{validation}$, is defined similarly to Equation 8.1.
- Pick the model whose error on the validation sample is the lowest, then make predictions on the holdout sample.
- If the typical error on the holdout sample is about the same size (no more than about 10-20% larger) as the error on the validation sample, we can say the model generalizes well.

A typical split of the original data is 60/20/20. This means that out of every 100 observations in the original dataset, 80 are reserved for training (20 of which are set aside for validation, with 60 being used to build the model), and 20 are reserved for the holdout.

Having a larger validation sample typically gives you a more accurate idea of the generalization error at the cost of having less precision regarding the coefficients. Having a smaller validation sample yields more precise estimates of coefficients at the cost of underestimating the generalization error.

There is an additional consideration regarding splitting the data that is important for logistic regression models. It is best that all three subsamples have the proportions of each level of y be about the same. Intelligent construction of the subsamples can "stratify" them in such a way that they meet this condition. With random splits (the kinds used in this book), the proportions of each level will be close, but not necessarily equal, to the frequency in which they appear in overall data.

8.2.3 Repeated K-fold cross-validation

The estimated generalization error, $RMSE_{validation}$, found on the validation sample can be quite sensitive to the particular set of individuals who happened to be contained in it. To minimize this sensitivity, **K-fold cross-validation** is used.

In K-fold cross-validation, the training data is randomly split up into K equally sized chunks. See Figure 8.3.

In round one of the procedure, the last chunk is used as the validation set, and the coefficients of the model are estimated using the remaining training data. Let us call the error on this validation sample $RMSE_{validation1}$. In round two of the procedure, the second-to-last chunk is reserved as the validation sample, and the coefficients are estimated using the remaining training data. Let us call the error on this validation sample $RMSE_{validation2}$.

The procedure continues until each chunk serves as the validation set once. For the model in question, the "typical" error on the validation sample is taken to be the average of the K errors.

$$RMSE_{Kfold} = \frac{1}{K}(RMSE_{validation1} + RMSE_{validation2} + \ldots + RMSE_{validationK}) \quad (8.2)$$

The value of K is a choice. The value $RMSE_{Kfold}$ tends to underestimate the true generalization error when K is smaller, but the computational time is shorter. When K is larger, computing takes longer, but $RMSE_{Kfold}$ better estimates the true generalization error. Typically, $K = 5$ or 10. For small datasets, K may need to be even larger (so that coefficients are estimated on as much data as possible), and for large datasets, K can be even as low as 3.

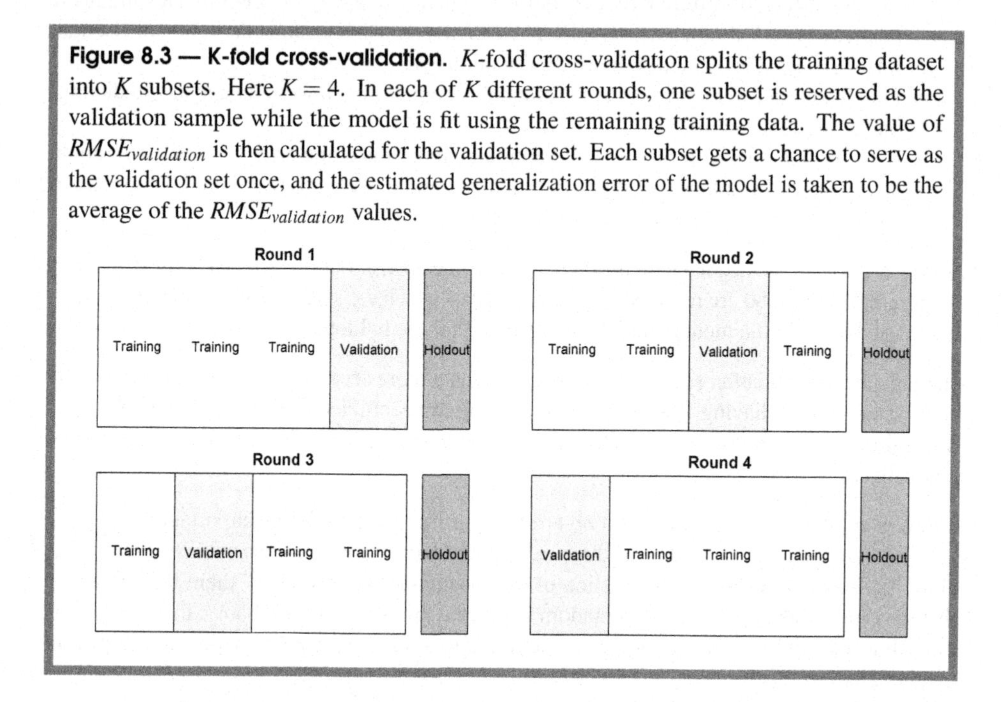

Figure 8.3 — K-fold cross-validation. K-fold cross-validation splits the training dataset into K subsets. Here $K = 4$. In each of K different rounds, one subset is reserved as the validation sample while the model is fit using the remaining training data. The value of $RMSE_{validation}$ is then calculated for the validation set. Each subset gets a chance to serve as the validation set once, and the estimated generalization error of the model is taken to be the average of the $RMSE_{validation}$ values.

One issue with K-fold cross-validation is that the validation error, $RMSE_{Kfold}$, is *still* somewhat sensitive to how the K-folds were randomly assigned. **Repeated K-fold cross-validation** somewhat alleviates this sensitivity by randomly reassigning the folds and repeating the procedure a number of times. Typically, a total of 10 repeats are performed, and the final estimate of a model's generalization error is the average of the estimates from each K-fold cross-validation.

$$RMSE_{repeatedKfold} = \frac{1}{10}\left(RMSE_{Kfold1} + \ldots + RMSE_{Kfold10}\right) \tag{8.3}$$

One special case worth mentioning is when $K = n_{train}$, the number of cases in the training sample. For each of the n_{train} rounds, only a single case serves as the validation sample. This is referred to as **leave-one-out** cross-validation. Remarkably, $RMSE_{LOO}$ (the estimated generalization error from leave-one-out cross-validation) can be computed from the model using the *entirety* of the training dataset (i.e., it is not necessary to actually fit each individual model). The value $RMSE_{LOO}$ is often referred to as the **predicted residual sum of squares**, or **PRESS**.

8.2.4 One standard deviation rule

In descriptive modeling, models with AICs within 2 of each other were, for all intents and purposes, equivalent—there are no statistical reasons to prefer one over the other. Likewise, models whose estimated generalization errors are "close" to each other predict similarly enough that there is little reason to choose one instead of the other. How close do the errors need to be for two models to be considered equivalent?

When we perform repeated K-fold cross validation, we get 10 estimates for the validation error ($RMSE_{Kfold1}, \ldots, RMSE_{Kfold10}$). Their average serves as the final value of the validation error, while their standard deviation gives an idea for its uncertainty.

The **one standard deviation rule** says that two models with validation errors within one standard deviation of each other are essentially equivalent. There is no solid reason for preferring one over the other. Thus, pick the *simplest* model whose error is at most one standard deviation above the smallest error.

For example, imagine we are comparing three models. Their values of $RMSE_{Kfold}$ are:

repeat:	1	2	3	4	5	6	7	8	9	10	Avg	SD
Model 1	4.8	4.7	4.8	4.7	4.2	4.1	4.8	4.1	4	4.4	4.46	0.33
Model 2	4.9	4.7	4.4	4.9	4.5	4.6	4.7	4.1	4.4	4.6	4.58	0.24
Model 3	5.4	5.2	5.5	4.6	4.6	5.4	5.1	5.1	5.2	4.6	5.07	0.35

Model 1 has the lowest validation error at 4.46. However, the standard deviation of the estimates is 0.33. Thus, any model with an error of $(4.46+0.33) = 4.76$ or less has essentially the same validation error. Model 2 is in this range, but Model 3 is not. Thus, we could pick either Model 1 or Model 2 as the final predictive model. If these models differed in complexity or in the number of variables, we would pick the simpler one.

8.3 Finding the model with the lowest validation error is unnecessary

Before diving into examples of predictive model building, let us study some properties of how the process works—how well do we expect the selected model to perform? In other words, will the model that we select really predict the best of all the models in the candidate set on new data?

For consistency, models in this section will be compared to each other by their validation error calculated from repeated K-fold cross-validation. We will take $K = 5$ and perform 10 repeats.

Ideally, all 2^k possible models are considered (as in Section 7.3.1), and the one with the smallest validation error is selected. Unfortunately, repeated K-fold cross-validation can be extremely time-intensive. Search procedures, which add or subtract a variable from the model one at a time, can be used to save time.

8.3.1 Example - Body Fat

The `BODYFAT` dataset has a total of 252 cases with 13 predictors. Let us randomly choose 200 to be the training sample and 52 to be the holdout sample. With no interactions, an "all possible" procedure requires looking at $2^{13} \approx 8000$ models. While finding the AICs of these models is an easy task in a descriptive modeling context, the computational time for repeated K-fold cross-validation is large.

Figure 8.4 — All possible models applied to the BODYFAT dataset. The generalization error (as estimated via repeated K-fold cross-validation) for each model is plotted against the number of variables it contains. Only the 30 top-performing models are plotted at each number of variables to keep the graph from being cluttered.

The dotted horizontal line represents the lowest validation error seen over all the models, and the solid line connects the models with the lowest errors for a given number of predictors. The "best" model has eight variables, but there are many other models that perform comparably. Overfitting is apparent when the error starts to increase and too many variables are added.

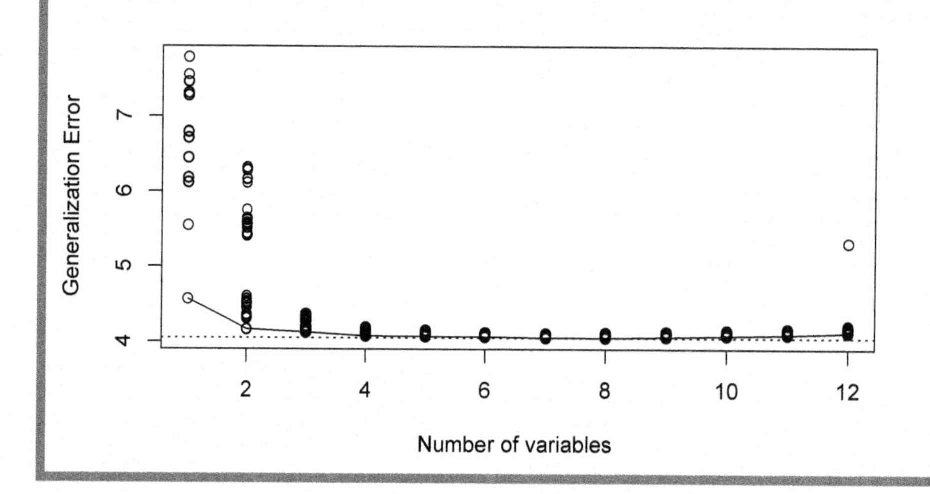

Figure 8.4 shows the validation error for each model vs. its number of variables. As with many datasets, there are a multitude of models (containing anywhere between 6 and 10 predictors) that are comparable in terms of their performance. In fact, there are dozens of models that are essentially indistinguishable from each other according to the one standard deviation rule. Any of them make a fine choice.

The model with the overall smallest validation error has eight variables. However, since this error is just an *estimate* of its true generalization error, we cannot *guarantee* this model will be the one that performs the best on genuinely new data. In fact, when we use this model to make predictions on the holdout sample, it actually ranks 137th in predictive accuracy out of the 326 models considered. See Figure 8.5. Note: it could be the case that on a different holdout sample the model would end up predicting the best.

Based on all the data available to the model (the training set), our sophisticated model-building algorithm ends up selecting a model that predicts "just alright." There is really no way to tell in advance what model will end up generalizing best to new data we collect, so we just choose one of the multitude of good models and hope for the best.

Although the selected model is not the best, its performance is still pretty good. Its error is only 3% higher than the best-performing model on the holdout sample. Further, it does generalize well since the error on the holdout sample is no more than 10-20% above the validation error.

Figure 8.5 — Estimated vs. actual generalization errors for BODYFAT. For each model in a candidate set, the estimated generalization error from repeated K-fold cross-validation is plotted vs. the actual generalization error on the holdout sample. The diagonal line is when both quantities are equal. The models with the smallest values of the validation error (to the left of the plot) underestimate the generalization error on the holdout sample by about 5%, i.e., the models' estimates are overconfident.

The best-performing model as gauged from repeated K-fold cross-validation is the point on the very far left. There are over 100 other models that perform better on the holdout sample since their generalization errors are lower. It is typical that the model with the lowest validation error performs worse on the holdout sample than other models.

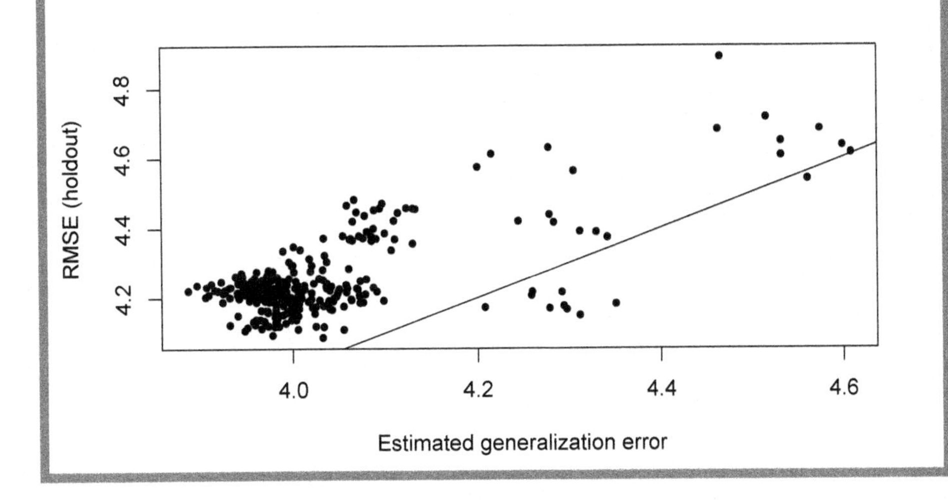

8.3.2 Example - Product Launch

The `LAUNCH` data has a total of 652 cases with over 400 predictor variables. The goal is to predict the profit of a newly released product four months after its release. Since an "all possible" procedure is infeasible, in this example we consider only the first 15 predictors in the data. Figure 8.6 shows the validation errors (as gauged by repeated K-fold cross-validation) of many candidate models vs. their number of predictors.

The behavior of the validation error versus the model's complexity is similar to what we saw in the `BODYFAT` dataset. The error quickly decreases as the first few variables are added to the model, then the validation error plateaus, then begins to slightly increase as too many variables are added and the model becomes overfit.

The model with the lowest validation error has nine predictors ($RMSE_{validation} = 0.280$), but there are dozens of equivalent models according to the one standard deviation rule. In fact, the difference in validation errors between the "best" performing model and the "100th best" is less than 0.003 (about 0.6%).

When the selected model makes predictions on the holdout sample, it ranks 175th out of 249 nearly equivalent models according to the one standard deviation rule. As with the `BODYFAT` example, the model selected using the training set is the one that "lucked out" during repeated

K-fold cross-validation and does not actually generalize the best (but we had no way to choose the one that did).

However, this model is still useful. The lowest $RMSE_{holdout}$ is observed to be 0.302, while the selected model has $RMSE_{holdout} = 0.315$, a difference of less than 5%. The model's generalization performance is adequate since the percentage increase in error from the validation to holdout sample is $(0.315 - 0.280)/0.280 = 12.5\%$.

Figure 8.6 — "all possible" procedure applied to the LAUNCH dataset. The estimated generalization error (as gauged by repeated K-fold cross-validation) for each model is plotted against the number of variables contained in the model. To reduce clutter, only the 20 best-performing models at each number of predictors is shown. The dotted horizontal line represents the lowest error across all models, and the solid line connects the models with the lowest errors for a given number of predictors. A model with nine variables has the lowest error overall, but dozens of other models are equivalent according to the one standard deviation rule. There is a hint that overfitting begins to occur after about 12 variables are in the model.

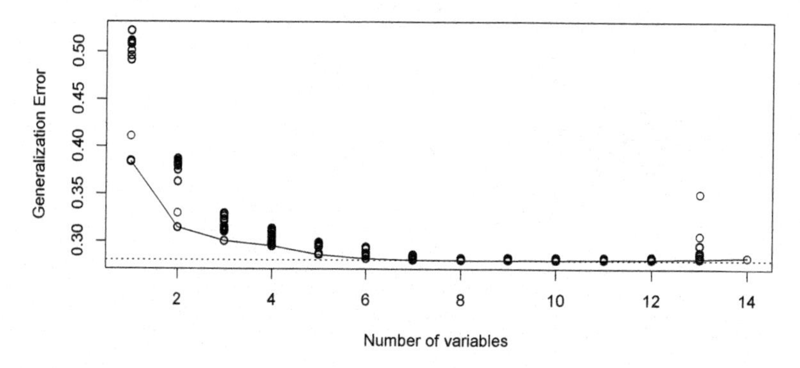

The estimated generalization error from repeated K-fold cross-validation is now plotted vs. the actual generalization error on the holdout sample. The diagonal line represents when both quantities are equal. For the best-performing models (far left; smallest estimated generalization errors), the actual value of $RMSE_{holdout}$ is noticeably larger than $RMSE_{validation}$, but only by at most about 15%. The best-performing model from the "all possible" procedure (far left point) has a larger generalization error than other similarly performing models on the holdout, but not by much. Again, this is typical.

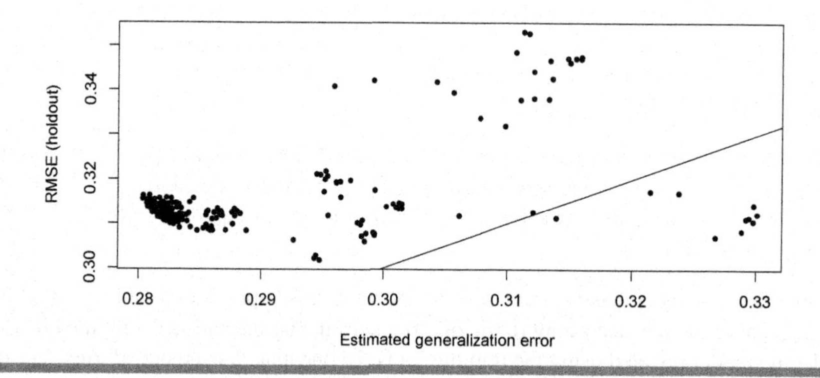

8.4 Search procedure for linear regression models

There are often a multitude of models that have essentially the same validation error (according to the one standard deviation rule) and that have comparable generalization errors on the holdout sample. Since the model with the *lowest* validation error is just one of many acceptable models, there is really no need to run the "all possible" procedure to find it. Besides, it rarely performs the best on the holdout sample anyway. This is good news, since the "all possible" procedure is extremely computationally intensive.

Instead, let us conduct a search for a good model in the same vein as we did for building a descriptive model (Section 7.3.2). Once again, the validation error will be measured via repeated K-fold cross-validation ($K = 5$ and 10 repeats).

- Given the current model, calculate the validation errors of the models obtained by adding/removing a single predictor.
- Augment the model by whichever move yields the smallest validation error.
- Continue until the model no longer improves.

The search procedure does not guarantee finding the model with the *lowest* possible validation error. It does not even necessarily find a model with a smaller validation error than a model that minimizes the AIC. Nevertheless, the model found by the search procedure is usually adequate.

In the following examples, the initial model will be the full model with no interactions and the search will only remove variables from the model. Although later adding in a predictor that had previously been removed can sometimes improve the model, the computational time saved by never considering such an option is significant.

Example - census

The CENSUS data contains 38 potential predictors (an "all possible" approach is out of the question for this large a problem). Let us randomly assign 20% of the data to be the holdout sample and take the training sample to be the remaining cases. Figure 8.7 shows the validation error vs. the number of predictors in the model for models considered during a search.

The model with the lowest validation error has 29 predictors. The one standard deviation rule says that all models whose errors are within one standard deviation of the smallest error are essentially equivalent. Consequently, we can choose a model with only eight predictors.

In R

```
set.seed(1337)
selected <- sample(nrow(CENSUS),round(0.80*nrow(CENSUS)))
TRAIN <- CENSUS[selected,]
HOLDOUT <- CENSUS[-selected,]
MODELS <- build.model(ResponseRate~.,data=TRAIN,method="backward")
MODELS$CVtable
  NumPred EstGenError   SD
   4       26.47 1.08
   5       25.11 1.16
   6       24.56 1.04
   7       24.20 0.85
+  8       23.95 0.94 <- simplest (CV error within one SD of lowest)
   9       23.78 0.98
.....
   28       22.97 1.05
*  29       22.94 1.03 <- lowest CV error
   30       22.97 1.15
```

The selected model contains information about the age and racial makeup of the block group as well as what type of households it contains.

In R

```
summary(MODELS$bestmodel)
                      Estimate Std. Error t value Pr(>|t|)
(Intercept)          6.531e+01  1.328e+00  49.189  < 2e-16 ***
Age65plus            2.021e-01  1.653e-02  12.223  < 2e-16 ***
Whites               4.075e-02  5.098e-03   7.993 1.90e-15 ***
RelatedHH           -2.301e-01  2.128e-02 -10.812  < 2e-16 ***
MarriedHH            4.404e-01  2.674e-02  16.469  < 2e-16 ***
NoSpouseHH           2.161e-01  1.753e-02  12.332  < 2e-16 ***
MedianHHIncomeCity -2.368e-05  4.908e-06  -4.825 1.47e-06 ***
RentingHH           -1.705e-01  9.150e-03 -18.635  < 2e-16 ***
MobileHomeUnits     -7.057e-02  8.612e-03  -8.194 3.80e-16 ***
```

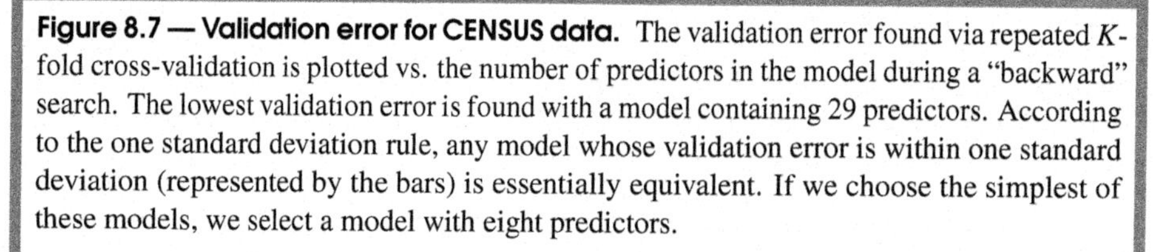

Figure 8.7 — Validation error for CENSUS data. The validation error found via repeated K-fold cross-validation is plotted vs. the number of predictors in the model during a "backward" search. The lowest validation error is found with a model containing 29 predictors. According to the one standard deviation rule, any model whose validation error is within one standard deviation (represented by the bars) is essentially equivalent. If we choose the simplest of these models, we select a model with eight predictors.

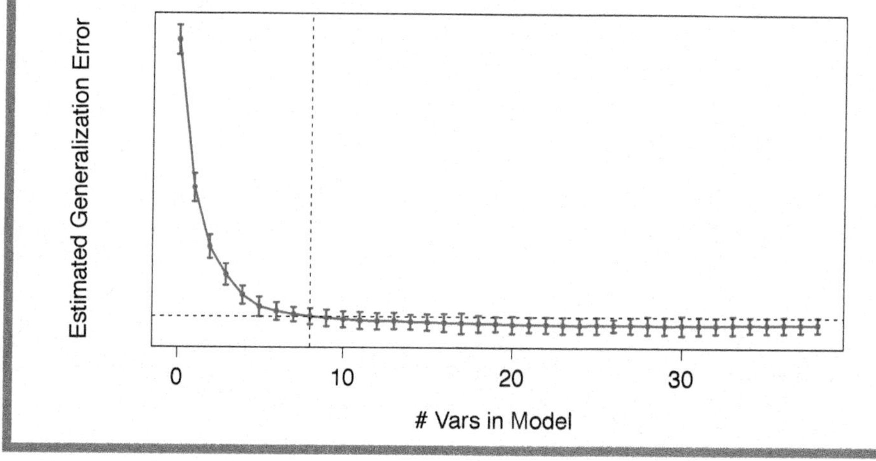

It is interesting to see how well this model predicts on the holdout sample compared to other models. For the AIC search, we begin at the full model and do not allow for the possibility of interactions. Below is a table of the generalization errors for *this particular holdout sample.*

In R

```
M.naive <- lm(ResponseRate~1,data=TRAIN)
M.cv <- lm(MODELS$bestformula,data=TRAIN)
M.full <- lm(ResponseRate~.,data=TRAIN)
M.fullint <- lm(ResponseRate~.^2,data=TRAIN)
M.aic <- step(M.full,scope=list(lower=M.naive,upper=M.full),trace=0)
generalization.error(M.cv,HOLDOUT)
```

Method	$RMSE_{train}$	$RMSE_{holdout}$
Naive	7.52	7.42
Crossvalidation	4.88	5.03
Full Model (no interaction)	4.72	4.93
Full Model (all interactions)	3.71	5.85
AIC search	4.73	4.94

The naive model represents the "no model" scenario where we predict the response rate to be the overall average. The error of the selected model is much lower (at 5.03 vs. 7.42), so it represents a vast improvement. Interestingly, the errors of the full model with no interactions and the model found via AIC search are lower than the selected model, but by no more than 2%. The full model with all two-way interactions is overfit and has an error much larger than the selected model.

If we try a different training/holdout split, the full model has a lower error than the selected model nearly 98% of the time. This is consistent with our model-building analysis. The full model does have a validation error within one standard deviation of the lowest value, so it too is considered acceptable. However, we err on the side of simplicity and choose simpler models when possible. These may not always perform the best, but we do guard ourselves against overfitting.

8.5 Model building for logistic regression

When building a predictive logistic regression model, the criterion for what makes a "good" model is not as well-defined as it is with linear regression. Should we be comparing misclassification rates (i.e., accuracies), false positive rates, or false negative rates? In general, the answer to this question is context specific.

- Goal: predict whether someone has a rare and fatal disease. Criterion: low rate of false negatives (person has the disease but model says the person does not).
- Goal: predict whether someone would be interested in a product. Criterion: low rate of false negatives (person would be interested but model says the person is not).
- Goal: predict whether an email is safe of junk. Criterion: low rate of false positives (email is safe but model says it is junk).
- Goal: predict whether a handwritten letter is an "r" or an "n." Criterion: low misclassification rate (each error is equally undesirable).

For example, let us consider the `PIMA` dataset. The goal is to predict whether a woman has diabetes. Let us use the **accuracy** as the criterion for evaluating a model.

The accuracy is the percentage of observations predicted correctly. The misclassification rate is the percentage of observations predicted incorrectly. The accuracy and misclassification rate add up to 100%.

Figure 8.8 shows the estimated generalization accuracy (by repeated K-fold cross-validation) vs. the number of predictors in the model. The figure also displays the estimated accuracy vs. the accuracy achieved on the holdout sample. The selected model has `Glucose`, `BloodPressure`, `BodyFat`, and `Age` as predictors. As we have seen before, the selected model (highest estimated accuracy) is not the one that actually performs the best on the holdout sample.

Figure 8.8 — Accuracy of predictive models for PIMA diabetes. The top panel shows the validation accuracy (gauged from repeated K-fold cross-validation) for the best-performing models for each number of predictors. The dotted horizontal line represents the highest accuracy seen over all models, and the solid line connects the models with the highest accuracy for that number of predictors. The "best" model found has four variables, but there are many other models that perform comparably. With only 60 observations in a validation fold, many models differ in the number of correct predictions by only one or two.

In the bottom panel, the validation accuracy is plotted vs. the actual accuracy on a holdout sample. The diagonal line represents when both quantities are equal. Many of the models with the highest estimated accuracy (points on right) are overly optimistic—the actual accuracy on the holdout is lower. The selected model (highest estimated accuracy; point farthest to the right) has a lower accuracy on the holdout sample than other similarly performing models, but not by much. These results are typical.

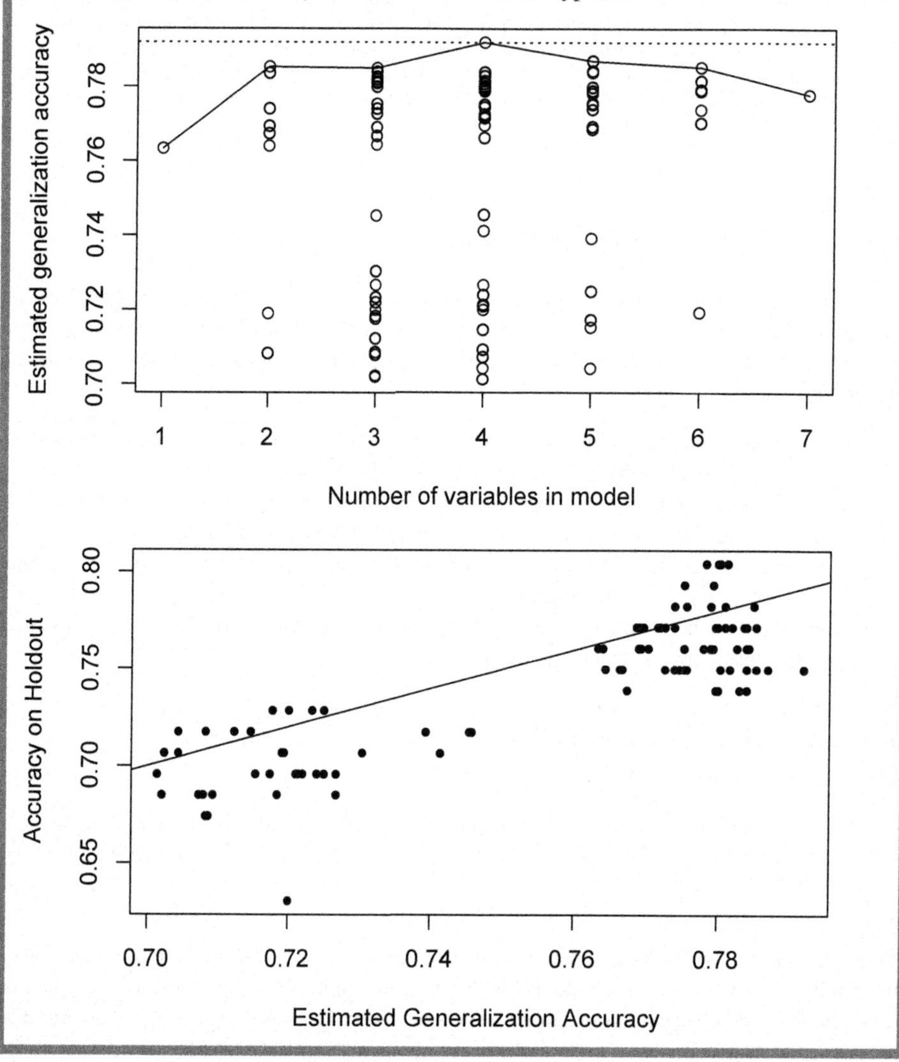

The "all possible" approach is not advised except when the dataset is small. The amount of time required to fit a logistic regression (much longer than the time required for a linear regression) combined with the time required to perform repeated K-fold cross-validation can be immense.

Search procedures (which work similarly to the ones used to build predictive linear regressions) can be used to speed up the process. Variables are added to or removed from the model based on what improves the accuracy the most.

When the search procedure terminates, a report is given that lists (for a given number of predictors) the best-performing model, its validation accuracy, and the standard deviation of the accuracy. It is recommended to follow the one standard deviation rule and to choose the simplest model that has an accuracy no smaller than one standard deviation below the largest value.

Building a predictive logistic regression model can be extremely time-consuming. For many problems, a different kind of model called a random forest typically achieves much higher accuracy at a fraction of the time. See Chapter 9. However, when the probability of the level of interest does indeed change according to the logistic curve (which can be rare), logistic regression models work extremely well.

Example - Wine

The `WINE` dataset records 11 characteristics of various vintages of wine and whether they are gauged as high or low quality by experts. Let us randomly pick 20% of the 2700 total cases to be in the holdout sample. The search procedure will start with the full model and will eliminate the "worst" predictor variable at each step.

Figure 8.9 displays the estimated generalization error (essentially the average misclassification rate) of models vs. the number of predictors in the model. The model with the lowest error has 8 predictors, but any of the models containing between 5 and 11 predictors have errors within one standard deviation and are thus acceptable.

In R

```
set.seed(1337)
train.rows <- sample( 1:nrow(WINE),0.80*nrow(WINE) )
TRAIN <- WINE[train.rows,]
HOLDOUT <- WINE[-train.rows,]
MODELS <- build.model(Quality~.,data=TRAIN)
MODELS$CVtable
  NumPredictors EstGenError          SD
              4   0.1354501 0.004343246
+             5   0.1340321 0.005169063 (selected by 1 SD rule)
              6   0.1311026 0.004110603
              7   0.1300709 0.004556201
*             8   0.1296769 0.004804376 (lowest error overall)
              9   0.1298714 0.004407623
             10   0.1298476 0.004302225
             11   0.1304916 0.003673292
```

Figure 8.9 — Validation errors for WINE dataset.

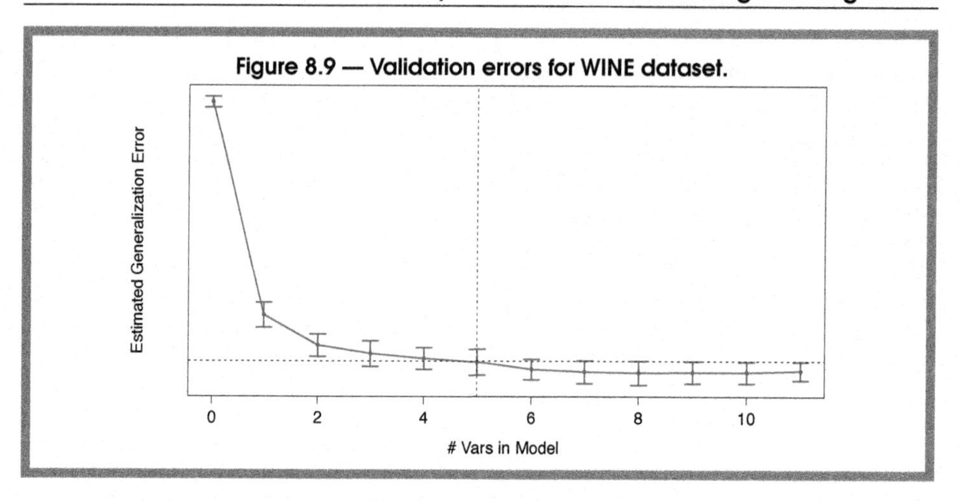

Let us choose the simplest model using the one standard deviation rule. The resulting model has five predictors.

In R

```
summary(MODELS$bestmodel)
                    Estimate Std. Error z value Pr(>|z|)
(Intercept)        338.67706   77.44120   4.373 1.22e-05 ***
volatile.acidity    -9.84831    0.77567 -12.697  < 2e-16 ***
residual.sugar       0.23141    0.03044   7.602 2.92e-14 ***
density           -353.80771   77.17957  -4.584 4.56e-06 ***
sulphates            3.05116    0.54161   5.634 1.77e-08 ***
alcohol              1.16501    0.11657   9.994  < 2e-16 ***
```

It is interesting to see how well this model predicts on the holdout sample compared to other models. Below is a table of the number of misclassifications on this *particular* holdout sample (results may vary for a different training/holdout split).

In R

```
M.naive <- glm(Quality~1,data=TRAIN,family="binomial")
M.cv <- glm(MODELS$bestformula,data=TRAIN,family="binomial")
M.full <- glm(Quality~.,data=TRAIN,family="binomial")
M.fullint <- glm(Quality~.^2,data=TRAIN,family="binomial")
M.aic1 <- step(M.cv,scope=list(lower=M.naive,upper=M.full),direction="both")
M.aic2 <- step(M.cv,scope=list(lower=M.naive,upper=M.fullint),direction="both")
generalization.error(M.naive,HOLDOUT)
generalization.error(M.cv,HOLDOUT)
generalization.error(M.full,HOLDOUT)
generalization.error(M.fullint,HOLDOUT)
generalization.error(M.aic1,HOLDOUT)
generalization.error(M.aic2,HOLDOUT)
```

Method	# Misclassifications on Holdout (out of 540)
Naive	214
Cross-validation	103
Full Model (no interactions)	93
Full Model (all interactions)	64
AIC search (no interactions)	91
AIC search (with interactions)	70

The selected model has a disappointing performance and has the most misclassifications except for the naive model. Interestingly, the full model with all two-way interactions (which is typically very overfit) has the fewest misclassifications. Models with a low AIC also do well. They are closer to "the truth" than others, and it looks like in this case, having as realistic a model as possible has paid off.

In this example, considering interactions is critical. Since logistic regression combined with repeated K-fold cross-validation is such a computationally intensive process, search procedures often cannot consider them.

8.6 Further issues

Ideally, any method for building a predictive model should have the following features:

- The method should consider interactions between predictor variables.
- The method should be able to handle categorical predictors.
- The method should estimate generalization errors of models (repeated K-fold cross-validation seems to be the best way).

Unfortunately, no routine in `R` outside of `build.model` in package `regclass` as of this writing can do all three. Interactions are usually not considered due to time constraints (the number of possible models, and even the number of possible moves in a search, is simply too large).

Further, categorical variables and K-fold cross-validation do not work well together. The issue is that there is a chance that not all levels of the categorical variable will be represented in a training fold, especially if some levels are rare. When a level is present in the validation sample but not in the training sample, the level is combined with the referenced level. `build.model` allows K-fold cross-validation with categorical variables.

Another way to obtain a sophisticated predictive model with interactions and/or categorical variables is to build the model as if you were constructing a descriptive model (minimize the AIC) and to hope for the best. Although this type of model is constructed with no specific regard to how well it generalizes, it should be decent (though often somewhat overfit) because in some sense it is closer to "the truth" than other models.

Alternatively, you can abandon regression entirely and try a different modeling approach like a partition model or random forest, which will be discussed in the following chapter.

8.7 Summary

Predictive modeling is an extremely important task and is one of the techniques that can give businesses an edge over the competition. Philosophically, predictive modeling is easier than descriptive modeling because it is a "hack job"—as long as the model makes accurate predictions, it does not necessarily matter how "close" it is to reality. However, building a predictive model can be so computationally challenging (because of repeated K-fold cross-validation) that the overall number of models we can consider is restricted.

The key to effective predictive modeling is to choose a model based on how well it predicts data it has not seen before. Overfitting is the biggest concern for predictive models. A model is overfit when it has, in effect, memorized the quirks present in the collected data that do not exist in a general setting. A model that is overfit will predict values on the current data quite well (whose answers we already knew), but it can give wildly inaccurate predictions on new data (whose answers we really want to predict).

The standard procedure for building a predictive model is to split the original data into training (where the model is fit) and holdout samples. K-fold cross-validation is used on a model fit using the training data to estimate the generalization error. This estimate can then be compared to the actual generalization error on the holdout sample. A rule of thumb is that if the generalization error on the holdout is not more than 10-20% larger than what was estimated, the model generalizes well.

Often, after we have fit a multitude of models, we find that the validation errors for many models will be comparable. The one standard deviation rule says that all models whose validation errors are within one standard deviation of the smallest value are essentially equivalent. We typically choose the simplest of these models to guard against overfitting.

One of the biggest lessons in predictive modeling is that the model that *actually* predicts the best on genuinely new data will most certainly *not* be the one you have selected (regardless of the method used to make the selection). However, the procedures outlined in this chapter in some sense give you the best shot at coming up with a "decent" model given the data to which you have access.

8.8 Using R

The standard commands for building a predictive model are `step` (in the base package), `regsubsets` (in the `leaps` package), `glmulti` (in the `glmulti` package), `bestglm` (in the `bestglm` package), and `rfe` (in the `caret` package). However, only the latter two will perform cross-validation to estimate generalization errors, and both have drawbacks: `bestglm` does not incorporate interactions or categorical variables with more than two levels, and `rfe` only performs a backward search.

`build.model` in `regclass` is designed as a catch-all function to build any type of model, regardless of the predictors or any logical issues arising from multi-level categorical variables. This function converts the data frame into a form with which `bestglm` will work behind the scenes. The command takes the following arguments:

In R

```
build.model(form,data,type="predictive",Kfold=5,repeats=10,seed=NA,...)
```

- `form` is a model formula for the most complex model under consideration, e.g., `y ~ .^2`
- `data` is the name of the data frame that contains the data.
- `type` is either `"predictive"` or `"descriptive"`. If a predictive model is desired, models are judged on the estimated generalization error from repeated K-fold cross-validation. If a descriptive model is desired, models are judged on AIC.
- `Kfold` and `repeats` are optional arguments telling how repeated K-fold cross-validation should be performed.
- `seed` is an optional argument that *should* be set for predictive models. Since K-fold cross-validation is a random procedure, in order to reproduce the results it is necessary to make sure the random number seed has been set.

- `...` are additional arguments accepted by `bestglm`. By default, the "all possible" procedure is attempted, but this can be changed by passing `method="forward"`, `method="backward"`, or `method="seqrep"`. If you wish to restrict the number of variables in the model, you can pass `nvmax=8` (for example, if you wanted only up to eight variables).

Typically, the results of `build.model` should be given a name such as

`MODELS <- build.model()`. Once this has been done, you may access:

- `MODELS$bestmodel` - the best-fitting model (simplest model with acceptable generalization error). Typically, you will want to do `summary(MODELS$bestmodel)` to see the coefficients. Note: due to an oddity in `bestglm`, the formula for this model will name the response as y, regardless of what the name of *y* actually was.
- `MODELS$bestformula` - the best-fitting model's formula. You can use this to fit the model on the training data, e.g., `M.cv <- lm(MODELS$bestformula,data=TRAINING)`.
- `MODELS$CVtable` - a table giving the number of predictors, estimated generalization error, and standard deviations for various models.
- `MODELS$predictors` - a list giving the names of the predictors in the models corresponding to the list in `CVtable`. To access the predictors in the best model with five predictors, do `MODELS$predictors[[5]]`.

8.9 Exercises

1: Let's build a good predictive model for the bicycle demand data `EX7.BIKE`. Since the worth of a predictive model is based on how well it generalizes and predicts *new* data, it may or may not be the same model that minimizes the AIC in the previous chapter's exercise.

a) Using `set.seed(2015)`, split the data into a (70%) training and (30%) holdout sample. Using `head()`, print out the first row of your training dataset and confirm that it corresponds to a Saturday with a demand of 2132.
b) Using `build.model()`, find a good predictive model for `Demand`. Do not consider interactions, and add `seed=2015` for reproducibility.
   1) How many variables are in the model with the lowest estimated generalization error?
   2) What three predictors are in the model selected by the one standard deviation rule?
c) Rerun `build.model()`, but now allow for the possibility of having interactions between the three variables in the model selected by the one standard deviation rule in (b2) (make sure the seed is still 2015). Do we need to incorporate any of these interactions into the model? In other words, does the model with the lowest generalization error contain an interaction?
d) Find the generalization errors on the holdout sample for the full model (no interactions), full model (with interactions), and the model using only the three predictors selected by the one standard deviation rule from (b2). Which of these models ends up performing the best on the holdout sample? Which model is "overfit"? Note: when fitting these models, be sure to use `data=TRAIN` in your `lm()` statements and not the entirety of the dataset! You may ignore warnings (the full model with interactions has a few coefficients that can't be estimated).

2: Let's build a good predictive model for the catalog order data `EX7.CATALOG`. Since the worth of a predictive model is based on how well it generalizes and predicts *new* data, it may or may not be the same model that minimizes the AIC in the previous chapter's exercise.

a) Using `set.seed(2015)`, split the data into a (75%) training and (25%) holdout sample. Using `head()`, print out the first row of your training dataset to confirm that it corresponds to a customer where `Buy` is `No` and `DaysSinceLastPurchase` is 603.

b) Using `build.model()`, find a good predictive model for `Buy`. Do not consider interactions, and add `seed=2015` for reproducibility.
   1) How many variables are in the model with the lowest estimated generalization error?
   2) What two predictors are in the model selected by the one standard deviation rule?

c) Rerun `build.model()`, but now allow for the possibility of having interactions between the variables in the model selected by the one standard deviation rule in (b2) (make sure the seed is still 2015). Do we need to incorporate any of these interactions into the model? In other words, does the model with the lowest generalization error contain an interaction?

d) Find the generalization errors on the holdout sample for the full model (no interactions), full model (with interactions), and the model selected by the one standard deviation rule from (b2). Which of these models ends up performing the best on the holdout sample? Is this the model that had been selected by `build.model`?

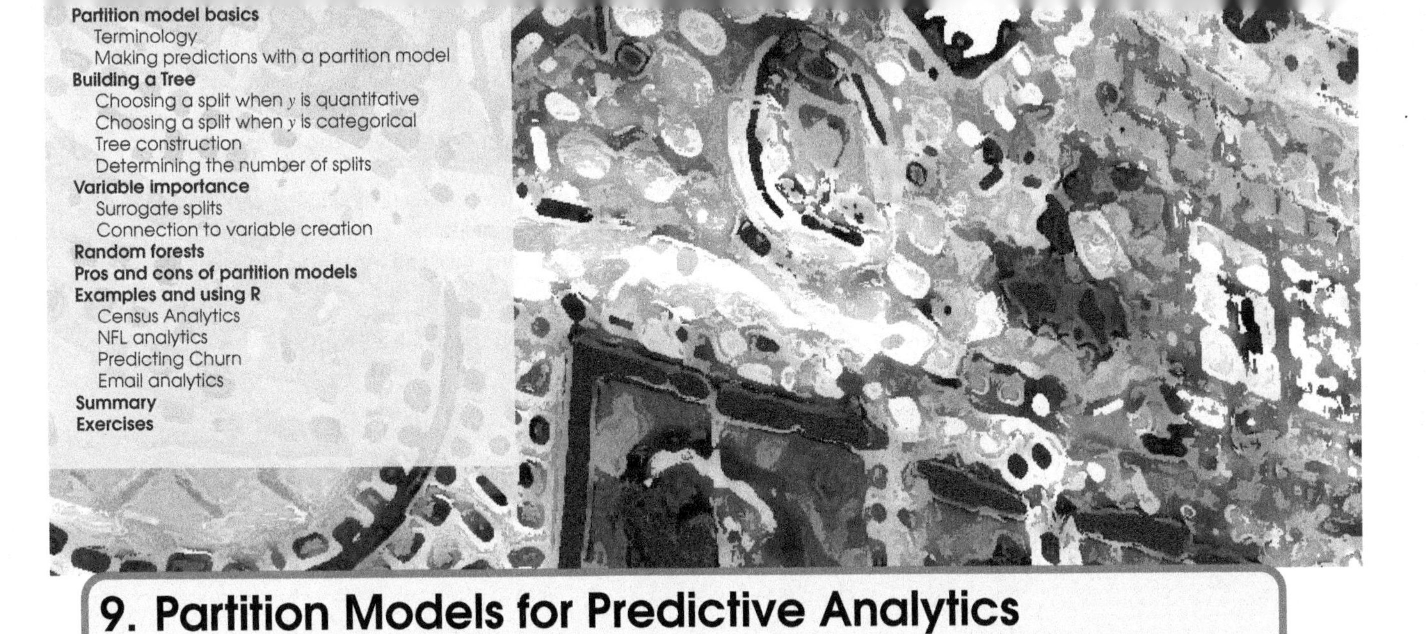

Partition model basics
- Terminology
- Making predictions with a partition model

Building a Tree
- Choosing a split when y is quantitative
- Choosing a split when y is categorical
- Tree construction
- Determining the number of splits

Variable importance
- Surrogate splits
- Connection to variable creation

Random forests

Pros and cons of partition models

Examples and using R
- Census Analytics
- NFL analytics
- Predicting Churn
- Email analytics

Summary

Exercises

9. Partition Models for Predictive Analytics

Linear regression models assume that the world functions in a very specific way: the average value of some quantity of interest (y, e.g., sales) is essentially a weighted sum of other quantities (x's; e.g., advertising, region, price). Though x and y are arbitrary quantities (they can be transformations or functions of the original measurements like $\ln(sales)$, $\sqrt{price}$, $(sales/price)^2$, etc.), the fundamental assumption of linearity between y and x is very restrictive. What if the world just doesn't work this way? For example, consider Figure 9.1.

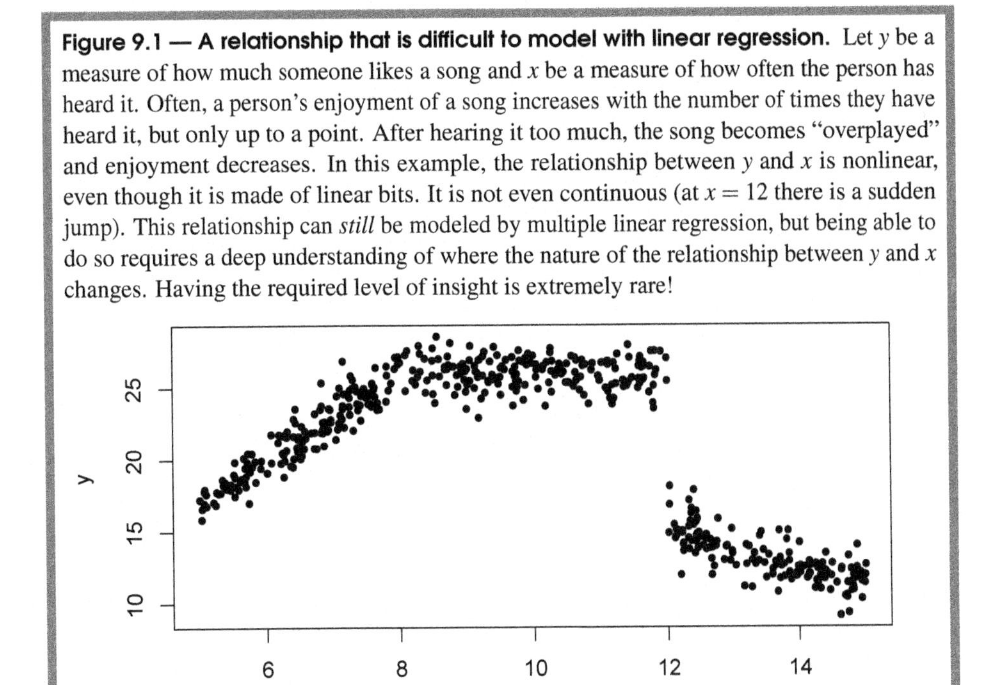

Figure 9.1 — A relationship that is difficult to model with linear regression. Let y be a measure of how much someone likes a song and x be a measure of how often the person has heard it. Often, a person's enjoyment of a song increases with the number of times they have heard it, but only up to a point. After hearing it too much, the song becomes "overplayed" and enjoyment decreases. In this example, the relationship between y and x is nonlinear, even though it is made of linear bits. It is not even continuous (at $x = 12$ there is a sudden jump). This relationship can *still* be modeled by multiple linear regression, but being able to do so requires a deep understanding of where the nature of the relationship between y and x changes. Having the required level of insight is extremely rare!

In Figure 9.1, the relationship between y and x is complex and nonlinear, changing in nature over the range of x in the plot. When $x \leq 8$, the relationship looks positive and linear. For $8 < x < 12$, there looks to be no relationship between x and y (y stays nearly constant), and for $x > 12$, the relationship is negative and linear.

Remarkably, this relationship can *still* be modeled with a linear regression, albeit with a very clever definition of variables. Let:

$$r_1 = \begin{cases} 1, & \text{if } x \leq 8 \\ 0, & \text{otherwise} \end{cases} \qquad r_2 = \begin{cases} 1, & \text{if } 8 < x < 12 \\ 0, & \text{otherwise} \end{cases} \qquad r_3 = \begin{cases} 1, & \text{if } x \geq 12 \\ 0, & \text{otherwise} \end{cases}$$

One can think of r_1, r_2, and r_3 as indicator variables that encode the region of x to which the individual belongs. Then, one can write the model as:

$$y = r_1 \times (\beta_0 + \beta_1 x) + \beta_2 r_2 + r_3 \times (\beta_3 + \beta_4 x) + \varepsilon$$

To see this, consider the cases where:

- $x \leq 8$. The values of r_2 and r_3 are both equal to zero while $r_1 = 1$, so the model becomes $y = \beta_0 + \beta_1 x$ (a straight line).
- $8 < x < 12$. The values of r_1 and r_3 are both equal to zero while $r_2 = 1$, so the model becomes $y = \beta_2$ (a constant).
- $x \geq 12$. The values of r_1 and r_2 are both equal to zero while $r_3 = 1$, so the model becomes $y = \beta_3 + \beta_4 x$ (a straight line).

Rewriting the equation and defining x_0, x_1, etc., appropriately, we get:

$$y = \beta_0 r_1 + \beta_1 (x \times r_1) + \beta_2 r_2 + \beta_3 r_3 + \beta_4 (x \times r_4) + \varepsilon$$

$$y = \beta_0 x_0 + \beta_1 x_1 + \beta_2 x_2 + \beta_3 x_3 + \beta_4 x_4 + \varepsilon$$

Thus, it turns out that we can indeed write y as a weighted sum of *some* predictor variables, so the relationship between y and x *can* be modeled with a linear regression!

Regression really does provide an extremely flexible framework that can model a wide range of complex relationships. However, to model y effectively, sometimes it is required to have deep insight into exactly *what* needs to be used as predictor variables. Sometimes, the problem is easy and y has a linear relationship with the measured quantities in the data. Other times, transformations and interactions must be used or entirely new variables must be created. For problems with many variables, it is almost assured that *any* model you construct will be missing some important component.

One can avoid some of these difficulties by approaching the problem from a different angle. Instead of imposing some functional form and equation on the relationship between y and the predictor variables, we can instead use a simple set of rules to predict y. The following rules model the relationship in Figure 9.1 fairly accurately:

$$y = \begin{cases} 17, & \text{if } 5 \leq x \leq 6 \quad 21, \ \text{if } 6 < x \leq 7 \quad 24, \ \text{if } 7 < x \leq 8 \\ 26, & \text{if } 8 \leq x < 12 \quad 14, \ \text{if } 12 < x \leq 14 \quad 12, \ \text{if } x > 14 \end{cases}$$

Figure 9.2 shows this rule-based model, and it looks reasonable (though far from perfect). In effect, a rule-based model abandons any particular form (linear, quadratic, logarithmic, etc.) for the relationship between y and the predictors. Instead, it splits up the possible values of x's into intervals and predicts y to be the average value of y among all individuals in that interval.

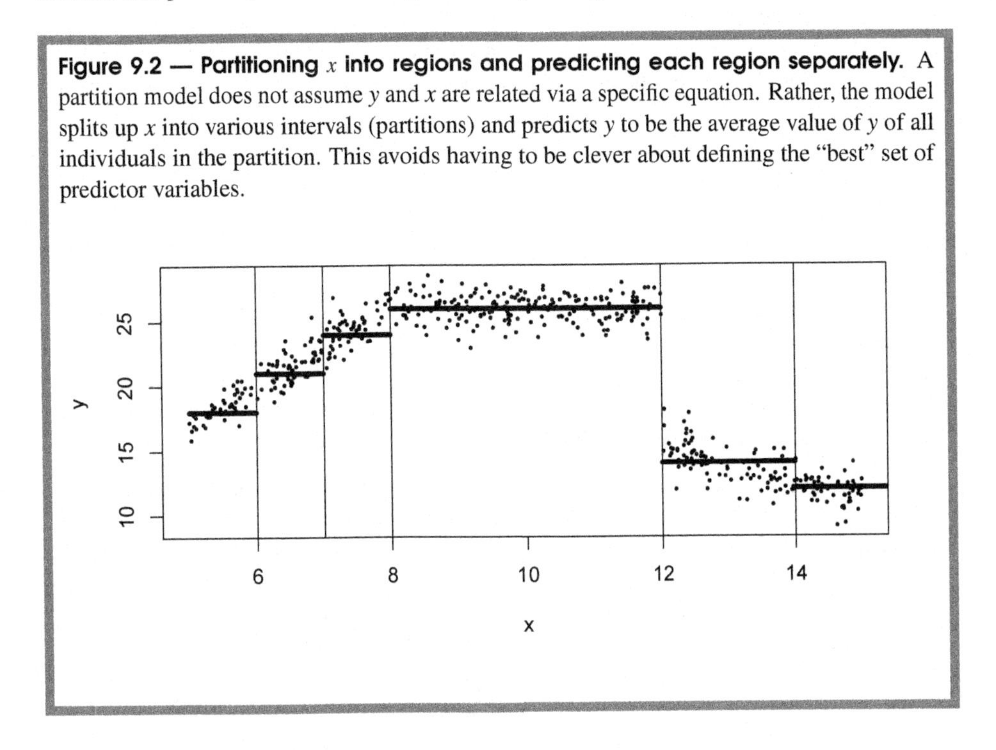

Figure 9.2 — Partitioning x into regions and predicting each region separately. A partition model does not assume y and x are related via a specific equation. Rather, the model splits up x into various intervals (partitions) and predicts y to be the average value of y of all individuals in the partition. This avoids having to be clever about defining the "best" set of predictor variables.

Rule-based models are called **partition models**. The rules split up the **data space** (the possible combinations of x) into a set of regions called partitions (e.g., $0 < x_1 < 2$ and $5 < x_2 < 5.5$). Essentially, the model figures out a way to group similar individuals into clusters.

Buying into the "birds of a feather flock together" mentality, the model assumes that the values of y among the individuals in a partition are typical of the y-values in that region of the data space. Thus, a reasonable way to predict y is to take the average value of y among the individuals in the partition. All individuals in the partition have the same predicted value for y, and this value will vary from partition to partition.

In this chapter, we will explore the use of partition models for predictive modeling. How do we determine the partitions and the set of rules that predict y the "best"? These partition models are often called **classification and regression trees** (**CART** for short) for reasons that will be clear shortly.

On many modern datasets, it turns out that rule-based models are typically more effective than regression. Why? The linearity assumption in a linear regression model (or logistic curve in a logistic regression model) tends to be overly simplistic and restrictive, and it is difficult to select or invent the most appropriate set of predictors. Further, a partition model more effectively captures the subtle interactions that are almost always present in real relationships.

9.1 Partition model basics

A partition model splits up the data space into regions called **partitions**, then predicts a common value of y for every individual in the region. Consider Figure 9.3. Two diagonal lines have split the data space into four partitions (though one partition contains no individuals). These lines have equations:

- $x_2 = 1.5 - 1.8x_1$
- $x_2 = -0.3 + 2.3x_1$

We can determine to which region an individual belongs by seeing whether it is above or below each line.

Figure 9.3 — Partition model. Two diagonal lines have partitioned the data space (possible combinations of x_1 and x_2) into four regions. y is a quantitative variable on the left and a categorical variable (circle vs. triangle) on the right. In both cases, the y-value of an individual is displayed at that individual's combination of x_1 and x_2.

To predict the values of the two new individuals (the starred points) on the left, we take the average value of y of all other individuals in the partition. To predict the level of the new individuals on the right, we look at the proportion of each level among all other individuals in the partition. The starred point at $x_1 = 0.3$, $x_2 = 0.6$ would be predicted to be a triangle since the majority of individuals in the partition are triangles. The starred point at $x_1 = 0.4$, $x_2 = 0.2$ has a 50% chance to be either shape since half of the individuals are circles and half are triangles.

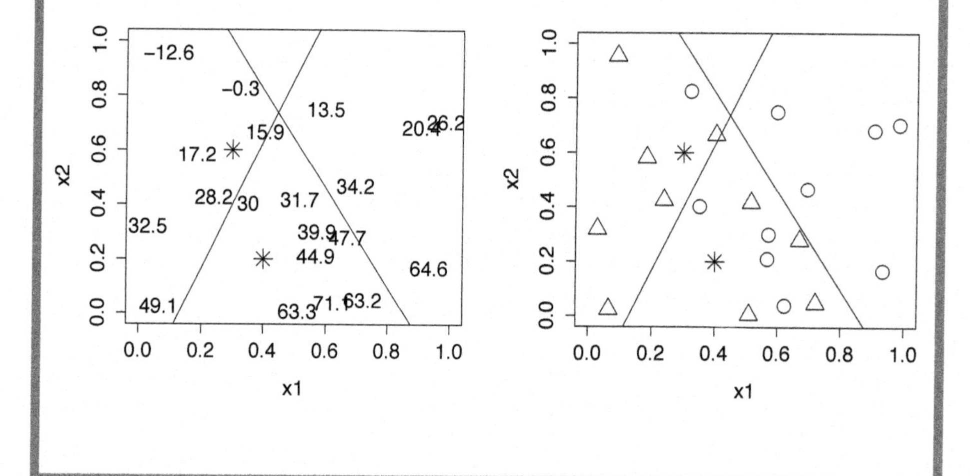

For example, to be in the partition on the far left, the individual must be *below* the line $x_2 = 1.5 - 1.8x_1$ but *above* the line $x_2 = -0.3 + 2.3x_1$. Thus, the lines represent two decision rules:

- Is an individual's value of x_2 bigger or smaller than $1.5 - 1.8x_1$?
- Is an individual's value of x_2 bigger or smaller than $-0.3 + 2.3x_1$?

Depending on the answers to these questions, each observation is neatly assigned to one of the four partitions.

Each partition uses a *single* predicted value for y, regardless of where in the partition the prediction is taking place. To predict a value of y for a partition, the y-values of all other individuals in the partition are considered.

> If y is quantitative (numerical like sales, GPA, etc.), then the predicted value is the *average* of the y-values of every individual in the partition.
>
> If y is categorical, the predicted *probability* of each level can be taken to be the proportion of individuals in the partition with that level (often, this probability is slightly modified to take into account the overall frequencies of each level in the data). The predicted *level* is whatever level has a probability greater than 50% (usually the majority level).

C The starred point in the left partition in Figure 9.3 has a predicted value of y equal to the average of $-12.6, -0.3, \ldots, 49.1$, which equals 18.6. Its predicted probability of being a triangle is about 86% since six out of seven individuals in the partition are triangles. In fact, *any* individual in the left partition (regardless of its location) has these same predicted values.

The other starred point has a 50% chance of being a triangle and a 50% chance of being a circle since the proportions of each shape are the same.

The output of a partition model is a set of regions (partitions) of the data space. Each of these partitions can be described by a set of rules. Sticking with our example in Figure 9.3, we can write:

- If $x_2 \leq 1.5 - 1.8x_1$ and $x_2 > -0.3 + 2.3x_1$, then the individual is in the left partition.
- If $x_2 \leq 1.5 - 1.8x_1$ and $x_2 \leq -0.3 + 2.3x_1$, then the individual is in the bottom partition.
- If $x_2 > 1.5 - 1.8x_1$ and $x_2 > -0.3 + 2.3x_1$, then the individual is in the top (empty) partition.
- If $x_2 > 1.5 - 1.8x_1$ and $x_2 \leq -0.3 + 2.3x_1$, then the individual is in the right partition.

It is much easier to visualize these rules using a decision tree.

Figure 9.4 — Partition model as decision tree. The four partitions in Figure 9.3 made by the two diagonal lines can easily be presented as the following decision tree.

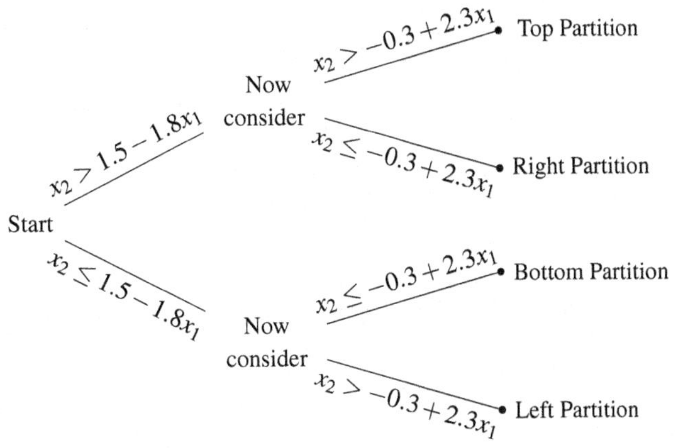

Typically, partitions and decision rules are constructed so they only involve *one* variable at a time, e.g., $x_1 \geq 2$ vs. $x_1 < 2$. For example, consider Figure 9.5. The goal is to determine whether an individual has made a purchase (triangle) or not (dot) based on x_1 and x_2 (income and distance to the store). The figure shows that 100% accuracy can be obtained by splitting the data space into four partitions represented by the decision rules:

If $x_1 \leq 0.5$ and $x_2 > 0.4$, predict "triangle"   If $x_1 \leq 0.5$ and $x_2 \leq 0.4$, predict "dot"
If $x_1 > 0.5$ and $x_2 > 0.6$, predict "dot"   If $x_1 > 0.5$ and $x_2 \leq 0.6$, predict "triangle"

These rules are displayed in the form of a decision tree. First, x_1 is considered. Its size determines what branch of the tree will be followed. Then, x_2 is considered. Based on x_2, the final partition and prediction is chosen. Even though there are four partitions (and thus four rules), we only had to consider two of them when making a prediction. In a way, a decision tree provides a more compact representation of the set of decision rules.

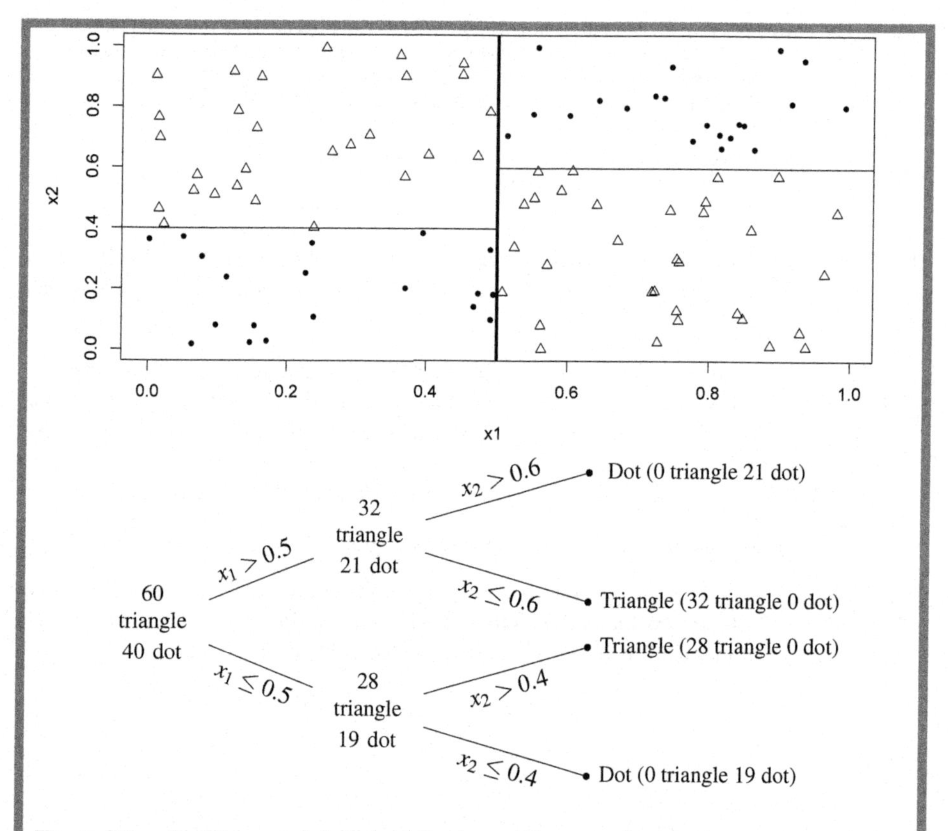

Figure 9.5 — Partition model as decision tree. The type of point (dot or triangle) can be predicted perfectly if the data space is split into four specific partitions. The four rules, "if x_1 is less than 0.5 and x_2 is less than 0.4, then predict dot," etc., describe the partitions and are easily visualized with a decision tree. Starting at the very left, follow the branches according to the values of the x's until reaching a "leaf" or terminal node. The predicted probability of each level can be taken to be the relative proportion of individuals in the partition with each level (perhaps modified by the overall frequency of each level in the data).

The tree can be enhanced to give an idea of what each partition looks like by labeling each node with the average value of y or the proportion of individuals with each level of y. In Figure 9.5, the "base" of the tree represents the naive model where all the data is in one big partition. In this case, there are a total of 60 triangles and 40 dots in the data, so we could predict a 60% chance of being "triangle" and a 40% chance of being "dot." Since "triangle" has the higher probability, the predicted level for all individuals is "triangle," giving a misclassification rate of 40%.

The first decision (whether x_1 is bigger or smaller than 0.5) essentially splits the partition in two. One partition has 32 triangles and 21 dots, while the other has 28 triangles and 19 dots. If this was our model, it would be a poor one since every individual is still predicted to be a triangle (majority in both partitions). Each branch for these two partitions splits them in half again. In the end, we have four partitions. These last two splits make classification perfect since each "leaf" of the tree has 100% of one class.

9.1.1 Terminology

The tree is called a **regression tree** if y is a quantitative, numerical variable (though the technique has nothing to do with regression). It is a **classification** tree if y is categorical and the goal is to predict the probability of each level (the individual is assigned to whichever level has more than 50% probability).

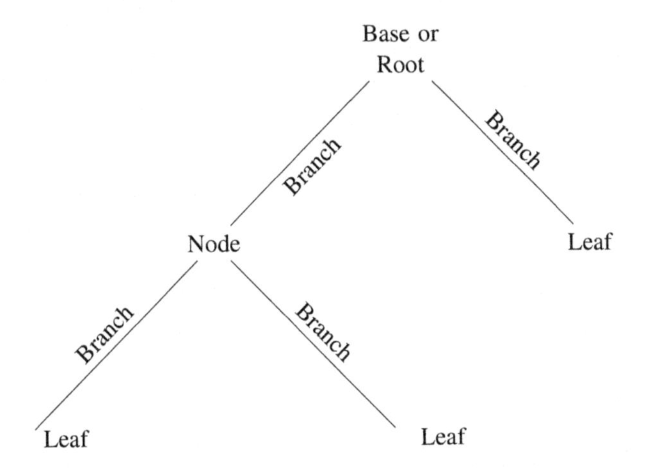

Trees are made of **nodes** and **branches**. A node is a partition of the data space and represents a group of "similar" individuals who all satisfy a set of conditions (e.g., $x_1 < 5$, gender = male, and $x_2 \geq 10$). A pair of branches coming off of a node represents a decision rule, e.g., $x < 5$ vs. $x \geq 5$ or Color = red vs. Color = not red. A pair of branches thus splits a partition in two.

The tree begins at the **base node**, or **root**. This partition contains all the data, and we can think of it as the "naive" model. Recall that the naive model predicts an individual's value of y to be the overall average value of y (if quantitative) or the majority level (if y is categorical). For example, imagine a partition model is being used to predict whether a shopper buys and there are 30 "buy" and 70 "not buy" in the data. The naive model will predict all individuals to have a 70% chance of not buying, and thus will classify all of them as "not buyers."

A node is called a **parent node** if branches leave from it. The two nodes that come off a parent are referred to as **child nodes**.

A **terminal node**, or **leaf**, is a node that has no further splits. These are the set of nodes that represent the final set of partitions of the data space and are used for prediction and classification. All other nodes are intermediate in the sense that they serve only to guide us down the tree during the sequence of decisions toward the leaf.

9.1.2 Making predictions with a partition model

To make a prediction, start at the root of the tree and follow the branches down according to the relevant decision rule until a leaf is reached. If y is quantitative, the predicted value is the average value of y of all individuals in the leaf. If y is categorical, the predicted probability of each level is the proportion of individuals in the leaf with each level[1]. The predicted level is whichever one has the higher probability. See Figure 9.6 and Figure 9.7 for examples.

Figure 9.6 — Predicting a quantitative y (GPA) with a partition model. The goal is to predict college GPA from high school GPA and ACT score. To make a prediction for a person with a high school GPA of 3.5 and an ACT score of 24, we start at the base node. The first rule involves high school GPA, and we head to the left since HS < 3.79. The next rule also involves high school GPA, and we head off to the right since HS ≥ 3.44. We continue off to the left (since ACT < 27.5), then off to the right (since ACT ≥ 23.5). The predicted college GPA is 3.18, which is the average college GPA of all 90 individuals in this partition.

Note: sometimes, not all variables are used to make the prediction, e.g., imagine predicting college GPA when HS GPA is 3.0. We head to the left at the base (HS < 3.79), then left again at the next node (HS < 3.44) to reach a leaf where the predicted college GPA is 2.98. ACT score did not turn out to be relevant for this prediction!

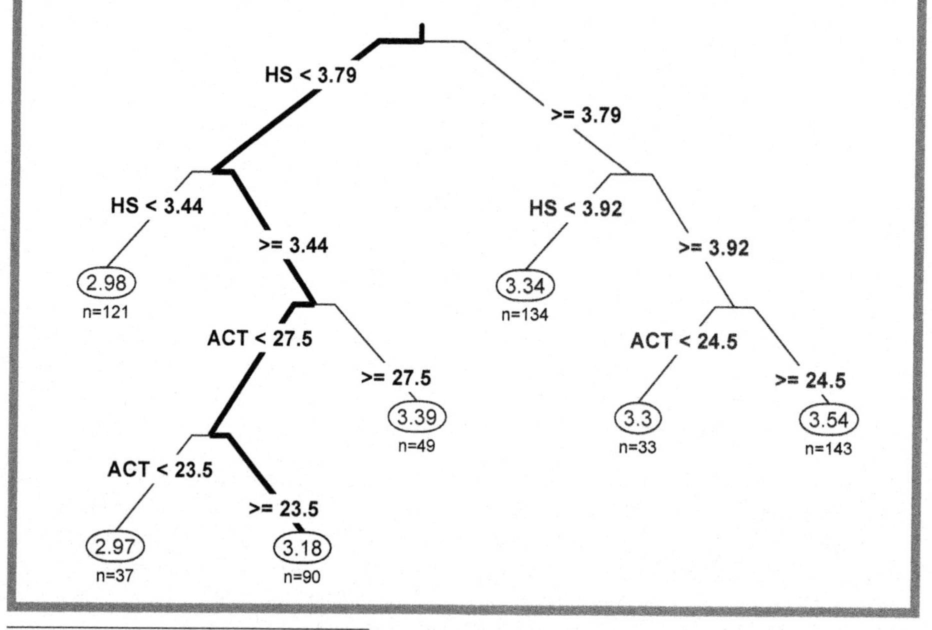

[1] Often, the *prior* probability of each level is taken into account when making predictions. For example, if the data contains 99% of level A and 1% of level B, and if a partition contains individuals with an even mix of levels A and B, the predicted probabilities can be modified to take into account level B's rarity. Further, if a certain type of error (e.g., false negative) is particularly detrimental, the predictions can be modified to make the error of interest less common.

Figure 9.7 — Predicting a categorical *y* (success of new product) with a partition model. The goal is to predict whether a new product will succeed or fail six months after release based on the product type (A, B, C, D) and the number of units sold per store three months after launch (SoldWeek). To make a prediction for a product of type B that has SoldWeek = 4, the bolded path is followed. We first consider SoldWeek. It is ≥ 2.1, so we head to the right. Next, we consider Category. It is A, B, C, so we head to the left. Finally, we reconsider SoldWeek. It is ≥ 3.2, so we head to the right. In the leaf, about 25% of the 71 products failed while 75% of the products succeeded. This new product is predicted to succeed.

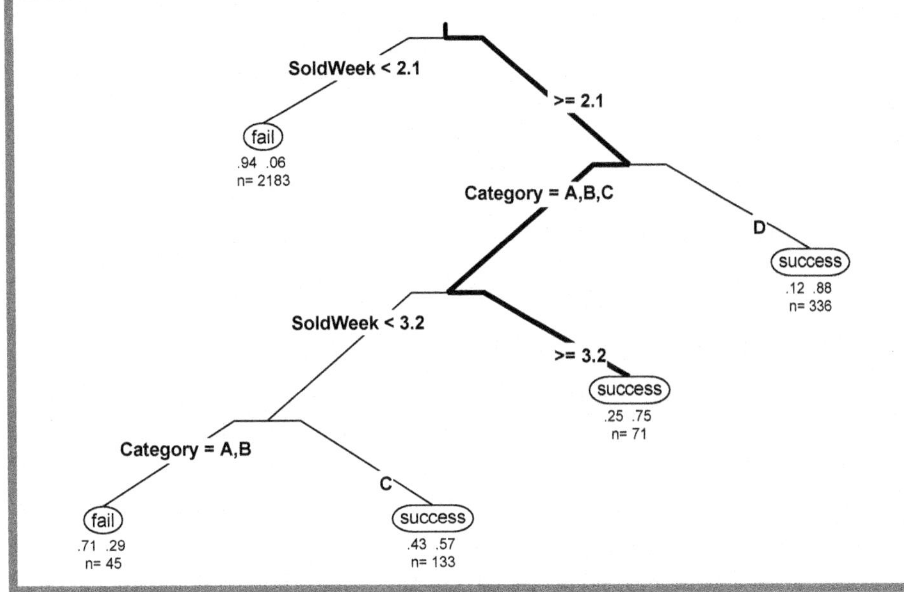

Often, not all variables are used to make the prediction. In Figure 9.6, the goal is to predict the college GPA of someone based on his or her high school GPA and ACT score. For "low" high school GPAs (less than 3.44), the predicted value is 2.98, regardless of ACT score (none of the decision rules involve ACT score along the path from the base node to the leaf).

> Since some variables may be considered only along specific paths, a partition model naturally incorporates interactions between variables without having to define new variables to do so.

In the GPA example, the tree implicitly incorporates the interaction between high school GPA and ACT score—whether ACT "matters" depends on the student's HS GPA. For low HS GPAs (less than 3.44), ACT score is irrelevant. For high HS GPAs (at least 3.92), ACT score plays an important role.

When categorical variables are predictors, two or more levels may be treated together in a decision rule. For example, in Figure 9.7, one of the splits is on the item's product category. If it is level A, B, or C, the branch leads us to the left. If the level is D, the branch leads us to the right. Thus, the tree (at this point) is treating categories A, B, and C the same. Following the A/B/C branch, there is another split on product category later on—A or B leads us to the left and

C leads us to the right. Thus, the tree treats product category as having three effective levels: "A or B", "C", and "D."

> Partition models are able to spontaneously combine levels of a categorical variable. Reducing the effective number of levels of a categorical variable is something that comes naturally to a partition model, but it would require substantial effort in a regression model.

9.2 Building a Tree

We have seen that a partition model is basically a set of rules that can be easily visualized by a decision tree. Thus, the only choices in a partition model are *what set of rules should be used.* In other words, how should the data space be partitioned? To simplify construction, standard practice is to consider only basic rules such as "If $x_1 < 1$ and $x_2 \geq 3.5\ldots$" instead of rules like "If $x_1 - 2x_2 \leq 0.5\ldots$" so that the partitions will always be rectangles. Rules that use more than one variable take too much computational time to develop, and they do not seem to substantially increase the performance of the model in general.

9.2.1 Choosing a split when y is quantitative

To build a tree, we must first define what makes a good rule (commonly referred to as a split). What makes one rule better than another? When y is a quantitative variable, rules that decrease the sum of squared errors (SSE) of a partition are good.

Recall that the predicted value for any individual in a partition is just the average value of y among the individuals in that partition. Thus, the sum of squared errors (SSE) for a partition is defined to be the sum of the squared differences between individuals' y-values and the average y-value in the partition.

$$SSE_{partition} = \text{sum over all individuals in the partition of } (y_i - \bar{y})^2$$

The *decrease* in the sum of squared errors for a proposed split (new rule) is the difference between the sum of squared errors of the "parent" partition and the sum of squared errors of the two resulting "child" partitions.

$$\text{Decrease in } SSE = SSE_{parent} - (SSE_{child_1} + SSE_{child_2}) \tag{9.1}$$

> The "best" split of a partition and best new rule will be the one that decreases the sum of squared errors the most.

There is no shortcut for finding the best new rule to add to the tree—*every* possible way of splitting a partition must be considered! To make the process a bit quicker, only certain values for splits are attempted. These values are the midpoints between each unique value of x found in the partition. For example, if the unique values of x are 1, 5, and 10, then possible splits are

$x \leq 3$ vs. $x > 3$ and $x \leq 7.5$ vs. $x > 7.5$. If there is more than one predictor variable, the optimal split for *each* of the variables is found, then the absolute best rule splits the partition and is added to the tree.

Choosing the optimal split for a partition occurs after an exhaustive consideration of all possible ways to make the split—all possible values of each possible variable. Whichever new rule gives the largest decrease in the sum of squared errors is added to the tree and used to then split the partition.

Aside 9.1 — Calculating SSE reduction when y is quantitative. Imagine a partition contains the following five individuals and the proposed split is $x \leq 2.5$ vs. $x > 2.5$.

y	0	5	5	4	9
x	1	2	3	4	5

The parent partition has $\bar{y} = (0+5+5+4+9)/5 = 4.6$, so

$$\begin{aligned} SSE_{parent} &= (0-4.6)^2 + (5-4.6)^2 + (5-4.6)^2 + (4-4.6)^2 + (8-4.6)^2 \\ &= 4.6^2 + 0.4^2 + 0.4^2 + 0.6^2 + 3.4^2 = 33.4 \end{aligned}$$

The first child has $\bar{y} = (0+5)/2 = 2.5$, while the second child has $\bar{y} = (5+4+9)/3 = 6$. This gives

$$SSE_{child_1} = (0-2.5)^2 + (5-2.5)^2 = 12.5 \qquad SSE_{child_2} = (5-6)^2 + (4-6)^2 + (9-6)^2 = 14$$

The reduction in SSE of the proposed split is $33.4 - (12.5 + 14) = 6.9$.

An alternative rule is $x \leq 1.5$ vs. $x > 1.5$. The reduction in SSE of this split can be shown to be $33.4 - (0 + 14.75) = 18.75$. Thus, the rule $x \leq 1.5$ vs. $x > 1.5$ is better than the rule $x \leq 2.5$ vs. $x > 2.5$.

For example, imagine that we are making a predictive model for college GPA using HS GPA, ACT score, and gender. How should the first split (of the base partition) be made so that the resulting sum of squared errors is the smallest? Should it be HS GPA < 3.5 vs. HS GPA ≥ 3.5? ACT < 28 vs. ACT ≥ 28? Male vs. female, etc.? For each predictor, we need to exhaustively consider every single possible split, then see which works best.

Figure 9.8 shows the sum of squared errors of the two resulting child partitions when the parent is split on each value of each variable. We see that the "best" split uses high school GPA and the optimal decision rule is HS GPA < 3.795 vs. HS GPA ≥ 3.795. The sum of the resulting SSEs of the two child partitions is about 107, much lower than had we split on ACT (113) or gender (116).

9.2.2 Choosing a split when y is categorical

When y is a categorical variable, splits that decrease the overall **impurity** of the partition are good. There are a few ways to measure impurity, but the Gini index is the default in many software packages, including R.

Figure 9.8 — Decrease in sum of squared errors of partitions when predicting college GPA. Each decision rule, e.g., HS GPA < 3.0 vs. HS GPA ≥ 3.0, yields a different decrease in the sum of squared errors (Equation 9.1). We want to find the split that gives the largest SSE reduction: $SSE_{parent} - (SSE_{child_1} + SSE_{child_2})$. In this case, the best decision rule is HS GPA < 3.795 vs. HS GPA ≥ 3.795. Splitting on gender or any value of ACT does not improve the tree nearly as much.

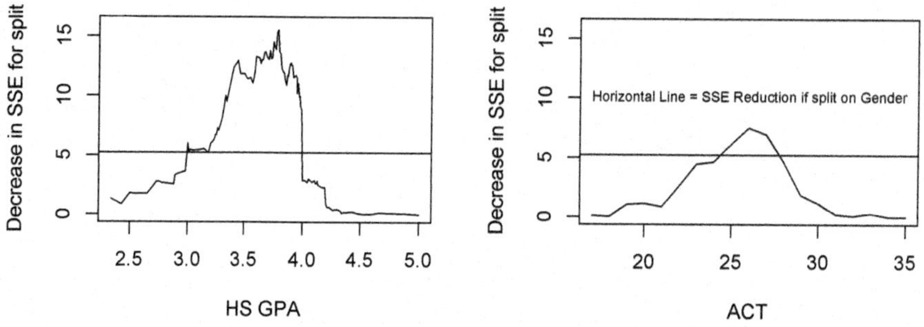

For a particular partition containing n cases, let there be n_A individuals with level A and n_B individuals with level B. The impurity of the partition is defined to be $1 - (n_A/n)^2 - (n_B/n)^2$. Note that if all y-values in a partition are the same, then the impurity is equal to 0 as you would expect. If a partition has equal amounts of both levels, the impurity is 0.5.

(C) Imagine flipping a coin to classify an individual in the partition as A or B. If the coin comes up heads (with probability n_A/n), the individual is classified as having level A. If the coin comes up tails (with probability n_B/n), the individual is classified as having level B. The impurity is the probability that a randomly picked individual is misclassified using this scheme.

The impurity is also called the Gini index and should not to be confused with the misclassification *rate* in a partition, which equals either n_A/n or n_B/n, whichever value is lower.

The equations for the impurity of a partition and the decrease in impurity for a split are rather involved:

$$\text{Impurity of Partition} = 1 - \left(\frac{n_A}{n}\right)^2 - \left(\frac{n_B}{n}\right)^2 \tag{9.2}$$

$$\text{Decrease in Impurity} = Impurity_{parent} - \frac{(n_{child_1} \times Impurity_{child_1}) + (n_{child_2} \times Impurity_{child2})}{n_{parent}} \tag{9.3}$$

The "best" split of a partition will be the new rule that decreases the impurity the most. Again, there is no shortcut for finding the optimal split—every new rule involving every possible predictor must be considered.

Figure 9.9 shows how the first split for the PRODUCT dataset is chosen. The goal is to predict whether a new product will succeed or fail (Outcome) six months after release based on the product type (Category, levels A, B, C, D) and the number of units sold per store three months after launch (SoldWeek13). The impurities for each split in the variable SoldWeek13 and on Category (A, B, C, D) are calculated. The lowest possible impurity is when the split is done on SoldWeek13 at a value of 2.09.

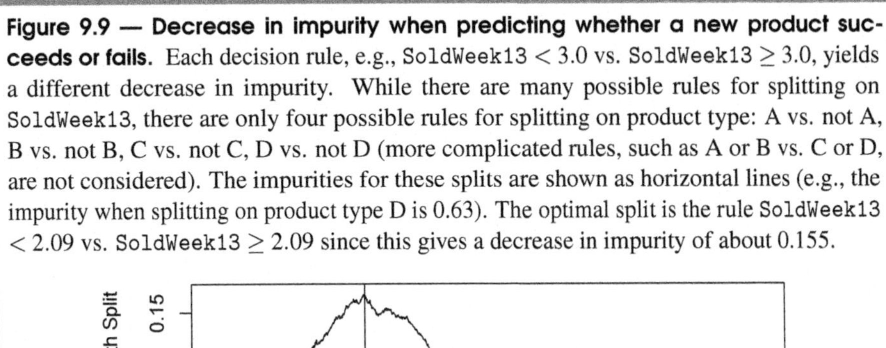

Figure 9.9 — Decrease in impurity when predicting whether a new product succeeds or fails. Each decision rule, e.g., SoldWeek13 < 3.0 vs. SoldWeek13 ≥ 3.0, yields a different decrease in impurity. While there are many possible rules for splitting on SoldWeek13, there are only four possible rules for splitting on product type: A vs. not A, B vs. not B, C vs. not C, D vs. not D (more complicated rules, such as A or B vs. C or D, are not considered). The impurities for these splits are shown as horizontal lines (e.g., the impurity when splitting on product type D is 0.63). The optimal split is the rule SoldWeek13 < 2.09 vs. SoldWeek13 ≥ 2.09 since this gives a decrease in impurity of about 0.155.

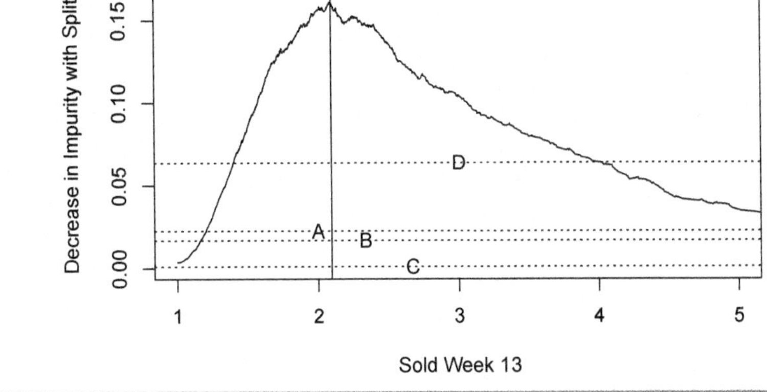

9.2.3 Tree construction

The tree is grown *recursively*—every step of the algorithm uses the results of the step that came before it. In fact, these models are often referred to as **recursive** partition models.

When the procedure begins, all individuals are in the base node. All ways of splitting it are considered exhaustively (every single value for every single variable), then the optimal rule is added to the tree and the optimal split is made. This splits the base node into two child nodes. The process is then repeated on each child node. The optimal way of splitting each child is determined, then whichever split gives the biggest decrease in SSE or impurity is taken. Refer to Figure 9.10.

On the surface, it may seem like the computational requirements for the procedure increases as the tree grows larger. After all, the optimal split for *each* partition has to be found before a new rule can be added. In reality, each split takes progressively *less* time than the split before it! After split i there are $i+1$ total partitions. The optimal splits for all but the two newest children have previously been calculated. Thus, every additional split requires only two additional exhaustive searches. Since the number of individuals in a partition decreases after every split, the time required to find the optimal split decreases.

Aside 9.2 — Calculating decrease in impurity when y is categorical. Imagine a partition has the following five individuals and the proposed split is $x \leq 2.5$ vs. $x > 2.5$.

y	A	B	A	B	B
x	1	2	3	4	5

The impurity of the parent partition ($n = 5$, $n_A = 2$, $n_B = 3$) is:

$$1 - (2/5)^2 - (3/5)^2 = 0.48$$

The impurity of the first child ($n_{child_1} = 2$, $n_A = 1$, $n_B = 1$) is:

$$1 - (1/2)^2 - (1/2)^2 = 0.50$$

The impurity of the second child ($n_{child_2} = 3$, $n_A = 1$, $n_B = 2$) is:

$$1 - (1/3)^2 - (2/3)^2 = 4/9$$

Thus, the decrease in impurity is:

$$0.48 - \frac{2(0.50) + 3(4/9)}{5} = 0.013$$

After repeating this calculation for the other three ways of splitting the data, we find the optimal split is $x \leq 3.5$ vs. $x > 3.5$, which gives a decrease in impurity of 0.22.

In theory, the tree can be grown so that each leaf contains only one observation. In this case, the tree would give a perfect fit to the data (much like a regression using any $n - 1$ predictor variables will give a perfect fit), but it would probably not generalize well to new data. There is some "optimal size" for a tree that needs to be determined.

9.2.4 Determining the number of splits

Adding another branch to the tree (a new rule to the model) is like adding an additional predictor in a regression: the sum of squared errors (or impurity) of the model always decreases. For predictive modeling, we do not care how well the model fits the collected data (we know those y-values already). Rather, we want a model that generalizes well to *new* data.

After adding too many branches and too many rules, the tree becomes overfit—the tree essentially memorizes the quirks in the collected data and will not predict new observations very well.

Let us choose the size of a tree to minimize its expected generalization error. This can be estimated using repeated K-fold cross-validation. Review Section 8.2.3, which introduces the technique in the context of predictive regression models.

The size of a tree is measured not by the number of splits or rules, but rather by a **complexity parameter**, or **cp**. The complexity parameter provides a threshold for how much the tree must improve in order to justify the addition of another branch or rule.

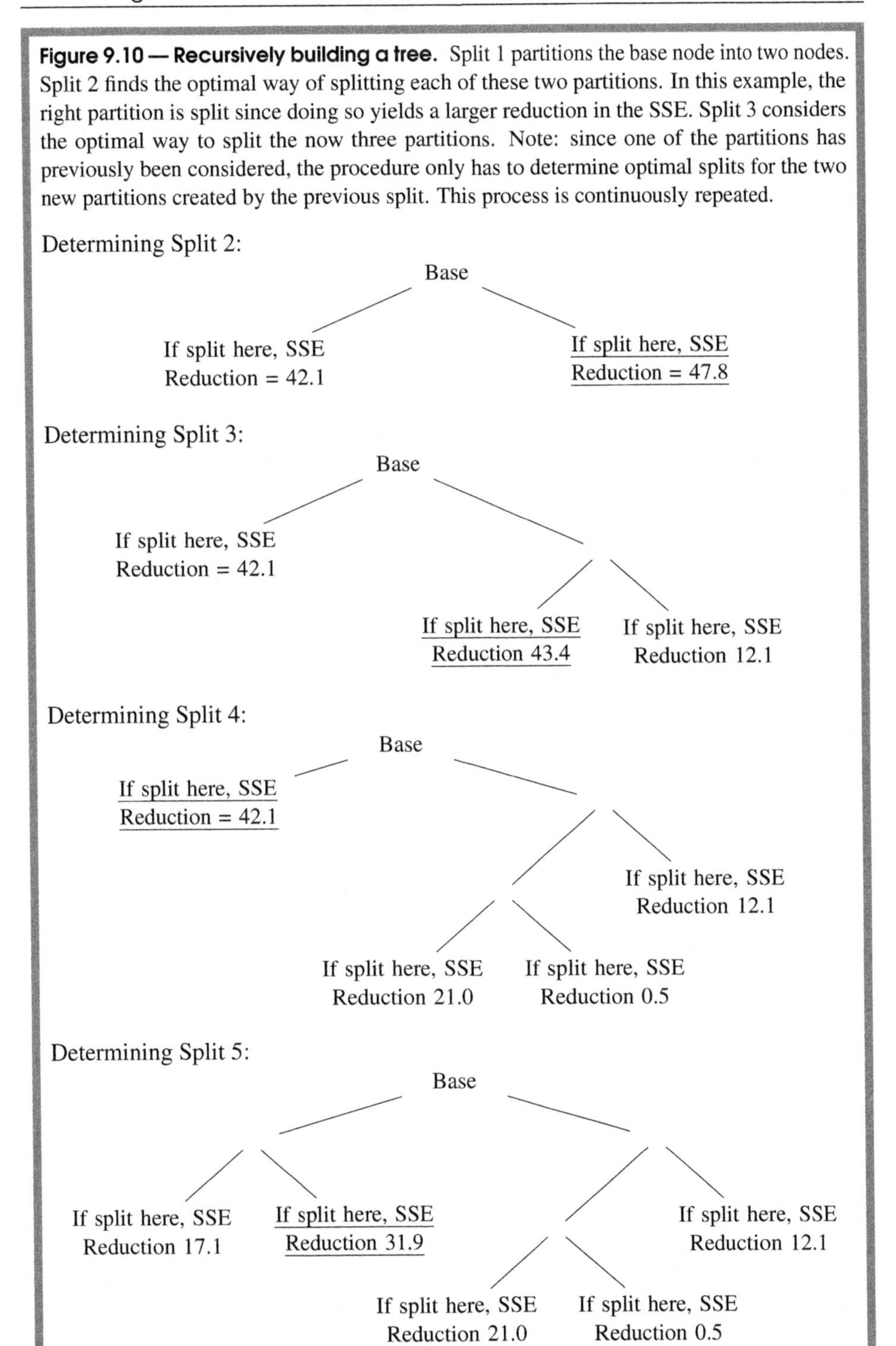

Figure 9.10 — Recursively building a tree. Split 1 partitions the base node into two nodes. Split 2 finds the optimal way of splitting each of these two partitions. In this example, the right partition is split since doing so yields a larger reduction in the SSE. Split 3 considers the optimal way to split the now three partitions. Note: since one of the partitions has previously been considered, the procedure only has to determine optimal splits for the two new partitions created by the previous split. This process is continuously repeated.

When y is quantitative, the value of cp tells us how much the value of R^2 (which is related to the sum of squared errors) must increase to justify an additional rule to the model. When y is categorical, the value of cp is related to the impurity. Smaller values of cp give more complex trees with more rules.

The procedure for choosing the "correct" size of the tree is as follows:

1. Build the tree to a very large size (e.g., take $cp = 0$).
2. At each step in the tree's growth, keep track of its estimated generalization error, number of splits, and complexity parameter (the amount by which R^2 increased or the impurity decreased as the most recent rule was added).
3. Plot the estimated generalization error vs. the complexity parameter of the tree.
4. The "optimal" complexity parameter is the one that gives the smallest estimated generalization error. If the one standard deviation rule is used, the "best" value is the largest cp whose generalization error is at most one standard deviation above the smallest value.
5. Note: the final selected tree is most likely *not* the one that will actually predict the best on new data. As with a predictive regression model, the chosen tree is the "best we can do" given the collected data, and it is impossible to anticipate exactly what model will be the best in the future.

Figures 9.11 through 9.13 show the estimated generalization error vs. the size and complexity of the partition models predicting college GPA and whether a customer opens a new account (`ACCOUNT` data). In both cases, the generalization errors decrease initially as the trees begin to grow. The trees eventually become overfit as "too many" rules are added. The optimal complexity parameter can either be found graphically or using the **complexity table**.

Since the estimated generalization error is found with repeated K-fold cross-validation, a random procedure, it is possible to come up with a different optimal tree if the procedure is repeated. This is one of the drawbacks of any predictive model-building procedure—the "optimal" tree is really just the optimal model for a *particular* set of validation samples. Thus, it is genuinely impossible to choose the absolute *best* model. This would require glimpsing into the future to see what the new values of y will be. In predictive modeling, we settle for one (of many) "good" models and hope for the best.

9.3 Variable importance

A variable can appear more than once in a tree or not at all. Likewise, some sequences of branches may utilize a particular variable while others may not. How can we obtain an idea of how useful a particular variable is for predicting y? One way is to count up the total sum of squared error reduction (or impurity reduction) when it is the splitting variable.

While this may gauge the importance of the variable to the tree, it may miss how useful the predictor "could" be for predicting y. For instance, imagine predictors x_1 and x_2 are highly correlated and are both highly associated with y (along with other predictors). When the tree "wants" to split by using the information contained in x_1 or x_2, the split will likely involve x_1 half the time and x_2 the other half. If the reductions in sum of squared errors due to x_1 or due to x_2 are counted up, they will be about half of what they would have been had one of those predictors been omitted. The importance of each variable will thus be about half of what it "should" be.

Figure 9.11 — Choosing size of the tree (quantitative). The model predicts college GPA from high school GPA, ACT, and gender. The plot below shows the estimated generalization error (found from repeated K-fold cross-validation) vs. the size and complexity parameter (cp) of the tree. The corresponding complexity table is presented as well. Note: the generalization error presented in the table is the error *relative to the naive model* (a tree with no splits that predicts y as the overall average $\bar{y}$ in the data). The tree becomes overfit as too many rules are added to the model, and the generalization error starts to increase.

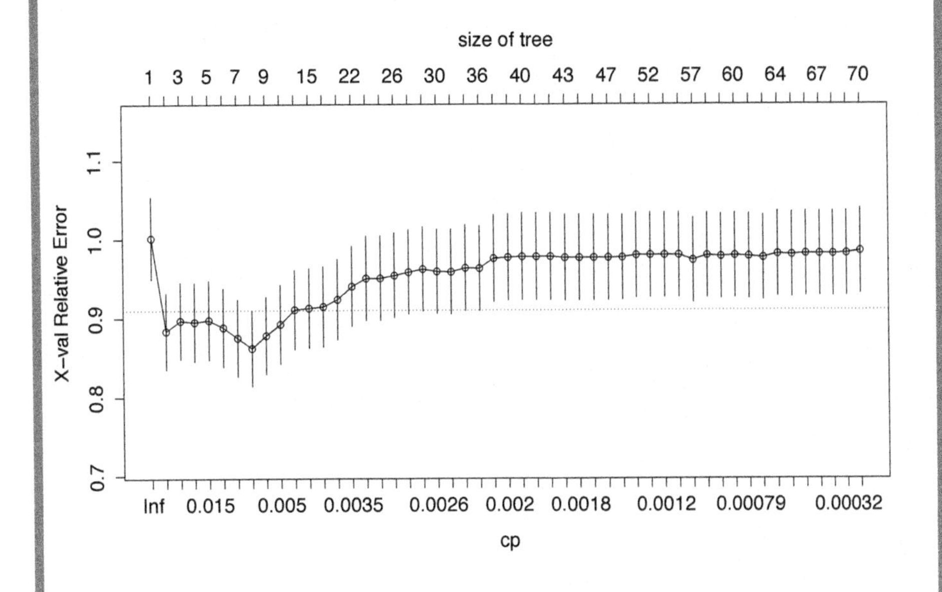

In R

```
set.seed(1337)
TREE <- rpart(CollegeGPA~HSGPA+ACT+Gender,data=EDUCATION,
              control=rpart.control(xval=10,minbucket=5,cp=0))
plotcp(TREE)
getcp(TREE)
                CP nsplit rel error    xerror       xstd
     0.1276366183      0 1.0000000 1.0015458 0.05183727
1SD* 0.0272972629      1 0.8723634 0.8835465 0.04836107
     0.0203523454      2 0.8450661 0.8968067 0.04875749
     ....
     0.0094775234      6 0.7822168 0.8749689 0.04869493
min* 0.0068238932      7 0.7727393 0.8617896 0.04788277
     0.0053610161      8 0.7659154 0.8779853 0.04885854
```

The lowest estimated generalization error occurs when the tree has eight partitions (seven splits) and a cp parameter of 0.0068 (see Figure 9.12). However, simpler trees look to be sufficient. The one standard deviation rule says that any tree whose error is within one standard deviation of the lowest is acceptable. A dotted line is drawn at one standard deviation above the lowest error, so any tree with an error below the dotted line is fine. The simplest tree we can choose has only a single split (two partitions).

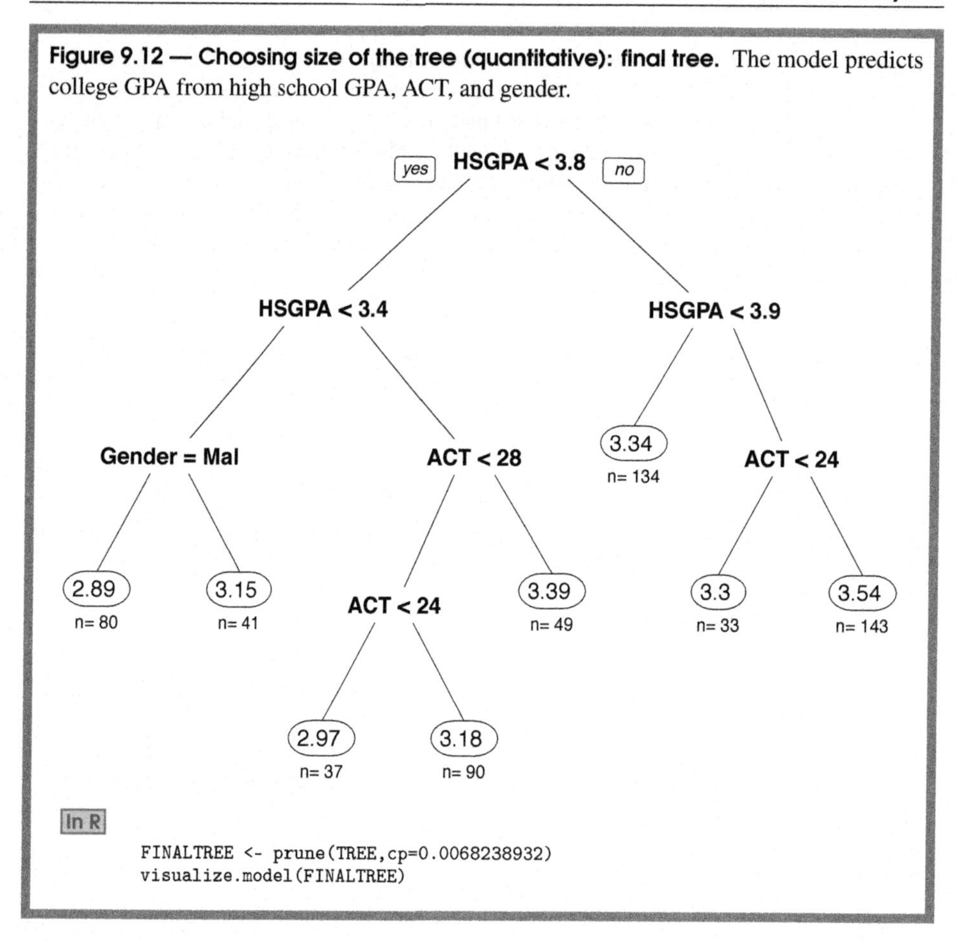

Figure 9.12 — Choosing size of the tree (quantitative): final tree. The model predicts college GPA from high school GPA, ACT, and gender.

```
FINALTREE <- prune(TREE,cp=0.0068238932)
visualize.model(FINALTREE)
```

9.3.1 Surrogate splits

The solution to this problem is to calculate a **surrogate split** for each splitting variable.

> Imagine x is the splitting variable. The surrogate variable for this split is the variable that best predicts x using a partition model with a single split. Note: this one-split partition model is completely unrelated to the tree being built to predict y.

For example, consider Figure 9.14, which shows the final partition model for the `ACCOUNT` dataset (predicting if someone will open a new account). The first split uses someone's savings balance. The surrogate variable for this split is the variable that best predicts savings balance (when using a partition model with a single split). In this case, the surrogate variable is someone's checking balance. Thus, every time savings balance shows up in the tree, checking balance is credited with some variable importance as well.

The overall importance of a predictor is a weighted sum of the decrease in sum of squared errors (or impurity) for the splits where it is either the splitting or surrogate variable. A variable that does not even appear in the tree can actually have a relatively high importance.

Figure 9.13 — Choosing size of the tree (categorical). The model predicts whether someone opens up a new account from how long he or she have been at the bank, checking and savings balances, income, etc. The plot shows the estimated generalization error (found from repeated K-fold cross-validation) vs. the size and complexity parameter (cp) of the tree. The corresponding complexity table is presented as well. The tree noticeably becomes overfit once too many (more than about 14) partitions are added—the estimated generalization error starts to increase as the complexity of the tree grows.

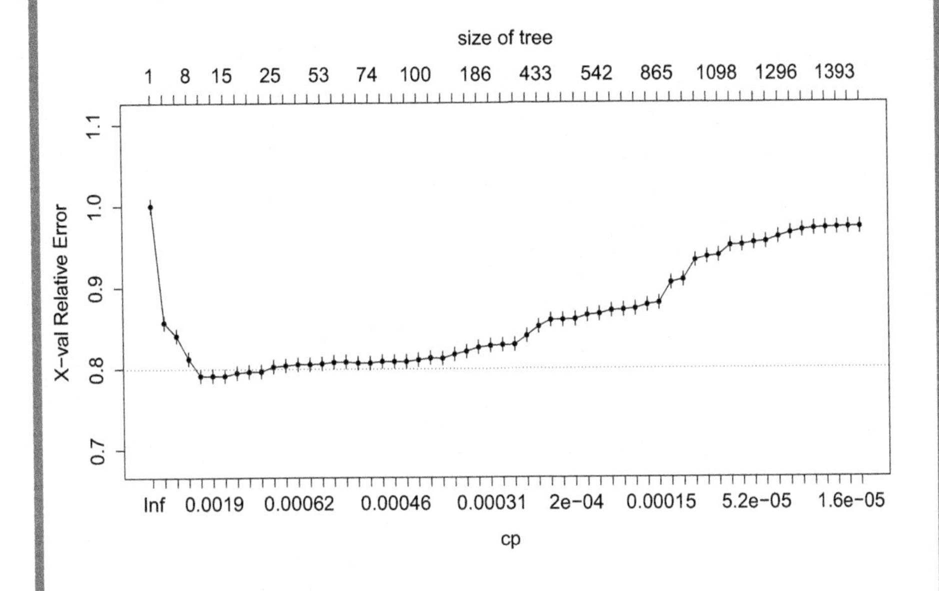

In R

```
set.seed(2015)
TREE <- rpart(Purchase~.,data=ACCOUNT,
              control=rpart.control(xval=10,minbucket=5,cp=0))
plotcp(TREE,pch=20)
getcp(TREE)
                CP nsplit rel error    xerror        xstd
     4.674577e-03      7 0.8103800 0.8120580 0.008374470
1SD* 2.636941e-03     11 0.7862879 0.7910823 0.008306908
     1.438332e-03     13 0.7810140 0.7912022 0.008307302
min* 1.318471e-03     14 0.7795757 0.7909625 0.008306514
     1.018818e-03     15 0.7782572 0.7947980 0.008319075
```

The lowest estimated generalization error occurs when the tree has 15 partitions (14 splits) and a cp parameter of 0.0013. According to the one standard deviation rule, we could choose a slightly simpler tree with only 11 splits. See Figure 9.14.

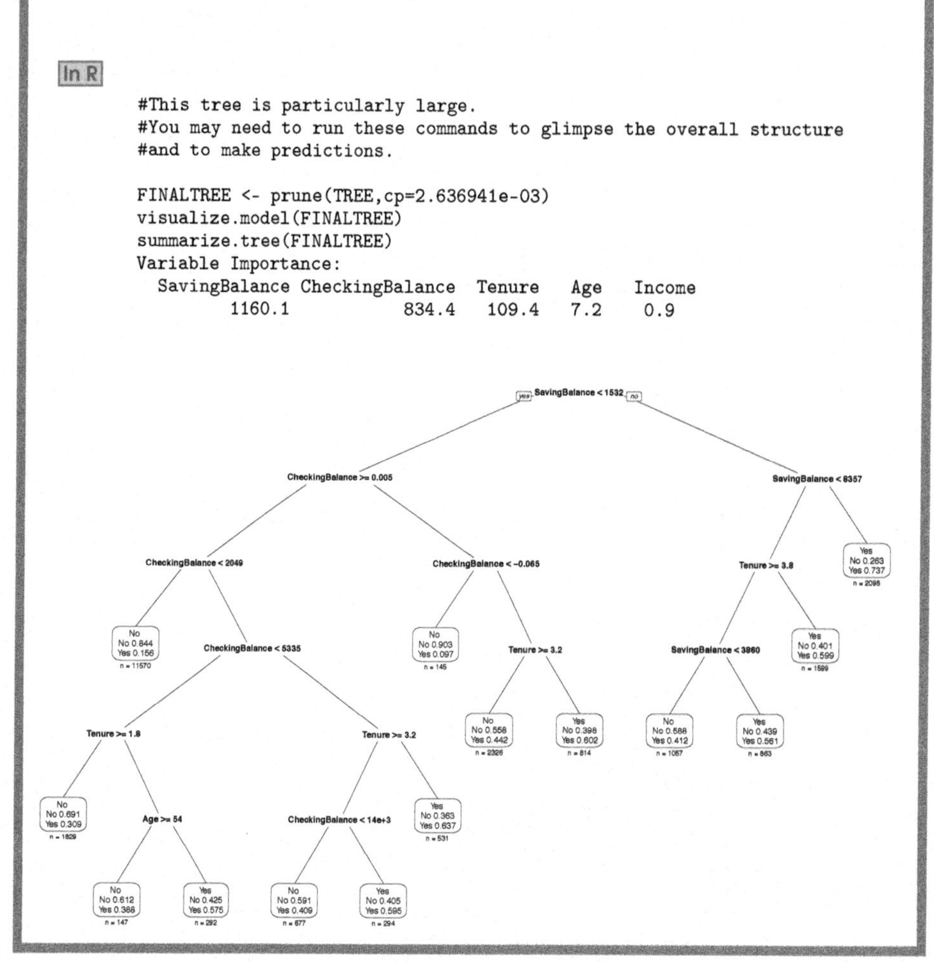

Figure 9.14 — Final model for ACCOUNT data. Savings and checking account balances are indeed the most important variables, and their presence is prominent near the base of the tree. Someone's tenure at the company appears three times, age once, and income not at all. Each variable's importance is listed below. Savings and checking balances are by far the most important variables. Notice that even though income is not in the tree, it still has a (very small) bit of importance. This is because it must have been a surrogate split for at least one of the variables in one of the branches.

In R

```
#This tree is particularly large.
#You may need to run these commands to glimpse the overall structure
#and to make predictions.

FINALTREE <- prune(TREE,cp=2.636941e-03)
visualize.model(FINALTREE)
summarize.tree(FINALTREE)
Variable Importance:
  SavingBalance CheckingBalance  Tenure   Age   Income
         1160.1           834.4   109.4   7.2      0.9
```

Also in Figure 9.14 is a list of the variable importances. The most important variable is savings balance, with an "importance" of 1160. However, only the *relative* values (not actual values) of the importance matter here. The importance of checking balance is 834, about 72% (834/1160) of the importance of savings. Income has only 0.08% (0.94/1160) of the importance of checking balance. In this case, these numbers roughly match the frequencies in which the variables appear in the tree. Income (the least important variable) doesn't appear in the tree, but it still has some importance due to the fact that for at least one split it acts as a surrogate.

9.3.2 Connection to variable creation

At the beginning of the chapter, we saw that a discontinuous, nonlinear relationship (Figure 9.1) could still be modeled with a linear regression with a clever choice of variables. Alternatively, a partition model could provide a reasonable approximation to the relationship.

$$y = \begin{cases} 17, & \text{if } 5 \leq x \leq 6 \quad 21, \text{ if } 6 < x \leq 7 \quad 24, \text{ if } 7 < x \leq 8 \\ 26, & \text{if } 8 \leq x < 12 \quad 14, \text{ if } 12 < x \leq 14 \quad 12, \text{ if } x > 14 \end{cases}$$

In this example, the data space is split into six total partitions. Imagine treating the partition to which the individual belongs as a *characteristic* of that individual, i.e., a level of a categorical variable. Then, we can write the partition model *as* a regression equation with a single categorical predictor variable. For the above example:

$$y = 17 + 4x_1 + 7x_2 + 9x_3 - 3x_4 - 5x_5$$

Here, $x_1, x_2, \ldots, x_5$ are indicator variables encoding to which partition the individual belongs. The "reference" level we can take to be when $5 \leq x \leq 6$.

$$x_1 = \begin{cases} 1, & \text{if } 6 < x \leq 7 \\ 0, & \text{otherwise} \end{cases} \quad x_2 = \begin{cases} 1, & \text{if } 7 < x \leq 8 \\ 0, & \text{otherwise} \end{cases} \quad x_5 = \begin{cases} 1, & \text{if } x > 14 \\ 0, & \text{otherwise} \end{cases}$$

Thus, at its core, building a partition model can be viewed as a fancy technique for *variable creation*. Once the partitions have been defined, the model essentially predicts y using the partition identities as levels of a categorical variable.

If one is willing to assume that the difference between individuals' values of y and the average value of y in the partition are Normally distributed (with the same standard deviation), then the regression model framework can be used to provide confidence intervals for coefficients or to provide prediction intervals for new individuals.

9.4 Random forests

As we will see in a few examples, a classification or regression tree is typically a relatively weak predictor of y—regression models often have smaller generalization errors. The goal of a **random forest** is to combine the results of many individual trees and hopefully turn a multitude of weak predictors into a single strong predictor. As the name suggests, a forest consists of a few hundred or more trees. However, the individual trees in a random forest differ from a tree in a partition model in significant ways.

- Each tree is constructed using a *random* sample of the training data. This "alternative" training set is generated by randomly picking (with replacement) observations from the original training data. Some cases will appear more than once in the alternative training set, while others will not appear at all. Typically, about $2/3$ of the original training cases end up being present in any given alternative training set.

- When a new rule is to be added to the tree, only a *subset* of predictors are chosen as candidates for splitting variables. In a partition model, every variable is considered when finding the best split. The predictors that are considered for a tree in a random forest are randomly re-selected for each split. Typically, if k is the number of available predictors, then $k/3$ predictors are chosen for consideration if y is quantitative or $\sqrt{k}$ if y is categorical.
- The tree is grown to the maximum possible size, i.e., until each leaf contains only a single observation. There is no pruning back to a simpler tree with an optimal complexity parameter.

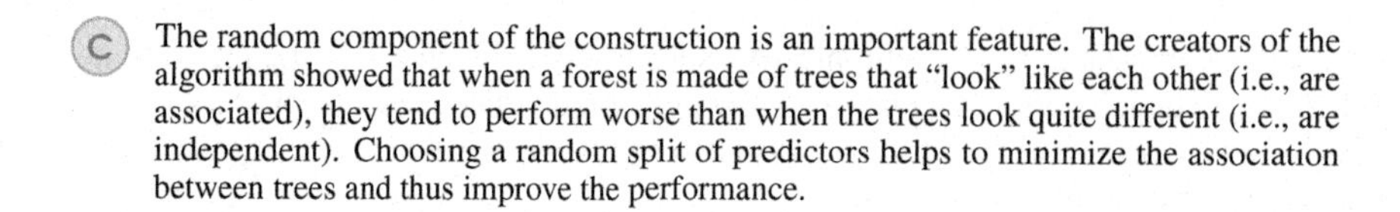
The random component of the construction is an important feature. The creators of the algorithm showed that when a forest is made of trees that "look" like each other (i.e., are associated), they tend to perform worse than when the trees look quite different (i.e., are independent). Choosing a random split of predictors helps to minimize the association between trees and thus improve the performance.

After every tree in the forest has been built, predictions are made by combining the predictions of the individual trees. If y is quantitative, the predicted value is the average of the predicted values from each tree. If y is categorical, the predicted probability of a level is the proportion of trees that predict that level (the case is classified as whichever level has the highest probability).

Random forests also have some features that are very useful:

- Increasing the number of trees does not decrease the performance of the algorithm (in fact, the more trees, the better). Many other advanced algorithms become "overfit" when a model becomes more complex.
- An unbiased estimate of the generalization error is found automatically during construction with no need to perform cross-validation. The $\approx 1/3$ of the original training set that is left out when making the artificial training set is used to estimate the error.

Random forests are on the cutting edge of predictive modeling and are often more successful than regression techniques and other advanced models, especially when y is a categorical variable. In fact, they are one of the top-performing techniques and are often used as baselines for data competitions such as the ones on `kaggle.com`.

9.5 Pros and cons of partition models

Partition models and random forests have many advantages over regression models.

- They are faster to develop on large datasets with many variables.
- They handle categorical variables without creating new indicator variables.
- They are not as sensitive to outliers.
- They naturally incorporate complex interactions between variables (x_2 may have different splitting rules depending on the values of x_1).
- They are equation-free and approachable when the number of rules is small.

Random forests tend to perform much better than single partition models. However, they have a few key drawbacks:

- They often lack interpretability. It's not possible to say "larger values of x are associated with larger values of y," etc. How y and x vary together is hidden in the tree.

- They do not perform as well as regression models when regression is actually an appropriate model (e.g., linear relationships between y and the predictors).
- A partition model is usually overfit (even when cross-validation is used to determine its size). Random forests do not typically overfit.
- There are no tests of significance about predictors.
- There is no way to immediately find confidence/prediction intervals for new data.
- Splitting procedures have a slight bias toward splitting on categorical variables with many levels.
- The entire tree structure can be sensitive to a single observation. While the predicted values may not change much when a new point is added to or deleted from the data, the decision rules can change drastically. This is not an issue for random forests since there are so many trees.

9.6 Examples and using R

Let us walk through a few examples in predictive analytics to illustrate the successes and failures of the regression, partition, and random forest frameworks. In R, fitting a partition model or random forest is very easy.

- Set the random number seed. Since the estimated generalization error of a tree is found using K-fold cross-validation (a random procedure), it is important to prime the random number generator for reproducibility. Any integer will do.

```
set.seed(1337)
```

- Fit the initial (overly complex) tree. In the code below, `xval` gives K for the K-fold cross-validation and `minbucket` gives the minimum number of individuals allowed to be in a partition (a partition cannot be split if it has this many or fewer individuals).

```
TREE <- rpart(y~.,data=DATA,control=rpart.control(xval=10,minbucket=5,cp=0))
```

- Examine the CP table of the tree to see how many rules and splits it should contain (typically using the one standard deviation rule).

```
getcp(TREE)
```

- Prune the tree down to the relevant complexity (copy/paste the relevant value of cp from the CP table).

```
FINALTREE <- prune(TREE,cp=)
```

- Visualize the tree and examine variable importance.

```
visualize.model(FINALTREE)
summarize.tree(FINALTREE)
```

- Find the generalization error on the holdout sample (called `HOLDOUT`).

```
generalization.error(FINALTREE,HOLDOUT)
```

- To fit a random forest, first set the random number seed (so that the forest can be reproduced). Specify the number of trees (the more, the better) with `ntree`. Note: there are optional additional arguments that can be added (such as the number of randomly selected variables to consider at each split), but the defaults are typically fine. If you want to know the relative importance of each predictor, be sure to say `importance=TRUE`.

```
FOREST <- randomForest(y~.,data=DATA,ntree=,importance=TRUE)
summarize.tree(FOREST)
generalization.error(FOREST,HOLDOUT)
```

9.6.1 Census Analytics

The census dataset (CENSUS) examines characteristics of block groups (on average about 39 blocks containing a total of 600-3000 people). The quantity of interest is the response rate, which is the percentage (0-100) of households that returned the census form (as required by law) by the deadline. Households that do not mail in the form are visited by workers who must conduct interviews to get all the necessary information. It is useful to predict the response rate so that the government can more efficiently allocate these follow-up workers.

In this particular set of the data, there are 3534 block groups and nearly 40 predictor variables, e.g., the percentage of the block group located in rural, suburban, or urban areas, the percentage of people who are female, information about the age and racial makeup, information about living arrangements (married, with kids, with related family), income levels, the percentage of houses owned, rented, vacant, or occupied, and the house value.

Let us randomly split the data into training and holdout samples, where the holdout has 1000 cases. How does the generalization error on the holdout sample compare for the regression, partition, and random forest models?

With so many potential predictors, finding an appropriate regression model takes a while. The partition model is built using the one standard deviation rule and ends up having nearly 100 splits. The random forest uses 500 trees.

Aside 9.3 shows the procedure in R, and Figure 9.15 gives a plot of the predicted vs. actual values and a summary of the importance of predictors and model performances. In short, the random forest has a smaller generalization error than the regression model, which in turn has a smaller generalization error than the partition model.

In this case, the random forest is the best performer with an error on the holdout sample that is 1.4% lower than that of the regression model. The partition model has the largest holdout error. It may be the case that a better regression model could be found if interactions were considered. However, the time required to build a predictive regression model with them is immense.

Census model	Regression	Partition	Forest
$RMSE_{holdout}$	4.678	5.443	4.612

9.6.2 NFL analytics

The goal of the NFL dataset is to predict the number of wins (from 2002-2011) over the course of a season (a maximum of 16) from more than 100 predictors such as offensive and defensive statistics (number of first downs, fumbles, rushing yards, etc.). Let us take the 2001 through 2009 seasons to be the training data and the 2010 through 2012 seasons to be the holdout sample. Note: this is an example where a model may need to change over time as the NFL evolves.

If coaches are willing to buy into cause/effect relationships, the most important variables in the model provide ideas of where coaches and players should improve. The variables that appear in a predictive model of course do not necessarily have cause/effect relationships with y (the regression equation is not a physical law), so we need to be careful not to overinterpret the variable's importance. If fumbles appear in the final model, it doesn't mean that having an additional fumble *causes* a team to lose the game, or that decreasing the number of fumbles will *cause* the team to win more games.

Aside 9.3 — Predictive model for CENSUS data. Building a predictive model involves splitting the data into training/holdout samples, trying out regression, partition, and random forest models on the training sample, then determining which predicts the best on the holdout sample. The random forest provides the best predictive model for this dataset.

The following code demonstrates the analysis using the `regclass` package. It is important to set the seeds to the numbers displayed or your results may be different.

In R

```
#Split data into training/holdout
set.seed(2015)
train.rows <- sample(1:nrow(CENSUS),2534,replace=TRUE)
TRAIN <- CENSUS[train.rows,]
HOLDOUT <- CENSUS[-train.rows,]
```

```
#Find a good regression model and get its generalization error
MODELS <- build.model(ResponseRate~.,data=TRAIN)
REG <- lm(MODELS$bestformula,data=TRAIN)
generalization.error(REG,HOLDOUT)
  $RMSE.holdout
  [1] 4.972701
```

```
#Find a good partition model
set.seed(1999)
TREE <- rpart(ResponseRate~.,data=TRAIN,
             control=rpart.control(xval=10,minbucket=5,cp=0))
getcp(TREE)
       1.218868e-03      98 0.2034760 0.4134933 0.01630070
  1SD* 1.216797e-03      99 0.2022572 0.4132245 0.01629810
       1.209061e-03     101 0.1998236 0.4137465 0.01633980
FINALTREE <- prune(TREE,cp=0.001216797)
generalization.error(FINALTREE,HOLDOUT)
  $RMSE.holdout
  [1] 6.196634
```

```
#Fit a random forest with 500 trees
set.seed(2020)
FOREST <- randomForest(ResponseRate~.,data=TRAIN,ntrees=500,
importance=TRUE)
generalization.error(FOREST,HOLDOUT)
  $RMSE.holdout
  [1] 4.798895
```

The random forest model has the lowest $RMSE_{holdout}$ in this instance. For this particular split of training/holdout samples, it is the "best" technique. Using a different random number seed and training/holdout split, the model with the lowest generalization error may change. In this case, the random forest is the winner for most training/holdout splits.

Figure 9.15 — Census models. A comparison of the predicted vs. actual values of the regression, partition, and random forest models shows a relatively good match, though some techniques perform better than others. The random forest ends up having the smallest error on the holdout sample at 4.80 compared to the regression at 4.97 (partition is much worse at 6.20). Further, it appears that the predictions made by the random forest have the highest correlation with the actual values in the holdout sample.

The most important variables deal with the fraction of renting and homeowner households, followed by who heads the household, a bit of racial information, and age information. The actual values of these numbers are not important. Only the relative sizes matter.

In R

```
summarize.tree(TREE)
HomeownerHH RentingHH   MarriedHH    RelatedHH    NoSpouseHH
58460.6878  46422.7281  38931.5221   33266.3025   30645.4989

summarize.tree(FOREST)
                      %IncMSE IncNodePurity
HomeownerHH         24.6771119    25844.1906
RentingHH           20.7783217    17906.1099
Whites              10.8700350    13743.5690
Age18to24            8.0380109    11374.9045
FemaleHH             9.0959563     8682.6433
MarriedHH            6.8370728     5654.3013
```

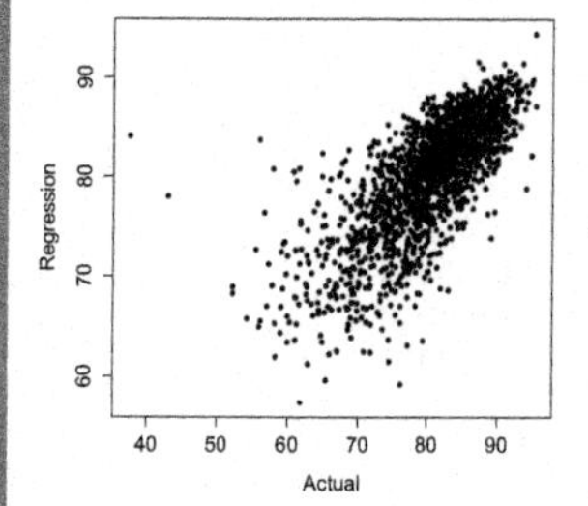

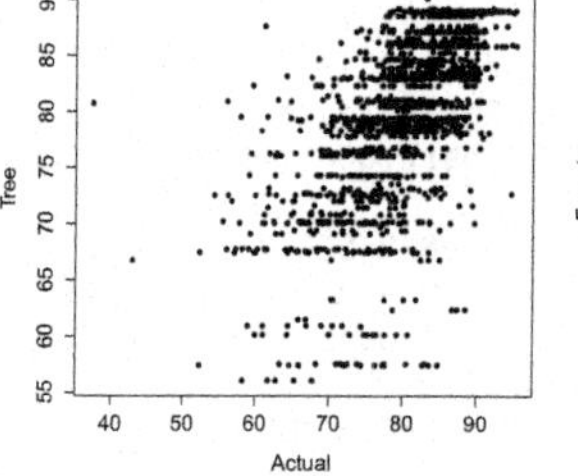

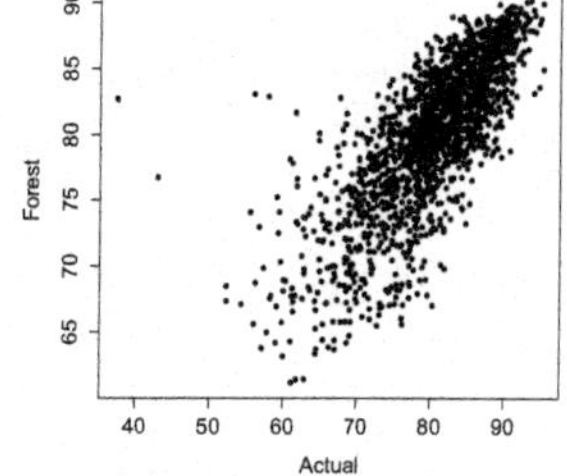

In R

```
#Predicted vs. Actual for regression model
r.predict <- predict(REG,newdata=HOLDOUT)
plot(r.predict~HOLDOUT$ResponseRate,pch=20,xlab="Actual",ylab="Regression")

#Predicted vs. Actual for partition model
t.predict <- predict(FINALTREE,newdata=HOLDOUT)
plot(t.predict~HOLDOUT$ResponseRate,pch=20,xlab="Actual",ylab="Tree")

#Predicted vs. Actual for random forest model
f.predict <- predict(FOREST,newdata=HOLDOUT)
plot(f.predict~HOLDOUT$ResponseRate,pch=20,xlab="Actual",ylab="Forest")
```

Aside 9.4 — Predictive model for wins of an NFL team. Building a predictive model involves splitting the data into training/holdout samples, trying out regression, partition, and random forest models on the training sample, then determining which predicts the best on the holdout sample. The regression model (even though it was found using AIC criteria) provides the best predictive model for this dataset.

In R

```
#Split the data into training (2002-2009) and holdout (2010-2012)
TRAIN <- NFL[1:256,]
HOLDOUT <- NFL[257:352,]

#Search for a regression model with a low AIC
naive.model <- lm(X4.Wins~1,data=TRAIN)
full.model <- lm(X4.Wins~.,data=TRAIN)
S <- step(naive.model,scope=list(lower=naive.model,upper=full.model),
          direction="both",trace=0)
generalization.error(S,HOLDOUT)
  $RMSE.holdout
  [1] 1.450349

#Partition model
set.seed(773)
TREE <- rpart(X4.Wins~.,data=TRAIN,
              control=rpart.control(xval=10,minbucket=5,cp=0 ))
getcp(TREE)
     0.009283856     13 0.16698333 0.4951381 0.04201773
1SD* 0.009197264     14 0.15769947 0.4537819 0.03931723
     0.008920294     15 0.14850221 0.4531876 0.03936330
     0.007352936     16 0.13958191 0.4507790 0.03936446
min* 0.006156838     17 0.13222898 0.4373007 0.03826602
     0.005773792     18 0.12607214 0.4472630 0.03891168
FINALTREE <- prune(TREE,cp=0.009197264)
generalization.error(FINALTREE,HOLDOUT)
  $RMSE.holdout
  [1] 2.076022

#Random Forest
set.seed(3388)
FOREST <- randomForest(X4.Wins~.,data=TRAIN,ntrees=500,importance=TRUE)
generalization.error(FOREST,HOLDOUT)
  $RMSE.holdout
  [1] 1.605111
```

How does the generalization error on the holdout sample compare for the regression, partition, and random forest models? In this case, due to the large number of predictor variables, let us choose the regression model with a low AIC with a search, starting with the naive model. See Aside 9.4 and Figure 9.16 for details.

In this case, the regression model outperforms the random forest. The relationship between the number of wins and the predictors (as we have seen) is quite linear. When a linear regression is appropriate, the regression will often outperform any tree-based models.

NFL model	Regression	Partition	Forest
$RMSE_{holdout}$	1.45	2.08	1.61

Figure 9.16 — NFL model. The selected partition model is the simplest one whose estimated generalization error is at most one standard deviation above the lowest error observed. In this case, the size of the tree has 14 splits.

A comparison of the predicted vs. actual values of the regression model (found via AIC search), partition model, and random forest shows a decent matchup. The regression model looks to have equal amounts of over- and underestimations of the actual number of wins. The random forest may have a bias—when the actual number of wins is low, the forest tends to predict slightly more wins, and when the actual number of wins is high, the forest tends to predict slightly fewer wins.

The winning model here is the regression with a $RMSE_{holdout}$ of 1.45 compared to 1.61 for the random forest and 2.08 for the partition model. The most important variable is the number of yards per point.

In R

```
summarize.tree(FOREST)
                                      %IncMSE IncNodePurity
X110.OffYdsPt                    1.3417366420   369.6006845
X26.OffPassAdjNetYdsperAtt       0.6775144703   219.8615284
X96.DefKickReturnsAlwd           0.5262466980   167.9376026
X111.DefYdsPt                    0.6133474423   139.6909223
X25.OffPassNetYdsperAtt          0.4515415886   129.1144124
X22.OffPasserRating              0.3031254801   101.1878065
X20.OffPassAdjYdsperAtt          0.2921377196    94.8601616
X89.DefPassAdjNetYdsperAttAlwd   0.3541799211    93.9429957
```

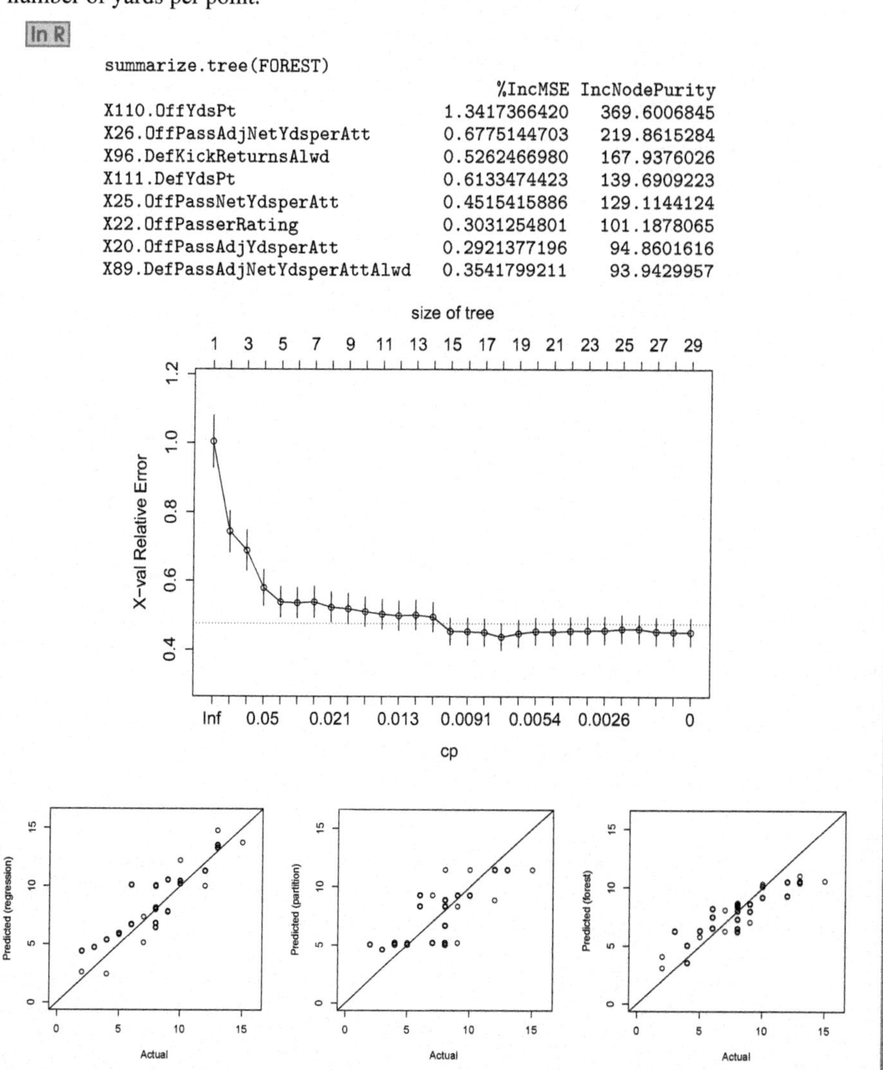

9.6.3 Predicting Churn

From the viewpoint of a bank or cell-phone company, a customer "churns" when he or she closes an account or does not renew a contract. Attrition analysis is a key focus for any customer-oriented company. Consider the CHURN dataset. We want to predict whether customers of a wireless company will churn at the end of their contract. The data contains details of 5000 customers, such as their usage (how many day minutes, night minutes, etc.), whether they have an international plan, and the number of customer service calls they have made.

Let us create a holdout sample of size 1000. As with our other examples, the regression model will be conducted via AIC search (starting with the naive model) to save time, the partition model will be the simplest one whose estimated generalization error is at most one standard deviation above the lowest value, and the random forest uses 500 trees. Aside 9.5 and Figure 9.17 show details of the search and models.

Figure 9.17 — Churn model. The selected partition model is the simplest one whose estimated generalization error is at most one standard deviation above the lowest error observed. In this case, the tree has 23 splits.

Based on the misclassification rate (or the false negative rate, i.e., fraction of customers who did churn but the model predicted otherwise), the random forest is the best model. Its misclassification rate is only 3.4% (logistic regression is 12.7%), and its false negative rate is 20% (logistic regression is 74%).

The four most important variables are the total number of minutes and amount spent during the daytime, the number of customer service calls, and whether the customer had an international plan.

In R

```
summarize.tree(FOREST)
                                       No MeanDecreaseGini
totaldayminutes             5.028119e-02        134.42849
totaldaycharge              5.031072e-02        129.07120
numbercustomerservicecalls  2.301567e-02        113.39942
internationalplan           1.971259e-02         84.38340
```

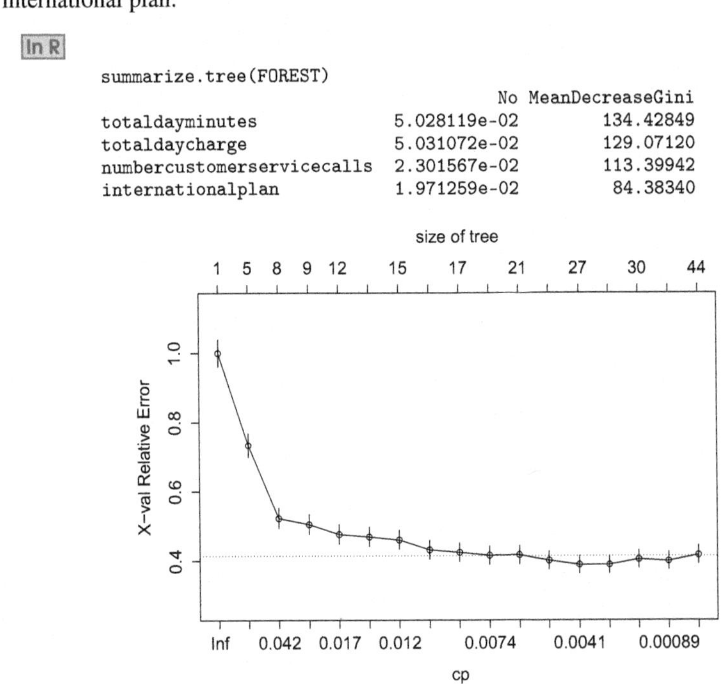

Aside 9.5 — Predictive model for CHURN. Building a predictive model involves splitting the data into training/holdout samples, trying out regression, partition, and random forest models on the training sample, then determining which predicts the best on the holdout sample. The random forest provides the best predictive model for this dataset.

In R

```
#Split data into training and holdout
set.seed(1337)
training.rows <- sample(nrow(CHURN),4000)
TRAINING <- CHURN[training.rows,]
HOLDOUT <- CHURN[-training.rows,]

#Regression model
naive.model <- glm(churn~1,data=TRAINING,family="binomial")
full.model <- glm(churn~.,data=TRAINING,family="binomial")
S <- step(naive.model,scope=list(lower=naive.model,upper=full.model),
          direction="both",trace=0)
generalization.error(S,HOLDOUT)
  $Confusion.Matrices$Holdout
                    Predicted No Predicted Yes Total
   Actual No                 834            18   852
   Actual Yes                109            39   148
   Total                     943            57  1000
   $Misclassification.Rates$Holdout
   [1] 0.127

#Partition model
set.seed(4242)
TREE <- rpart(churn~.,data=TRAINING,
          control=rpart.control(xval=10,minbucket=5,cp=0 ))
getcp(TREE)
        0.0071556351        19 0.3166369 0.4150268 0.02644586
        0.0053667263        20 0.3094812 0.4168157 0.02649927
   1SD* 0.0047704234        23 0.2933810 0.4007156 0.02601346
   min* 0.0035778175        26 0.2790698 0.3881932 0.02562750
        0.0026833631        27 0.2754919 0.3881932 0.02562750
FINALTREE <- prune(TREE,cp=0.0047704234)
generalization.error(FINALTREE,HOLDOUT)
  $CM.holdout
                    Predicted No Predicted Yes Total
   Actual No                 846             6   852
   Actual Yes                 44           104   148
   Total                     890           110  1000
   $misclass.holdout
   [1] 0.05

#Random forest
set.seed(9191)
FOREST <- randomForest(churn~.,data=TRAINING,ntree=500,importance=TRUE)
generalization.error(FOREST,HOLDOUT)
  $CM.holdout
                    Predicted No Predicted Yes Total
   Actual No                 847             5   852
   Actual Yes                 34           114   148
   Total                     881           119  1000
   $misclass.holdout
   [1] 0.039
```

The random forest has the lowest misclassification rate at 3.9%, followed by the partition model at 5% and the logistic regression at 12.7%. A more interesting quantity may be the number of false negatives—customers that are not predicted to churn but who churn anyway. These represent missed opportunities where the company may have been able to intervene to entice these customers to stay. The false negatives are the lower-left number in the confusion matrix. The logistic regression is particularly bad. The model fails to find 109 (74%) of the 148 customers who churned. The random forest only fails to find 34 (20%) of them. Overall, the random forest procedure is the clear winner. Not only does the procedure take less time than finding a decent logistic regression model, but it performs much better too.

9.6.4 Email analytics

In the early 1990s, junk mail filters were developed using word frequencies (e.g., mail, receive, offer, free, hello), punctuation frequencies (like !, $, #), and the number of capital letters in a row. The junk mail dataset (JUNK) has 57 total predictors. Let us randomly split the data into 1000 cases for the holdout sample and have the remaining 3501 for training. See Aside 9.6 and Figure 9.18 for details.

Figure 9.18 — JUNK mail model. The selected partition model is the simplest one whose estimated generalization error is at most one standard deviation above the lowest error observed. In this case, the tree has 38 rules. The two most important variables are the appearance of exclamation points and dollar signs. The most important word is "remove," perhaps because junk emails often say "to remove your email from the list...".

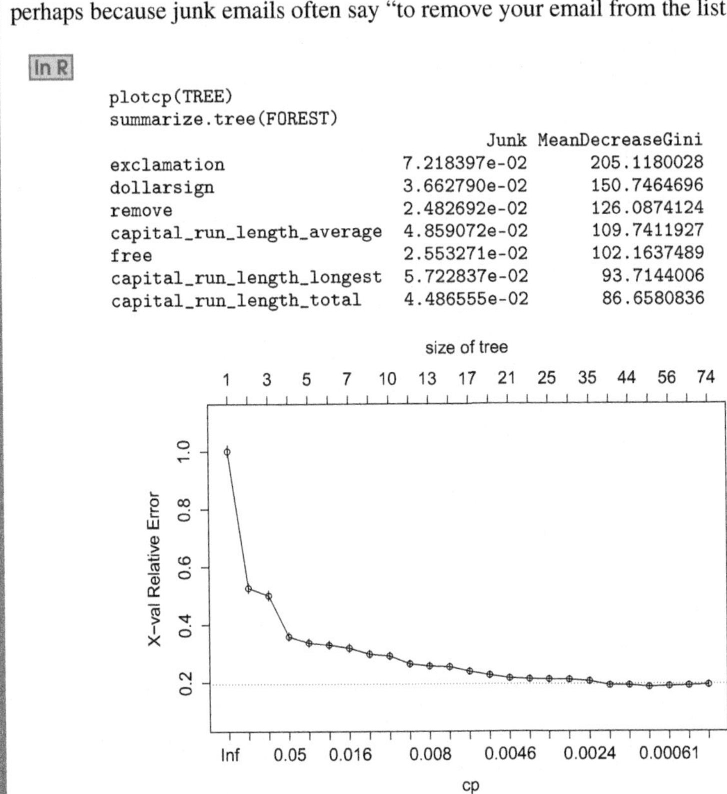

In R

```
plotcp(TREE)
summarize.tree(FOREST)
                                    Junk MeanDecreaseGini
exclamation                 7.218397e-02      205.1180028
dollarsign                  3.662790e-02      150.7464696
remove                      2.482692e-02      126.0874124
capital_run_length_average  4.859072e-02      109.7411927
free                        2.553271e-02      102.1637489
capital_run_length_longest  5.722837e-02       93.7144006
capital_run_length_total    4.486555e-02       86.6580836
```

Aside 9.6 — Predictive model for junk mail. Building a predictive model involves splitting the data into training/holdout samples, trying out regression, partition, and random forest models on the training sample, then determining which predicts the best on the holdout sample. The random forest provides the best predictive model for this dataset by far.

In R

```
#Split into training and holdout
set.seed(2020)
train.rows <- sample(1:nrow(JUNK),3501,replace=TRUE)
TRAIN <- JUNK[train.rows,]
HOLDOUT <- JUNK[-train.rows,]

#Logistic regression
naive.model <- glm(Junk~1,data=TRAIN,family=binomial)
full.model <- glm(Junk~.,data=TRAIN,family=binomial)
S <- step(naive.model,scope=list(lower=naive.model,upper=full.model),
          direction="both",trace=0)
generalization.error(S,HOLDOUT)
  $Confusion.Matrices$Holdout
                 Predicted Junk Predicted Safe Total
   Actual Junk              758             71   829
   Actual Safe               81           1230  1311
   Total                    839           1301  2140
  $Misclassification.Rates$Holdout
  [1] 0.07102804


#Partition model
set.seed(9382)
TREE <- rpart(Junk~.,data=TRAIN,
              control=rpart.control(xval=10,minbucket=5,cp=0 ))
getcp(TREE)
                CP nsplit rel error    xerror       xstd
     0.0028109628     31 0.14125088 0.2094167 0.01160341
     0.0021082221     34 0.13281799 0.2037948 0.01146089
1SD* 0.0017568517     38 0.12438510 0.1897400 0.01109301
     0.0014054814     43 0.11454673 0.1897400 0.01109301
min* 0.0007027407     47 0.10892481 0.1841181 0.01094095
     0.0005270555     55 0.10189740 0.1869290 0.01101735
FINALTREE <- prune(TREE,cp=0.0017568517)
generalization.error(FINALTREE,HOLDOUT)
  $CM.holdout
                 Predicted Junk Predicted Safe Total
   Actual Junk              744             85   829
   Actual Safe              100           1211  1311
   Total                    844           1296  2140

  $misclass.holdout
  [1] 0.0864486


#Random Forest
set.seed(4842)
FOREST <- randomForest(Junk~.,data=TRAIN,ntrees=500,importance=TRUE)
generalization.error(FOREST,HOLDOUT)
$CM.holdout
             Predicted Junk Predicted Safe Total
Actual Junk             771             58   829
Actual Safe              33           1278  1311
Total                   804           1336  2140

$misclass.holdout
[1] 0.04252336
```

The random forest has the lowest misclassification rate on the holdout sample at 4.3%. Second place is the regression model at 7.1%. The partition model has a misclassification rate of 8.6%. In practice, the most important type of error is when an email that is safe is predicted to be junk, a "false positive," so to speak (bottom left in confusion matrix). Of the 1311 safe emails in the holdout sample, the logistic regression flags 83 (6.3%) as junk, the partition model flags 100 (7.6%), while the random forest flags 33 (2.5%).

A follow-up analysis of the most important variables is interesting. Based on the random forest, the most important predictors are the fraction of characters in the email that are ! or $ (if you are old enough to have seen early junk mail, this seems reasonable), followed by the word "remove" (i.e., click here to remove yourself from this list) and the number of capital letters that appear all in a row.

9.7 Summary

Partition models are a new and exciting way to approach predictive modeling. Unlike linear or logistic regression models, they make no structural or distributional assumptions about the form of the relationships between y and the predictors. This allows them to be extremely flexible and general. For large or complex datasets, partition models are quicker to build, and random forests typically outperform regression techniques.

At its core, a partition model is just a set of rules. For example, if a person has a checking account, a savings account with more than $100, and a yearly income of less than $40,000, then the person has a 30% chance of being interested in a new account. These rules tend to group similar individuals together. As the expression goes: "Birds of a feather flock together." The strategy is to predict an individual's y-value using the y-values of that individual's "neighbors." A partition model just figures out what characteristics are important for grouping individuals together.

A single partition model is typically a fairly poor predictor of y. The random forests procedure creates hundreds of different partition models and combines their predictions to make (very often) a good predictor of y. By injecting randomness in the data and predictors each tree sees, the random forest procedure typically predicts better than regression models.

In a way, partition models (and other advanced techniques we have not discussed) are really the future of predictive modeling. Regression, which has been the focus of this course, was invented in a time before computers when datasets were small and relationships were fairly simple. While regression still can be quite useful for *describing* these simple relationships, it is typically not a technique that is competitive for predictive modeling. The biggest issue is that fitting a large number of regression models is very time-consuming, and estimating the generalization error is also quite slow.

Indeed, you may have wondered why the base package of `R` does not have procedures that conduct searches for regression models using estimated generalization error as the criterion for when a variable should enter or leave the model. The answer is that these days, this type of model is probably not the one that will be the most useful (and it takes too long).

9.8 Exercises

1: Use `EX9.BIRTHWEIGHT`. This dataset contains the birthweights of babies along with characteristics of the mother and father (including whether the mother smoked during preganancy). We want to predict `Birthweight`.

a) Because our aim is predictive modeling, the first step is to split the original data into training and holdout samples, specifying the random number seed (use 100 here) so that we can reproduce the results. Let's take 80% of the data to be training.
b) Use `build.model()` to find a good predictive regression model. Be sure to pass the argument `seed=1010` for reproducibility. Do not consider interactions. Fit this model and find its generalization error on the holdout sample. Would you say that it generalizes well?
c) Build a partition model, being sure to `set.seed(12)` immediately before using `rpart`. Use the cp suggested by the one standard deviation rule when pruning the tree. Look at a visualization of the tree, find the three most important variables to the tree, and find the generalization error of the tree. Would you say this model generalizes well?
d) Using your tree, predict the birthweight of a baby whose gestation period was 40, born to non-smoking Asian mother (height 60, weight 120) aged 26 with high school education who was married to an Asian man aged 26 (height 62, weight 140) with college education.
e) Construct a random forest using 1000 trees (this takes some time). Report the three most important variables in the forest and report its generalization error on the holdout sample. Note: immediately before running `randomForest()`, be sure to do `set.seed(2020)`.
f) Which technique gave the best predictive model? Is this model any *good* for making predictions? Note: 1 pound is about 454 grams (the units of birthweight). You may use your own judgment, but I would consider a useful model to typically get to within 0.5 lbs.

2: Use `EX9.NFL`, which is a part of the NFL analytics dataset (and contains statistics only from offense). The goal is to predict `Wins` (the number of wins in a season) based on characteristics of the team's performance over the course of a season.

a) Split the data into training/holdout samples like you did in #1 (use 100 as the random number seed). Use 75% of the data this time for the training sample.
b) Build the largest tree possible on the training data, run `getcp()`, and report the value of the optimal complexity parameter based on the one standard deviation rule. Note: as in #1 b, immediately before running `rpart()`, be sure to `set.seed(12)`.
c) Prune the tree to the optimal size using the `cp` you determined above. Look at a plot of the tree and also report the three most important predictors.
d) For the sake of illustration, imagine every predictor in the data equals 5. What would you predict for the number of wins in this case?
e) Report the generalization rate of your final tree on the holdout sample.
f) Construct a random forest using 1000 trees and report its generalization error on the holdout sample. Note: immediately before running `randomForest()`, be sure to do `set.seed(2020)`.
g) Using `build.model()` and the one standard deviation rule, find the best predictive model (exclude the possibility of interactions, and set the random number seed to 2015 in `build.model`). Even though a million models need to be fit, regression is fast, and it doesn't take that long. The best model will have four predictors. Fit it and report the generalization error on the holdout, noting that this time regression trumps the tree models.

3: Use `EX9.STORE`. This is part of a bank's transactional database and keeps track if customers had or had not shopped in each of 68 particular stores over the last 90 days. Let us predict whether a customer has shopped at `Store10`.

a) Split the data into 80% training and 20% holdout, using the random number seed 2015.
b) Build a partition model, being sure to `set.seed(12)` immediately before using `rpart`. Use the cp suggested by the one standard deviation rule when pruning the tree. Look at a visualization of the tree, find the three most important variables to the tree, and find the generalization error of the tree. Would you say this model generalizes well?
c) Using your tree, predict the probability that a customer shops at store 10 if he or she shops at stores 1-9 and 11-30 but not at stores 31-68.
d) Construct a random forest using 1000 trees. Report the three most important variables in the forest (are they the same ones as in the partition model?) and report its generalization error on the holdout sample. Note: immediately before running `randomForest()`, be sure to do `set.seed(2021)`.
e) Which technique gave the best predictive model? Is this model any *good* for making predictions? Note: imagine that "missed opportunities" are a bad kind of error. What percentage of people who shopped at store 10 does the model predict to have not shopped? Would you consider this "pretty good" in light of the fact that about half the people in the survey area shop at this store?

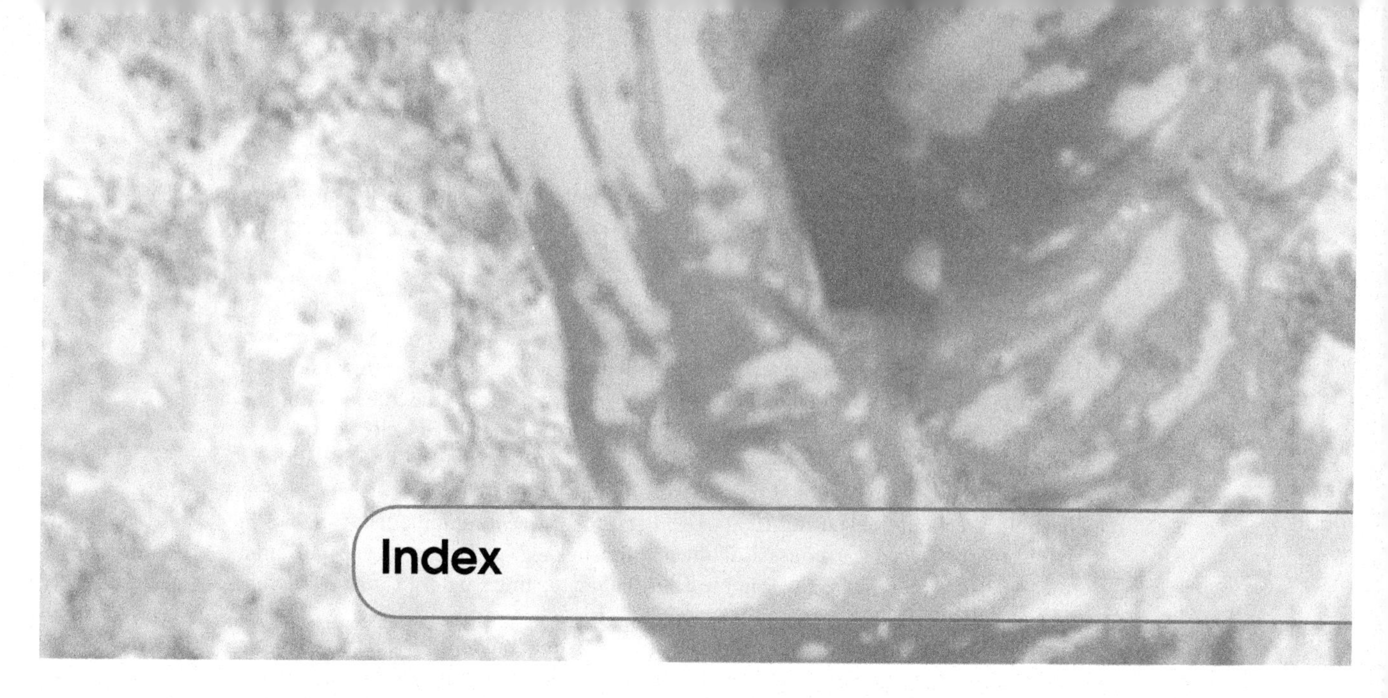

Index

-Symbols-

R^2, 85, 137
R^2_{adj}, 137, 138

-A-

Akaike information criterion (AIC), 255
all possible regression strategy, 257
ANOVA, 44
association, 15

-B-

binomial, 225
box plot, 19, 42

-C-

candidate set, 256
categorical variable, 17
census, 77, 84
classification and regression trees, 293
coefficient of determination, 58
complexity parameter *cp*, 304
complexity table, 306
conditional distribution, 16, 34
confidence interval, 91
confusion matrix, 236
contingency table, 33
Cook's distance, 179
correlation, 57
correlation matrix, 131

-D-

Data - ACCOUNT, 243, 306
Data - ATTRACTF, 41, 42, 46, 84, 199, 260
Data - ATTRACTM, 41, 60, 84, 209, 260
Data - AUTO, 23, 63, 65, 100, 106, 163
Data - BODYFAT, 63, 93, 145, 152, 162, 179, 182, 258, 266, 277
Data - BODYFAT2, 161
Data - BULLDOZER, 54, 135, 164, 211, 264
Data - BULLDOZER2, 213
Data - CALLS, 18, 28, 33, 38
Data - CENSUS, 281, 314
Data - CENSUSMLR, 167
Data - CHURN, 241, 244, 319
Data - DIET, 118
Data - DONOR, 62, 95, 105, 221, 249
Data - EDUCATION, 140, 204, 205
Data - faithful, 22, 24, 102
Data - FRIEND, 54
Data - FUMBLES, 54, 97
Data - JUNK, 321
Data - LARGEFLYER, 68
Data - LAUNCH, 273, 279
Data - MOVIE, 102, 107
Data - NFL, 84, 314
Data - OFFENSE, 157, 159
Data - PIMA, 232, 236, 283
Data - POISON, 230
Data - PRODUCT, 303
Data - PURCHASE, 231, 237
Data - SALARY, 80, 131, 143, 152, 161, 171, 173, 179, 193, 207, 258, 262
Data - SMALLFLYER, 68
Data - SOLD26, 169
Data - SPEED, 54
Data - STUDENT, 20–22, 24, 50

Data - SURVEY10, 63, 66, 100, 105
Data - SURVEY11, 30–32
Data - TIPS, 81, 104, 114–116, 139, 179, 195, 201
Data - WINE, 285
deleted studentized residual, 178
deviance, 234
direction, 54
discrepancy, 35
disturbance, 88
disturbances, 133

-E-

effect test, 203, 214, 243
extrapolation, 181

-F-

F test, 95
false negative, 236
false positive, 236
fitted values, 97
form, 54

-G-

gap, 20
generalization error, 273

-H-

heteroscedastic, 102
histogram, 19

-I-

identifier variable, 25
implicit regression equation, 173, 196, 201
impurity, 301
indicator variables, 194
influence, 177
influence plot, 179
interaction, 172, 206, 244
interaction plots, 174
interaction variable, 172
interquartile range, 23

-K-

K-fold cross-validation, 275
Kullback-Leibler divergence, 255

-L-

least squares, 83
leave-one-out cross-validation, 276
level of interest, 224
levels, 17
leverage, 177
Likert scale, 17
linearity, 55
log odds, 229
logistic regression, 223
lurking variable, 65, 147

-M-

Mahalanobis distance, 182
marginal distribution, 16, 33
maximum likelihood estimation, 227
mean, 23
median, 23
misclassification rate, 236
model hierarchy, 256
monotonic, 54
mosaic plot, 28
multicollinearity, 151

-N-

naive model, 86, 137, 236
nonlinearity, 55
Normal distribution, 20

-O-

one standard deviation rule, 277, 281, 306
outliers, 19, 58, 84, 176
overfitting, 272

-P-

p-value, 37, 40
partial F test, 157, 203
partition models, 293
Pearson's correlation, 57
permutation procedure, 36, 59, 93, 155
point estimate, 88, 111, 148
polynomial model, 164
power, 49
practical significance, 67, 95
PRESS, 276

-Q-

QQ-plot, 104
quantitative variable, 19

-R-

random forest, 311
rank-based tests, 48
recursive models, 303
reference level, 195
regression coefficients, 78

repeated K-fold cross-validation, 276
residual vs. predictor plots, 134
residuals, 83
residuals plot, 97
root mean squared error, 87

-S-

sample, 84
sampling distribution, 37, 90
scatterplot, 53
scatterplot matrix, 131
segmented bar chart, 18
simple linear regression, 75
simple linear regression model, 88
skewness, 19
Spearman's rank correlation, 62
standard deviation, 23
standard error, 89, 113, 148
statistical significance, 16, 40, 155
surrogate split, 308
symmetry, 19

-T-

time series analysis, 88
transformation, 225
transformation of variables, 104

-V-

validation sample, 274
variance inflation factor, 151

CPSIA information can be obtained
at www.ICGtesting.com
Printed in the USA
BVOW07s2305170118
505579BV00003B/65/P